ROOT STRENGTH

A HEALTH AND CARE PROFESSIONALS' GUIDE TO
MINIMIZING STRESS AND
MAXIMIZING THRIVING

ROOT STRENGTH

A HEALTH AND CARE PROFESSIONALS' GUIDE TO
MINIMIZING STRESS AND MAXIMIZING THRIVING

Shannon Dames, BN, MPH, EdD
Bachelor of Science in Nursing Professor
Health Professional Investigator for the Michael Smith Foundation
for Health Research/Lotte and John Hecht Memorial Foundation
Director of Research and Development for Roots to Thrive
Vancouver Island University
Nanaimo, British Columbia

ELSEVIER

ELSEVIER

Root Strength: A Health and Care Professionals' Guide to Minimizing Stress and Maximizing Thriving
ISBN: 978-0-323-77869-5

Managing Director, Global ERC: Kevonne Holloway
Senior Content Strategist (Acquisitions, Canada): Roberta A. Spinosa-Millman
Director, Content Development Manager: Laurie Gower
Content Development Specialist: Lenore Gray-Spence
Publishing Services Manager: Shereen Jameel
Copyeditor: Micheila Storr
Senior Project Manager: Umarani Natarajan
Design Direction: Julia Dummitt

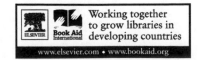

Working together
to grow libraries in
developing countries

www.elsevier.com • www.bookaid.org

Last digit is the print number: 9 8 7 6 5 4 3 2 1

To my mom, a cupcake amid a world of muffins that tend to be allergic to cupcakes. Rising again and again in the face of adversity - you've always embodied resilience, no matter the elements. It wasn't perfect, but it's enough. Enough to provide to me with the grit I needed to rise in the face of adversity, and the compost that fertilizes the beautiful garden I now have the pleasure of tending.

To my community, for teaching me that I am loved, and worthy to be my cupcake self. For celebrating the colors among us, providing the courage it takes to be authentic in this world.

And finally, to Elder Geraldine Manson. You've always been there to steady me when I lose my way, to remind me of who I am when I forget. Your wisdom and prayers continue to nurture the collective pilot light that is a lighthouse for many.

Table of Contents

About the Author

Dr. Shannon Dames was born and raised in Western Canada. For the past 20 years, she has lived and worked in Canada and the United States, wearing a variety of professional hats, including as a frontline nurse, administrator, educator, and researcher. She holds a master's degree in public health and completed her doctorate degree in education, focusing on the core factors that promote thriving communities of practice. Her current efforts centre on managing the barriers to individual resilience through medicine-assisted therapies and on the promotion of thriving cultures through intentional communities of practice.

Dr. Dames began this journey motivated to understand human BEing in a world that fixates on human DOing. To remember her inherent wholeness, and to co-create communities that can facilitate the same remembering in others. To collectively cultivate the conditions necessary to enable personal and professional thriving. She is a mother of two children, Piper and Beckett, whom she shares with Phillip Dames, her partner of 18 years. Most importantly, Shannon comes to this work as an equal, a fellow human and traveller on this journey. She joins countless others on this path, remembering how to connect inwardly and outwardly, to trust the process, and to co-create the safe spaces necessary for all humans to flourish.

Reviewers

Thomas F. Adams
Advanced Care Paramedic
Instructor of Primary Care Paramedicine
School of Health Sciences
College of the North Atlantic
Stephenville, Newfoundland and Labrador

Dr. Laura Armstrong, PhD, C. Psych
Associate Professor, Clinical Psychologist
School of Counselling, Psychotherapy and Spirituality
Saint Paul University
Ottawa, Ontario

Angie Arora, MSW, RSW
Professor
School of Community Services
Seneca College
Toronto, Ontario

Ralph Ashford, BA, MA
Professor
School of Justice and Community Development
Fleming College
Peterborough, Ontario

Kristin Barbour, RN, BScN, MN
Faculty—Saskatchewan Collaborative Bachelor of Science in Nursing Program
School of Nursing
Saskatchewan Polytechnic
Regina, Saskatchewan

Scott Blandford, BPA, MPA, DBA, IACP, IPSA
Assistant Professor
Public Safety Programs Coordinator
Faculty of Human and Social Services
Wilfrid Laurier University
Brantford, Ontario

Laura Bulmer, RN, BScN, MEd
Chair, Canadian Association of Continuing Care Providers (CACCE)
PSW Researcher/Advocate
Ontario Public Service Employees Union
Professor
Personal Support Worker Program
Sally Horsfall Eaton School of Nursing
George Brown College
Toronto, Ontario

Elizabeth P. Boynton, DVM
Professor
College of Veterinary Medicine
Western University of Health Sciences
Pomona, California

Nick Halmasy, MACP
Registered Psychotherapist
School of Justice and Community Development
Sir Sandford Fleming College
After The Call—First Responder Mental Health
Peterborough, Ontario

Heidi Holmes, RN, MScN, SANE, GNC
Professor
Faculty of Nursing
Conestoga College
Kitchener, Ontario

Suzie J. Kovacs, MSc, PhD
Assistant Professor
College of Veterinary Medicine
Western University of Health Sciences
Pomona, California

Manon Lemonde, RN, PhD, CON(C)
Associate Professor
Faculty of Health Sciences
Ontario Tech University
Oshawa, Ontario

Dr. Cheryl Pollard, RPN, RN, ANEF, PhD
Dean
Faculty of Nursing
University of Regina
Regina, Saskatchewan

Amy L. Ramsay, PhD
BAs in *Sociology, Religious Studies, and Women's Studies*; MA (*Education*);
MSc *Criminology*; MDiv; MTh; PhDs in *Criminal Justice and Management &*
Organization; EdS(c) *Doctor of Education, Specialist in Curriculum & Instruction*
Professor
Faculty of Human and Social Sciences
Sir Wilfrid Laurier University
Waterloo, Ontario;
Retired Police Sergeant
Ontario Provincial Police

Faith Richardson, DNP, RN
Ecotherapist, Clinician, Coach, Educator
North Island College
Port Alberni, British Columbia

Patricia L. Samson, MSW, PhD
Faculty of Social Work
University of Calgary
Calgary, Alberta

Mina D. Singh, RN, RP, BSc, BScN, MEd, PhD, I-FCNEI
Professor, Associate Director Research
School of Nursing
Faculty of Health
York University
Toronto, Ontario

Renée Sloos, BS, MSW, PhD, RSW
Postdoctoral Fellow
School of Social Work
York University
Toronto, Ontario

Caroline Tachejian, BA
Professor
Personal Support Worker Certificate Program
School of Nursing
Seneca College
Toronto, Ontario

Tracy Thiele, RPN, MN, PhD(c)
Registered Psychiatric Nurse
Canadian Federation of Mental Health Nurses
Winnipeg, Manitoba

Ann-Marie Urban, BScN, MN, PhD, RN, RPN
Associate Professor
Faculty of Nursing
University of Regina
Regina, Saskatchewan

Alice Villalobos, DVM
Fellow Emeritus National Academies of Practice
Private Practice Specializing in Oncology and End-of-Life Care for Animals
Hermosa Beach and Woodland Hills, California

Preface

How This Journey Came to Be

The content enclosed in this book represents the culmination of the journey I took to better understand why some of us who are caregivers thrive while others struggle to survive each day, despite similar work/life environments. The work began with a multidisciplinary group of caregivers with curriculum, organizational, and administrative expertise who identified a need among caregivers amid the rising tide of professional burnout in health care, finding little to no comprehensive, evidence-informed programs to address it. Motivated to address this need, we applied for and won a Michael Smith Foundation for Health Research REACH Award to develop a curriculum that would address the most significant assets (personal and contextual resources) that could bolster the ability to thrive amid highly stressful work environments. We developed the *Roots to Thrive* journey—the foundation of this book—as a supportive pathway for all caregivers to develop greater personal resilience, tying the theory to the experience of living it.

A Program of Research. The material within the book continues to evolve as we take in feedback from a variety of sources: those going through the program independently or in small informal pairs and groups, those taking part in workshops, contributing experts in the field, and those participating within a larger program of research. This journey is now intertwined with a program of research that investigates the impacts on caregivers' mental health and wellness scores, self-compassion, mindfulness development, perception of co-worker relationships, perceived satisfaction with one's career, and the impact on the brain as participants engage in this personal development work.

Decolonizing as We Go. This book uses terms and concepts that speak the language of the colonized system that many of us were born into, particularly in the Western world. The colonized systems that many have become conditioned to move within and contribute to continues to influence and inform us in countless ways. Often, the consequence of not assimilating is steep, threatening our need to be accepted, to feel valued, and to belong. Research, theory, hierarchies, and the like are upheld as gold standards that ensure we move forward in an informed and orderly fashion, but these pillars can also devalue the power of moving in a more heartfelt way, acknowledging the depth and breadth of knowledge we hold within us. The first part of the book speaks to the needs of the system, providing the theory and research that forms the foundation of this work, which in turn enables the buy-in necessary to invest ourselves in a more vulnerable, heartfelt way of being so that we can shake off the structures that hold us back.

Mitigating Cultural (Mis)appropriation. The theoretical underpinnings of this book align with several practices and frameworks that are embedded in other cultures less hindered by individualism. Because this book was developed within a Western culture—which is heavily influenced by individualism—there are several references to other ways of being found in more collectivist cultures. We have much to learn from cultures that recognize community and connection as a necessity of both surviving and thriving. The richness of these cultures promotes a greater understanding of human flourishing, upheld by values and rituals that promote inner and outer connection. The risk of including practices, readings, and frameworks from several cultures is the mounting tension (and rightly so) around cultural (mis)appropriation, whereby members of the dominant and advantaged culture appropriate from minority cultures. To mitigate this risk, I encourage readers to cultivate a deep understanding of the origin of the practices you take on as your own. Lean in to develop a genuine curiosity about its origin. Ask yourself how you relate to the originating culture and what your intentions are. By approaching these ways of being as an eager and appreciative learner, we are more likely to embody the humility and respect required to acknowledge those who carry these ways of being in the fabric of their being, honouring the wholeness of the practice, and preventing distortions that can occur when we do not consider the context from which a practice emerges.

Encouragement for the Journey

May we be like the diamond, pressed down time and time again, until all that is left is a shining gem, a beacon of light for all the world to see.

May we embark on this journey with the full and deep realization that the path that led us to today, the suffering we continue to feel, need not threaten us. Rather, these discomforts are a call to come home, to remember what has always been, so that we can awaken to our best, most authentic selves.

May we cultivate a community that can witness us in our essence, reminding us of who we are when we forget.

May we allow ourselves to believe and receive a felt sense of unconditional positive regard so fully that we can mirror the same inwardly and outwardly. From this place of safety and acceptance, we gain the courage to freely express our magnificent selves.

May we cultivate a love so deep within us that we can find the acceptance and compassion necessary to rest in our inner home—a safe place that comes to fill us so completely that it spills over, nurturing the planet and the precious beings that move upon it.

May we step into the river of life, letting go of the effort to calculate and control how and where it flows, surrendering to the point where we find joy in the journey itself, trusting in a benevolent and enriching end.

May we let go of the old belief systems that rely on willpower and perfectionism, fuelling so much unnecessary suffering.

Together, let us rewrite the old narratives that breed fear and shame, enabling us to use our past experiences, behaviours, and learnings as compost for the new growth germinating beneath the surface.

From this place of wholeness, may we celebrate the diversity of colours and ways of being among us.

Acknowledgements

This book represents a culmination of the work and wisdom of many talented researchers, authors, topical experts, and inspired change agents. Many thanks to those who spent many hours reviewing and editing, including Samantha Magnus, Alexa Garrey, Marti Harder, Tara Raymond, Graham Blackburn, Roisin Mulligan, Andrea Hunter, Wendy Young, Ryan Moyer, Crosbie Watler, Pam Kryskow, Gail Peekeekoot, Wes Taylor, and more!

Special thanks to:

My life partner, Phillip Dames. Thank you for your support as a co-parent, friend, and cheerleader. Most importantly, thank you for partnering with me to co-create a space for our family to feel and mirror unconditional positive regard for each other and for our community.

My colleagues and friends, Marnie Roper and Lori-Anne Demers. Your personal and professional contributions helped refine the essential elements of the journey described in this book. You are wise beyond your years and living examples of the magic that can happen when people live their calling authentically.

Dr. Crosbie Watler, for your inspired work in this text. Thank you for sprinkling compassion and holism into psychiatry. You are rewriting old and often unhelpful narratives. Your wise words and courageous way of being is a welcome beacon of light as we collectively find our way home.

About This Book

Root Strength: A Health and Care Professionals' Guide to Minimizing Stress and Maximizing Thriving is intended for those working in the caring professions, including (but not limited to):
- Health care students and practising professionals
- Students and practitioners in other caring professions, such as mental health providers
- First responders such as firefighters, police officers, paramedics, military personnel, medical evacuation pilots, dispatchers, nurses, doctors, personal support workers, emergency medical technicians, and emergency managers
- Veterinarians
- Social service workers

Root Strength is well suited for inclusion in courses of study such as
- Nursing courses
- Allied health courses in leading and managing, mental health, therapeutic communication, oncology, palliative care, critical care, forensics, and emergency, crisis, and trauma
- Veterinary medicine
- Psychology
- In-service training workshops
- Short courses in self-care for the caring professions and courses administered by local health authorities

Evolve for *Root Strength*

Located at http://evolve.elsevier.com/Dames/rootstrength, the Evolve website for this book includes
- Resources—Suggestions for YouTube links and relevant films, and links to TED Talks and related websites
- Thriving Toolkit—A collection of unique assessment/application activities related to each chapter in Part II

Elsevier eBooks

This exciting program is available to faculty who adopt a number of Elsevier texts, including *Root Strength: A Health and Care Professionals' Guide to Minimizing Stress and Maximizing Thriving*. Elsevier eBooks is an integrated electronic study centre consisting of a collection of textbooks made available online. It is carefully designed to "extend" the textbook for an easier and more efficient teaching and learning experience. It includes study aids such as highlighting, e-note taking, and cut-and-paste capabilities. Even more importantly, it allows students and instructors to do a comprehensive search within the specific text or across a number of titles. Please check with your Elsevier sales representative for more information.

The authors and contributors of the text recognize and acknowledge the diverse histories of the First Peoples of the lands now referred to as Canada. It is recognized that individual communities identify themselves in various ways; within this text, the term *Indigenous* is used to refer to all First Nations, Inuit, and Métis peoples within Canada.

In the text, gender-neutral language is used to be respectful of and consistent with the values of equality recognized in the *Canadian Charter of Rights and Freedoms*. Using gender-neutral language is professionally responsible and mandated by the Canadian Federal Plan for Gender Equality. Knowledge and language concerning sex, gender, and identity are fluid and continually evolving. The language and terminology presented in this text endeavours to be inclusive of all peoples and reflects what is currently acceptable, to the best of our knowledge, at the time of publication.

Coming to Know Through the Research

By developing congruence and sense of coherence, the two primary factors that promote thriving, we come to remember who we are from a place of wholeness, enabling us to access all our resources creatively and confidently. As a result, we gain a greater ability to navigate stimuli before they become chronic stressors. Once the potential threat is resolved, we are freed up to be with what is happening in the moment.

Jennifer's Journey

Professional caregiving is a career path that aligns with my beliefs and values. My experience thus far includes four years of work in the field. I continue to work on the frontline of health care in various positions. Although I work in a proud profession, I have come to learn that it is in some ways an underappreciated one.

I began my career in the acute care setting and have since transitioned to community care. Not only am I familiar with emotional exhaustion, but it was an embedded part of working in acute care. The combination of caring for acutely ill persons, insufficient staffing, and workplace stressors did not leave much room for prioritization of personal growth, health, and well-being. I have since learned invaluable tools that drive my pursuit of creating and enriching the health care milieu. I believe that confronting workplace challenges can create more understanding of the collaborative and interdisciplinary process.

Providing holistic and optimal care fostered a culture of working above our baseline with increased workload expectations. Working above my capacity was not sustainable; it eventually impacted my mental health and resulted in emotional and physical exhaustion. Systemic pressures to ensure we met patient care goals meant cutting corners and increasing frontline workloads. Environmental stressors such as limited equipment, social stressors such as requests for assistance from colleagues, leadership stressors such as pressures to meet care plan goals, and physical stressors related to the already arduous work—all took a heavy toll.

The combination of multifactorial stressors contributed to my experience of emotional and physical burnout. Like many individuals who enter caregiving fields, I continued to grit my teeth and endure. I worked in an environment that eventually led me to feel resentment, hostility, and a sense of dread. Reflecting on my conflict with the environmental milieu of acute care, I found an incredible need for a therapeutic milieu. I yearned for a culture that would foster and encompass a collaborative effort to heal and create an atmosphere that is both enriching and beneficial.

I resonate with those experiencing emotional exhaustion because I vividly remember periods where I would prioritize my work over my health and well-being. There were countless times where I have forgone my much-needed break to opt to care for clients who needed me instead. Only upon reflection would I come to realize that the institution and systems that guide our work also challenge our spirit. Frontline caregiving work is often an endless cycle in which we work ourselves into exhaustion, only to wake up and do it all over again. I eventually began to think that working as a professional caregiver was a thankless job, and I wanted to find avenues to reflect on and confront this notion.

I understand the challenges of working in the care delivery field, where we are under-resourced across all areas. These challenges take shape by way of limited staffing capability, lack of available equipment to help us complete our tasks, or reduced mentorship and educator access. To be set up for success, I needed to have tools of resilience—which I have come to understand as the willingness to be transparent and adaptable. Acknowledgment of this was paramount in my practice. The pressures to work under conditions where we were expected to meet a higher demand without adequate staffing contributed to challenges in maintaining safe practice. Constantly having to perform by the seat of my pants and scrambling to maintain safe care compounded my feelings of discontent. Working under pressure ultimately leads to more opportunities for mistakes and a decrease in frontline performance.

The art of professional caregiving should not have to equate to losing touch with my core self. With the cumulative workplace stress continuing to build, I felt deflated. I could not confidently perform at the level to which I strived daily. I came to a point where the exhaustion was beginning to impact my well-being. I could sense my core personality changing. I became short and quick to escalate over trivial conflicts. People close to me noticed this shift and commented on my well-being. It struck me that, systematically, the world of acute care settings had become unforgiving. The demands of acute care continued to move onward, and the work continued to pile up. Like a well-oiled machine, it would not stop when just one cog was not quite in place. The stressors of frontline caregiving gradually and insidiously permeated every aspect of my life. I found myself seeking solace in isolation and recoiling from social interactions that otherwise would have energized me.

Today, I feel that there are better ways to cope with the stressors that one cannot change. It is paramount to shift our perspective so that we can reflect on the institutions driving the pressures that in turn impact caregiving work. From a frontline perspective, I want to draw on strategies that can empower caregivers to recognize their agency. Through this acknowledgment, caregivers can act according to their capacity and can develop their resiliency to ensure they have the strategies for success and healthy coping. It is not exhaustion that compelled me to. Act—it was realizing that the system was a business that strived to meet goals, regardless of the consequences.

I want to challenge the notion of caregiving work as being thankless because I see opportunities to debunk the systemic structures that work to create an unsustainable work milieu. I see the opportunities for growth that encompass a vision that collaborates and inspires meaning into the notion of our work. The health care culture of putting our heads down to complete the work no matter the cost needs to be revitalized and re-envisioned to include a well-rounded and healthy practice.

Jennifer's Journey—*cont'd*

A work culture where contributions are not only appreciated but also valued by leadership and management is essential.

What motivates me to remain committed to this vital endeavour is the opportunity to participate in change-making strategies to prevent burnout and strengthen caregiver resiliency, with the intention of creating a work culture that promotes sustainable caregiving. The opportunity to hold space for frontline workers and represent a collaborative and forward-thinking approach motivates me to put in the work. I recognize that my privilege as a professional caregiver affords me the opportunity to challenge the status quo. In this role, I can breathe new meaning into what we can accomplish when we work collectively, and I am motivated to continue rising to this challenge.

Introduction: Humans First, Caregivers Second

As you live deeper in the heart, the mirror gets cleaner and cleaner.

Rumi

Human nature is complex, which makes weaving concepts such as resilience, stress, trauma, and coping into one inclusive framework is a lofty goal. However, at the risk of oversimplifying, it can also foster greater understanding of how one's orientation to self (congruence) and to the world (sense of coherence) impacts one's ability to thrive as humans in a complex world. I hope that readers will explore and expand their perspectives as they are led on this journey. I aim to provide enough theoretical and cognitive groundwork to lay a scientific foundation (manifesting as "The Roots to Thrive Theory"), but not so much that it distracts from the heart-centred nature of the work.

WHO IS THIS BOOK FOR?

This book is for all humans, as we are collectively bound by common human needs. Most of the research and statistics in this text apply to those who are providing professional caregiving services and are particularly vulnerable to high-stimulus and often trauma-laden workplaces. Caregivers includes those with a professional focus on serving others, be it in a health, welfare, protective, or safety function. While this broad audience may seem overly ambitious, there is common ground in the "I" beneath our professional roles. Thriving at work and home happens when we use our resources—congruence and sense of coherence. Doing so buffers us against external stressors, lowers our risk of mental and physical distress, improves co-worker relationships, increases job satisfaction, and reduces our tendency to rely on substances or distracting tasks to cope with stress.

WHO ARE CAREGIVERS?

In this work, caregivers are those charged with looking after others. The research within this book targets professional caregivers (nurses, physicians, social workers, educators, paramedics, care aides, veterinarians and animal care providers, dentists, law enforcement, etc.), but the principles also apply to those who provide care for dependents.

Although the content focuses on the psychological and spiritual well-being of individual caregivers, sustaining collective change requires that we also turn our attention to the broader system. As illustrated in Figure 1.1, people cannot bloom if the soil in which they are planted fails to provide essential nutrients and if the weather conditions constantly

threaten their well-being. Any lasting change requires supportive organizational structures that strive to minimize workplace stress and prioritize the cultivation of personal
resources—congruence and sense of coherence—to mitigate the impact of workplace stress
(Ruotsalainen et al., 2016).

Through the sections of the introduction that follow, I describe the roots of this book
as well as its central metaphor, core concepts, objectives (Appendix C), and applications.

HOW CAN YOU USE THIS BOOK?

There are a variety of ways to engage with this book. It can be used as a course text in postsecondary settings, as material for a professional development workshop, as a selection for
a book club or other small group, or by individuals who would rather work independently
or in pairs. Based on personality and opportunity, anyone in any setting can use the framework enclosed to begin tilling the soil and forging deeper roots both individually and collectively. Based on my experience with growing resiliency, the most effective way to forge
deeper roots is to engage in this work with others. You might do this with a peer you bring
on board or a mentor you admire. Whatever the case, the pace at which you will shift into
more helpful ways of being correlates with the development of trust in yourself and others.
As such, beneficial relationships provide a safe container to help you feel confident when
challenges inevitably come. Healthy relationships provide us with people who can remind
us of who we are when we forget as well as people who can serve as a more objective sound-
ing board when we feel ungrounded.

For those of us conditioned to rely more heavily on the thinking mind, coming to know
the research and theory behind the practices is a necessary step in cultivating a willingness
to invest in ourselves. For those motivated and ready to jump right in, the theoretical tun-
nel that precedes the experiential work may be an effortful barrier that erodes motivation.
With this understanding, I hope that each reader will feel empowered to use the work in a
way that feeds inspiration, enabling a certain ease whereby the reward outweighs the effort.

EQUITY AND CULTURAL SAFETY

While this work speaks to the common needs of all humans, the "priorities," the "how," the
"when," and whether various aspects are necessary to address will be influenced by several
factors including culture, values, beliefs, and circumstances; these factors act as the cultural
soil in which we have grown and from which we draw our strength. It is my greatest hope
that the theoretical underpinnings and suggested practices align in such a way that principles such as humility, celebrating diverse ways of being, and promoting personal **agency**
are underscored again and again.

The theoretical and experiential components of this work are heavily influenced by a
Western, individualist, and humanist framework. Despite the limitations implicit within
these contextual and cultural influences, the ultimate intention is to promote healing within
the context of communities characterized by **unconditional positive regard**. In this way,
we can evolve beyond an emphasis on the individual, expanding to enhance and underscore
the importance of connecting both inwardly and outwardly. Whether one begins inwardly
and pendulates outwardly, or begins outwardly and pendulates inwardly, the ultimate goal
is to promote a greater sense of connection, community, and belonging for all.

Human First

As the writer of this text, I come with the lived experience and pleasure of having served while wearing several personal and professional hats. As tempting as it is to hide under those hats, the "I" beneath them is the real impetus for this work. Like many, my story is full of hope and heartache. I left home at 15 and entered nursing at 18, dragging a good deal of baggage behind me. I spent many years wearing all the right hats and acquiring all the right awards, degrees, and promotions. As I journeyed through my health care career, like many, I learned about thriving and surviving through trial and error, navigating a range of terrains and roles. After toiling for many years to attain the right letters and hats, I have come to understand that accomplishments and titles have never and will never bring me lasting satisfaction, that blooming where I am planted is more about the journey than the destination, and that along the way I need a community of people that will witness and celebrate the real me and who can remind me of who I am when I forget. The "I" is more important than the hats we wear and the shoes we fill. My greatest hope is that we as caregivers, as humans who give care, come to realize that we, too, are worthy of care.

I am with you on this journey. We travel together. As caregivers, we wear a common hat, but more importantly, we share our common humanity. It is courage, faith, and possibility that propel us forward despite our fears, and it is self-compassion that reminds us to be gentle in the process. Understanding that there is messiness within the journey enables us to focus on progress rather than perfection. To change what we can and accept what we cannot. I promise you, the journey is worth the hardships you may find along the way. Beyond the storms, there are rainbows reminding us of the beauty within the process. At the end of each rainbow is a gift waiting to be opened, inviting you to step closer to your highest, most **authentic** self.

Let us not let our roles hide our humanity.

Caregiver Second

While caregiving involves wearing a variety of professional hats, I frequently refer to well-established cultural conditions in well-researched populations, such as physicians and nurses working in health care, but this is not meant to exclude other professions that are grappling with similar issues. While the hats may take on different forms, as professional caregivers, we have much in common.

While the research in this book centres on the profession of nursing, I use the term "care professionals" or "caregivers" to refer to physicians, nurses, care aides, dentists, first responders, police officers, and other disciplines that provide care to the public. One thing that many caregiver occupations have in common is stress. Workplace stress is a major issue among caregivers, with alarming consequences for caregivers' physical and mental health (Leiter et al., 2010). Many caregivers experience severe emotional exhaustion from workplace conflicts and stress (Laschinger et al., 2015; Parker et al., 2014).

In 2017, the Canadian Medical Association's National Physician Health Survey found that 49% of residents and 33% of physicians screened positive for depression, and 38% of residents and 29% of physicians for burnout (Simon & McFadden, 2017). In 2015, the Manitoba Nurses' Union launched a formal strategy to address the 64% of caregivers experiencing emotional exhaustion and the 52% experiencing critical incident stress and **post-traumatic stress disorder (PTSD)** (Manitoba Nurses' Union, 2015).

When our basic human needs go unmet, we experience chronic stress (emerging as anxiety and/or depression) until they are satisfied. As caregivers, we cannot thrive when we are distracted by the ominous cloud that haunts us when our basic human needs feel threatened. When unchecked, this form of chronic stress leads to **moral injury**, emotional exhaustion, and eventual burnout. According to the Centre for Addiction and Mental Health (CAMH, 2017), moral injury occurs when people or events transgress our moral values and beliefs. The moral and ethical dissonance that emerges from this form of injury disrupts our ability to trust ourselves and others. Events that can lead to moral injury include mistakes that cause harm, feeling unable to prevent harm, and feeling morally or ethically betrayed by peers and organizational leaders (CAMH, 2017).

With over 20 years of professional practice, I have burned out rather dramatically once, and I have spent plenty of time hovering on the brink of **burnout**. According to the research, I am not alone. Prolonged exposure to stress, fueled by feelings of insecurity, is a normal part of work for many caregivers. Burnout affects every care provider if not directly then indirectly, as they feel the ripple effects from struggling co-workers. As reflected in numerous studies, including Shier and Graham's (2015) research with social workers, when work environments fail to meet basic human requirements, it drives the ubiquity and severity of caregiver stress and ultimately erodes caregiver well-being. In turn, caregiver stress fuels addiction, anxiety, depression, suicide, and attrition rates among caregivers.

The Fallout of Burnout

One in every two Canadians will have, or have had, a mental illness by the time they are 40 years old (CAMH, 2019), and professional caregivers are at an even higher risk for mental illness. Studies show that 40% to 60% of professional caregivers face burnout at some point in their career (Olson et al., 2015; Rabb, 2014). In Canada, 500 000 people, representing 3% of working Canadians, miss work each day because of mental illness (CAMH, 2019). Health care providers are 1.5 times more likely to grapple with mental illness including burnout (Mental Health Commission of Canada, 2018). Additionally, a study completed in the United States found that caregivers acting as first responders are more likely to lose their life to suicide than in the line of duty (Heyman et al., 2018). Veterinarians also deal with an exceptionally high risk of burnout, which manifests as anxiety and depression, with one of six graduates having experienced suicidal ideation after leaving veterinary school (Nett et al., 2015). Another study that surveyed 10% of Canadian veterinarians found significantly higher burnout and compassion fatigue, anxiety, and depression and significantly lower resilience scores (Perret et al., 2020). In 2016, nurses made up 12% of WorkSafeBC mental health claims (British Columbia Nurses' Union (BCNU), 2019). While nurses represent much of the health care workforce (US Bureau of Labor Statistics, 2015), all caregivers are at risk for emotional exhaustion and burnout. For every dollar spent on Canada's health care system, about 70 cents of it is spent on human resources, not including education costs (BC Ministry of Health, 2014). The ultimate cost, the billions of dollars aside, is patient safety, as unhealthy health care providers are more likely to make errors, call in sick, and ultimately leave the profession, which exacts a huge financial toll in terms of recruitment and training.

Statistics vary widely in the research on caregivers who have left their place of employment or exited the profession altogether. With nurses, for example, attrition rates are at nearly 20% each year in Canada and the United States (Nursing Solutions Inc., 2018; O'Brien-Pallas et al., 2008). The attrition rates of novice caregivers are nearly double that of experienced nurses, with over half leaving because of co-worker-to-co-worker violence and the experience of long periods where they do not feel a sense of belonging (Mahli, 2013; McKenna & Newton, 2007; Thomas & Burk, 2009; Zarshenas et al., 2014). Looking at social workers as another example, high rates of burnout and attrition have been a trend for decades. Back in 2006, Siebert conducted a study of 1 000 actively practising social workers and found a current burnout rate of 39% and a lifetime burnout rate of 75%. Burnout was tied to personal factors such as one's trauma history, difficulty with childhood, and feeling responsible for client outcomes and occupational factors such as hours worked, heavy caseloads, supervisor support, and especially working in stressful, high-stimulus environments.

As a result of chronic stress, some caregivers will change work settings, some leave the profession altogether, and many remain in their workplaces despite their burned-out condition, impacting team morale and client care (Boamah & Laschinger, 2016; Currie & Carr Hill, 2012; Rush et al., 2013). The staff who take on the extra workload from unfilled vacancies or sick calls related to emotional exhaustion experience additional pressure to continue providing high-quality care with less time to do so. As a result, clients also suffer when staff work short, receiving more rushed and a reduced quality of care (Clark et al., 2007). Adding to issues of morale and quality care, the financial burden on the system is steep. When a caregiver resigns, a recruitment process must occur, followed by hiring and training of the new caregivers to fill the vacancy. In Canada, 10 years ago, it cost an average of $25 000 to replace a nurse and up to $64 000 to replace a specialized nurse (O'Brian-Pallas et al., 2008, 2010). In the United States, turnover costs are similar, ranging from $10 098 USD to $88 000 USD per nurse (Li & Jones, 2012). With inflation, these costs are higher now and continue to climb each year. Compounding high attrition costs, in 2014 the supply of Canadian registered nurses saw its first decline in two decades (Canadian Institute for Health Information [CIHI], 2015). In North America, current and compounding nursing shortages continue to cause alarm with an aging population (AACN, 2020; Chachula et al., 2015; CIHI, 2018).

While some professional caregivers leave the workplace because of burnout, many also stay—further contributing to toxic work environments. Most of us who have been in the field long enough are familiar with the symptoms of burnout and have contributed to workplace hostility as a result; these experiences have become a norm in today's health care culture. Burnout is recognized as an occupational hazard for many service-oriented professions that have ongoing and intense personal and emotional contact. In fact, the Canadian province of British Columbia recently extended presumptive PTSD coverage for mental health claims by all types of nurses (Providence Health, 2019).

Treatment-Resistant Mental Health Conditions

The prevalence of mental health issues among professional caregivers, including rates of PTSD and major depressive disorder (MDD), appears to be much higher than that in the general population. In a recent pre-pandemic study of Canadian nurses, 23% screened positive for PTSD and 36.4% for MDD (Stelnicki & Carleton, 2020). National estimates of annual prevalence rates for PTSD and MDD episodes in the general population suggest that Canadian nurses in particular experience these disorders at rates that are far greater than those in the general population (Statistics Canada, 2013). A wide range of preliminary evidence suggests that added stressors and traumatic events associated with the COVID-19 global health pandemic will only exacerbate this mental health crisis and related costs (Stelnicki et al., 2020). While the rates of mental illness among the general Canadian population remain concerning (Dückers et al., 2016), the disproportionately high rates of mental illness among health care providers are cause for greater alarm given their vital role in safeguarding the health and wellness of all Canadians.

As rates of PTSD and treatment-resistant depression grow, so too will their significant social and economic costs (Chiu et al., 2017; Vasiliadis et al., 2017), including increases in already astronomical direct health care costs as well as workplace burnout and absenteeism (Dyrbye et al., 2019; Laposa et al., 2003). For example, in British Columbia, nurses were responsible for submitting 12% of WorkSafeBC mental health claims in 2016 despite making up only 2% of the province's workforce (BCNU, 2019; CIHI, 2018). This is worrisome because a workforce of health care providers living with PTSD and/or treatment-resistant depression will directly contribute to reductions in patient safety and quality of care (Gong et al., 2014; Letvak et al., 2012; Welsh, 2009). Indeed, our ability to provide adequate health care to all Canadians rests upon our collective ability to provide adequate, efficient, and effective mental health support for our health care providers. Despite increasing expenditures, health care providers (McKinley, 2020) and others (Sunderland & Findlay, 2013) in Canada continue to express their need for additional support, suggesting that available treatments are insufficient. Bolstering this suggestion, estimates suggest that over one-quarter of people with MDD do not respond to treatment and are then classified as having treatment-resistant depression (Rizvi et al., 2014). Acknowledging the disproportionate impacts of PTSD on health care providers as well as the limits of available treatment options, the Public Health Agency of Canada (PHAC) recently prioritized the investigation of emergent and innovative interventions (PHAC, 2020).

Despite significant advances in treatment options for PTSD and/or treatment-resistant depression, many treatments continue to suffer from a host of limitations. As PTSD and treatment-resistant depression are often co-occurring, have notable symptom overlap, and may be treated with similar interventions (Campbell et al., 2007; Flory & Yehuda, 2015), they also suffer from similar treatment limitations. Indeed, the effects of various first-line pharmacological treatments for both PTSD and MDD are limited (Hoskins et al., 2015; Khan et al., 2012). For example, research has highlighted the inability of antidepressant medication to consistently demonstrate advantages over placebos (Fournier et al., 2010; Melander et al., 2003; Turner et al., 2008). Alternatively, psychotherapies suffer from limited patient engagement and high rates of nonresponse and premature discontinuation (Najavits, 2015; Rosen et al., 2016; Swift & Greenberg, 2012; Watkins et al., 2018). For example, studies indicate that nonresponse rates for **cognitive behavioural therapy (CBT)**—recommended as the first-line PTSD management choice (Katzman et al., 2014)—are reported to be as high as 50% (Green, 2013), and average recovery rates in intent-to-treat analyses have been reported to be as low as 40% (Hoge et al., 2014). In response, a host of recommendations have been made regarding optimal treatment modalities and needed innovations, including calls for treatment that is trauma informed (Bisson et al., 2007), that is community based instead of individual focused (Costa & Moss, 2018), and that combines pharmacological and psychotherapeutic interventions (Khan et al., 2012).

The Failing Promises of Modern Psychiatry

By Crosbie Watler, MD, FRCPC

This piece by Crosbie Watler, a Canadian thought leader and psychiatrist, speaks to the faulty conditions of the system that many of us have been taught to turn to for healing. According to the research, the status quo treatments are failing us. It's time to turn the corner, learn from our mistakes, and forge a new, evidence-informed, and spiritually enlightened path forward.

The last decade of the twentieth century was a heady time for modern psychiatry. Fluoxetine was released in the mid-80s, and many other so-called anti-depressants followed on its heels. Though never proven, we touted the neurotransmitter deficit model for depression and truly believed that we were on the threshold of a major breakthrough in psychiatry and neuroscience. In our collective excitement, we dubbed the 1990s "The Decade of the Brain."

Fast forward to the present day. Despite widespread and often indiscriminate pre-scribing, on a per capita basis, there are far more persons off work on disability for anxiety and depressive-related disorders than ever before. The increase continues and is exponential.

There are two myths at play that serve to perpetuate the status quo. First is the myth of *diagnosis* in psychiatry. In other areas of medicine, a diagnosis is a discrete, objectively verifiable condition. There remain many symptom clusters that fail to meet this standard. Lacking objective tests—much less treatments—the rest of medicine classifies these conditions as *syndromes.*

Examples of common syndromes include chronic fatigue syndrome and irritable bowel syndrome. In a desperate attempt to enhance the prestige of psychiatry—and as a requirement for billing the Health Maintenance Organizations (HMOs) in the United States—the American Psychiatric Association's *Diagnostic and Statistical Manual of Mental Disorders* (DSM) incorporates more diagnoses with each edition. The belief that psychiatric diagnoses are defined constructs, on par with diagnoses in other areas of medicine, is the myth at the core of modern psychiatric practice. Simply call-ing something a *disorder* does not make it real (Paris, 2015).

The image of a group of endocrinologists debating whether Type 1 diabetes should be a legitimate diagnosis is laughable, yet this is precisely how psychiatric "diagno-ses" are minted. If something is objectively real, we do not debate its existence, and what was truth does not simply become untruth with the next edition of the DSM. The DSM committee meetings provide forums for so-called experts to lobby for their pet "diagnoses," ones they feel comfortable treating and that will enhance their credibility and prestige.

Furthermore, if these diagnoses were real and credible, then why do psychiatrists so commonly disagree among themselves? It is common to hear reference made to a psychiatrist's particular "style." One psychiatrist's borderline personality disorder is another's bipolar type 2, with entirely different treatment protocols.

The Failing Promises of Modern Psychiatry—*cont'd*

Lacking consensus on diagnosis, it is no surprise that the trajectory of psychiatric patient care is highly variable, depending on the bias of the treating psychiatrist. Highly variable production systems operate at the expense of quality. And who bears the cost of a highly variable system of care? Certainly not the treating physician. Most physicians are paid for face time, not for outcome. This is akin to a contractor coming to your home and being paid for simply showing up.

If strike one—so to speak—is that our diagnoses are syndromes, then strike two is that our medical treatments lack efficacy. Given that we truly have no idea *what* we are treating in the first place, this should not come as a surprise! An embarrassing and rarely mentioned statistic is that our so-called *anti*depressants barely separate their impact from that of placebos. Furthermore, we've since learned that many negative studies were simply mothballed (Lancet, 2012).

What is truly incredible is that these medicines are still being marketed as *anti* anything. If our antidepressants and antipsychotics lived up to their lofty promise, most psychiatrists would be out of work and the "treatment-resistant" patients clogging our inpatient and tertiary care units would be promptly discharged. This, of course, is not the case.

Unfortunately, the public continues to drink from the punch bowl still being served by mainstream psychiatry. How many times have you heard a friend recounting a visit to the doctor?

"The doctor says I have a brain disease called major depressive disorder. There is not enough serotonin in my brain, apparently. He started me on Cipralex."

Two months later you ask how she is doing.

"Oh, that medication didn't work very well, I'm still off work. My doctor added a second medication, Wellbutrin, to 'boost' the first one, plus I'm on something to help me sleep ... insomnia is a side effect of Wellbutrin."

Two months later your friend stops by for a visit.

"My doctor thinks the reason my medications aren't working is that I might have bipolar disorder. He says there's a 'soft' type that's increasingly diagnosed these days. He added a mood stabilizer. I'm on four meds now and still off work. I'm starting to lose hope."

This scenario is played out countless times, day in and day out. As a boomer psychiatrist who was trained in the era of "biological psychiatry," I soon realized that we were not healing patients in any substantive way with our medications. We are instead creating lifelong mental health care *consumers*.

We prescribe mediocre treatments for phantom conditions. We cling desperately to the cloak of expertise and knowingness. We have become less interested in the complex personal stories that might explain a patient's suffering and inform non-pharmaceutical approaches. We are quick to identify "disorder" when the patient's challenge might be a natural and logical downstream manifestation of upstream and primary causes. This, to be fair, is a criticism that applies to other areas of medicine.

The conventional medical paradigm is rooted in the principle of specificity—a specific treatment for each discrete *disease*. In common parlance, *a pill for every ill*. We are in an era of increasingly specialized medicine, where the physician puts their organ

The Failing Promises of Modern Psychiatry—*cont'd*

of choice on a pedestal, often treating the downstream symptoms as the primary condition. When this fails—as it commonly does—psychiatrists often resort to desperate and toxic polypharmacy.

Such prescribing is often the result of *therapeutic despair* on the part of the treating physician. When a patient does not respond to treatment—and with the physician's ego on the chopping block—the doctor is desperate to *do something*, anything. It seems that uninformed action is deemed somehow better than inaction.

This demonstrates an all-too-familiar behavioural pattern and one not unique to the trades: *when the only tool one has is a hammer, everything looks like a nail.* The hammer in this case is the prescription pad. After many failed medication trials, the treating psychiatrist concludes that the problem lies with the patient, who is deemed "treatment resistant." The blame for treatment failure is projected onto the patient—*they* are treatment resistant.

What of the possibility that we are simply using the wrong treatments? Are we missing something? Rarely are these questions at the table. Curiosity and humility are simply thrown under the bus. Above all, do no harm? Also, under the bus. Despite all the claims for evidence-based and patient-centred care, the unavoidable and tragic conclusion is that the status quo works very well for the *industry of care*. For the patients? Not so much.

Much of what we do in clinical practice is simply "chasing smoke." We view the downstream symptoms as the primary condition. Any first-year medical student understands that fever is not a disease or disorder; it is a sign that there is something else amiss, something quite remote from the fever itself. In medicine—particularly in psychiatry—we often chase smoke.

The majority of those labeled as *depressed* are in fact *distressed* by the events in their lives and the stories they tell themselves about who they are. Predictably, they fail to respond to our pharmacopeia. Lost in the rush to increasingly specialized medicine is the appreciation for the human organism as a whole. We are the sum of our complex and interfacing systems, where symptoms in any one area might be secondary to remote *upstream* mediators. The overarching clinical question then becomes, "Is this symptom the chicken or the egg?"

In our search for a better paradigm, we might look to the wisdom of our ancient ancestors, from the Greeks, traditional Chinese, and yogi masters living thousands of years ago in India. These teachings share the view that there is far more to us than meets the eye. Am I my thoughts? Is it as simple as "I think, therefore I am?" Who am I, really? This question reflects our timeless quest for connection, identity, meaning, and purpose.

Connection with ourselves and with the world around us forms the bedrock of *spiritual health*. This new spirituality transcends specific religious affiliation and has spawned the phrase "spiritual but not religious." A holistic paradigm recognizes the importance of connectedness and is central to the Constitution of the World Health Organization (WHO), wherein "health is a state of complete, physical, mental and social well-being and not merely the absence of disease or infirmity." Social well-being flows from a sense that we are connected with ourselves and with the world around us.

The truth is, we have not evolved to live as we do. We evolved to live in clans, with myriad connections to others, with each member having a purpose that supported the whole. The price we have paid for the modern *lifestyle*, with all its conveniences and

The Failing Promises of Modern Psychiatry—*cont'd*

trappings of *success*, is profound disconnection. There is a pandemic of distress and existential despair. We have chased happiness for decades. Yet here we are. Bigger cars, monster homes, extravagant vacations, online shopping, cosmetic surgery … something, anything, to *make* us happy.

When our happiness remains elusive, we go to our doctor. We are then given a simple checklist that confirms *we are depressed*. Never mind that we really have no idea what depression *is* nor how it interfaces with normalcy. Recognizing this dilemma, the ancient Greeks created a boundary between *angst* and *melancholia*. Angst was a response to some life challenge and was inherent to normal human experience. Melancholia was a distinct, profound, and continuous depressive state that seemed independent of life circumstances.

Until the 1980s, a patient's depressive complaints were classified as being either *reactive* or *endogenous*. This parallels the ancient boundary between angst and melancholia. Reactive depressive symptoms were much less likely to respond to medication and were referred for psychotherapy. This important distinction was dropped from DSM-3 (1980). We are entering the fifth decade of an ever-expanded and overly inclusive concept of mental disorders. That this coincides with the introduction and aggressive marketing of novel "anti" depressants is no coincidence. We are in an era of medicalising *distress*, where most patients prescribed medications will fail to benefit (Melander et al., 2003). They will instead exhaust themselves going down rabbit holes that are proven and guaranteed to fail.

Elements of a Holistic Model
We tend to see only what we are trained to see or are comfortable managing. The decade of the brain has gotten us no closer to curing mental illness. Over the past decade there has been a dramatic decrease in the release of new psychotropic medications. It seems that even the pharmaceutical industry is throwing in the towel. Tweaking brain receptors, split off from the organism as a whole, is simply barking up the wrong tree. There is a better way.

The Body
The benefit of movement and exercise for our mental and physical well-being is widely recognized. We are all familiar with the saying "healthy body, healthy mind." A truly healthy body goes beyond the facade of one's appearance or BMI. Vital health is from the inside out. Central to this is the mind–gut connection. While the serotonin produced in the gut does not cross the blood–brain barrier, inflammatory cytokines certainly do, and as a result, they severely disrupt seratonin turnover. What triggers this inflammatory process? We need look no further than the modern Western lifestyle. The standard American diet (SAD diet) is inflammatory. The stress response is inflammatory.

Food as medicine is not a new concept. Hippocrates, considered by many to be the father of modern medicine, implored his patients, "Let food be thy medicine and medicine thy food." Beyond having passing familiarity with our national food guides, which are obsolete even as revised versions are published, today's doctors receive little or no training in nutritional health.

How many psychiatrists do a food diary with their patients? How many are aware that inflammation might be a significant perpetuating factor for a patient's depressive symptoms, much less test for it? How many can prescribe a specific nutrition plan that would support recovery and vital health? Beyond being passive recipients of *care*, how many psychiatrists call on their patients to be active partners in their holistic recovery plan? My patients are consistently amazed that a psychiatrist is asking them what they eat and sending them on their way with a lab requisition and a nutrition remediation plan.

The Mind

If our brains can be compromised by processes external to the blood–brain barrier, is the reverse also true? How do our thoughts and emotions impact our bodies? Living in the Western world, we are often in a state of heightened sympathetic tone—a state of fight, flight, or freeze. This adaptation is deeply wired into our brains and served us well for most of our evolutionary history, where imminent threats to life or limb were not uncommon. The threat would present itself, but once the threat was over—and if we survived—our nervous system would return to the restful state required for the body to heal and repair.

Modern-day threats no longer come in the form of the discrete and tangible tiger or rival tribesman. Today's threats come from having the luxury to sit and think, or more accurately put, to *ruminate* about all the potential calamities that might come our way. There is no such thing as *stress*, there is only the stress *response* to an external challenge. Life is challenging, but it does not have to be stressful—stress is a *possibility*.

Stress is a reflexive protective *response* at the level of our limbic brain—more specifically, the amygdala. In the absence of an objective threat to life or limb, the stress response is commonly triggered by *the stories* we tell ourselves—the so-called *amygdala hijack* (Goleman,1996). While we might not be able to completely eliminate the amygdala hijack, we can certainly influence what happens next. Rather than simply being along for the ride, we can learn to pause, witness, and reflect: *Am I using my brain, or is my brain using me?* (Tanzi & Chopra, 2013). We can redirect our minds from thoughts that are not serving us, recognizing that there is no such thing as stress in the external world—there is only the stress we *create* in response to life's daily challenges.

The stress response depletes the body in so many ways. As is the case with the SAD diet, stress is inflammatory. Chronic inflammation is an essential component of chronic diseases (Liu et al., 2017). Beyond its potential negative impact on mood, high levels of inflammation are commonly seen with PTSD along with a host of medical conditions, including coronary heart disease, diabetes, cancer, and dementia. Stress compromises our immune response and, in combination with our nutrient-poor SAD diets, heightens our susceptibility to disease. Even when not afflicted by a diagnosable illness, we feel depleted, lacking vital health.

A common presenting complaint is the patient claiming to have anxiety, or beyond that, an anxiety disorder. Generalized anxiety disorder is the diagnosis commonly applied. Rather than invoking yet another disorder, we might explore whether the anxiety *response* is a natural and logical consequence of dwelling on contexts beyond our immediate control. We do not classify tennis elbow as a disease. Tennis elbow is an overuse injury. Anxiety could be reframed as an overuse injury—overuse of the mind.

If I have my hand on a hot element, I can take Tylenol for the pain or I can take my hand off the element. If I have anxiety, I can take Lorazepam or I can learn mindfulness-based stress reduction. I can learn to meditate. I can evolve, giving up patterns that no longer serve me. I can take my power back, redirecting my mind from worrying

The Failing Promises of Modern Psychiatry—*cont'd*

about outcomes I cannot directly control. I can learn to quiet the mind, to think only when it serves me. I can experience the healing that comes from *alert thoughtlessness* (Tolle, 2005).

The Spirit

Spirit—herein defined as connection—is identifying with something beyond the material world, the world of *form* (Chopra, 2004). This connection has two poles—connection within (the *intra*personal) and without (the *inter*personal). We tend to be distracted by the noise around us, the external relationships. We feel hurt or rebuffed when we perceive some narcissistic injury. Brooding about how others treat us, we fail to recognize that we are our own harshest critic. We have incorporated so many messages both subtle and explicit. We cannot even remember where the story came from, yet we keep telling it:

> *"I am not enough."*
> *"I am a failure."*
> *"If others really knew me, they wouldn't like me."*
> *"I feel so guilty for my mistakes."*
> *"I hate myself."*

How is healing possible in such a toxic intrapersonal space? It is not. Without self-compassion, nothing else can take hold and flourish. Not CBT, not the next antidepressant trial, not even the whole-foods organic diet. After almost three decades of psychiatric practice, I continue to be amazed by the prevalence of self-loathing. In clinical practice, this is often the elephant in the room, akin to "Don't ask, don't tell." The patient is certainly not going to volunteer, "By the way doctor, I think you ought to know that I really hate myself." Conversely, the psychiatrist is unlikely to ask, "How do you feel about yourself?" Lacking their own self-awareness, the psychiatrist would be very uncomfortable knowing how to respond in any helpful way to a patient's intrapersonal despair.

Fundamentally, most of us have no idea who we are. How can we have compassion for something we do not know? Self-awareness is the foundation for self-compassion. Our sense of self is highly conditioned. We identify with our roles, relationships, successes, and failures. "I am a psychiatrist." No, I am not that. Psychiatrist is a temporary role I play in the movie of *My Life*. Who am I when I am not in that role? Whatever handle we identify with, does it capture the essence of who we are or is it something that can change? If "I am a success," then who am I when I fail?

We have become so identified with the *doing* that we have lost awareness of the *being* that is at our essence. On the day of our birth, we cannot avoid awareness of being. There is no inner dialogue or *story* telling us who we are or where we might be going. Undistracted by the thought stream, we are immersed in the silent witnessing that is our essential nature. This silent witnessing is central to the practice of meditation. From the stillness of *no mind*, we are content and whole. We are freed from the insatiable quest for something to *make* us happy.

Putting It All Together

Radical change requires radical action. Radical action is far-reaching and thorough—no stone is left unturned. Our treatments fail not because our patients are treatment resistant. Our treatments fail because they are not sufficiently radical. We are a complex

---

The Failing Promises of Modern Psychiatry—*cont'd*

interface of biological, psychological, social, and spiritual components. A radical inter-vention dictates treating all the components of health assertively and simultaneously. In this context, a model reliant on simple symptom checklists as evidence for *any* primary disorder is doomed to fail. How could it be otherwise?

Sources

Chopra, D. (2004). *The seven spiritual laws of success*. Amber-Allen Publishing/New World.

Goleman, D. (1996). *Emotional intelligence: Why it can matter more than IQ*. Bantam Books.

Liu, Y. Z., Wang, Y. X., & Jiang, C. L. (2017). Inflammation: The common pathway of stress-related diseases. *Frontiers in Human Neuroscience, 11*, 316. https://doi.org/10.3389/fnhum.2017.00316.

Melander, H., Ahlqvist-Rastad, J., Meijer, G., et al. (2003). Evidence b(i)ased medicine—selective reporting from studies sponsored by pharmaceutical industry: Review of studies in new drug applications. *British Medical Journal, 326*(7400), 1171–1173. https://doi.org/10.1136/bmj.326.7400.1171.

Paris, J. (2015). *The intelligent clinician's guide to the DSM-5*. Oxford University Press.

Tanzi, R. E., & Chopra, D. (2013). *Super brain: Unleashing the explosive power of your mind to maximize health, happiness, and spiritual well-being*. Harmony.

Tolle, E. (2005). *A new earth: Awakening to your life's purpose*. Dutton.

Responding to the Call: Forging a New Path Forward

For caregivers and their families and loved ones. For the populations they serve. For the future of public service and the wider systems we operate within. We can do better. We must do better.

There is a crisis in the health care system. It is not surgery wait times, federal transfer payments, antibiotic-resistant bacteria, or even opioid overdose deaths. The crisis is the epidemic of professional caregivers suffering from mental health conditions, caused or exacerbated by the toll that high stress, often trauma-laden positions exert. The statistics are alarming: as many as 94% of caregivers working in emergency and trauma-laden settings screen positive for PTSD (Iranmanesh et al., 2013). Nearly half of our professional caregivers screen positive for depression and report being unwell owing to work stress, which impacts morale, absenteeism, retention rates, and patient care (BMG Research, 2013; Chandler, 2012; Simon & McFadden, 2017).

Resiliency is important to enable thriving. As Confucius said, "Our greatest glory is not in never falling, but in rising every time we fall." Similarly, for this work, **resilience** is reflected in a way of being that views challenges optimistically, as opportunities to learn and grow. Resilience promotes an ability to adapt in the face of adversity, emerging from a benevolent orientation and a felt confidence that we have the resources and support system necessary to navigate challenges as they arise. On this journey, the two primary developmental assets that support a more resilient way of being are sense of coherence (Antonovsky, 1979) and congruence (Rogers, 1959).

To bolster resilience, we circle back again and again to the research, the conceptual frameworks, and several developmental practices that promote sense of coherence (mindfulness, gratitude, and optimism) and congruence (self-compassion, forgiveness, and resolving trauma). Workers who exhibit congruence and coherence generally feel positive about their contributions to the organization, are more effective and productive, and show less absenteeism (Dames, 2018; Salt et al., 2008; Steege & Rainbow, 2017; Steger et al., 2012). Furthermore, since Canadian workers spend an average of 10.5 hours working and commuting every day, promoting healthy behaviours at work is essential to decreasing the burden and cost of stress-related absenteeism, lost productivity, and disability claims (Bodenheimer & Sinsky, 2014; WorkSafeBC, 2018). Research shows that working on congruence and coherence with health care providers naturally impacts workplace culture, especially if employees are well supported by leaders (Dixon-Woods et al., 2014; Steger et al., 2012; West, 2018).

However, personal resilience is only one part of the equation. The other equally important part is the external work: contextual, cultural, and system resilience. We cannot expect to bloom where we are planted if the soil in which we find ourselves fails to provide the primary human requirements that enable us to flourish. For this leg of the journey back to personal wholeness, we focus on the inner work: personal resilience. Once we tend to resilience on the personal level, we are far more likely to feel empowered and resourced to enact the changes necessary on the contextual level.

CHAPTER 1

Root Strength: Sense of Coherence and Congruence

Who looks outside, dreams; who looks inside, awakes.

Carl G. Jung

Throughout the book, I use the metaphor of a tree to describe the relationship between caregivers and the external factors that drive stress and burnout in caregiving work (Figure 1.1). The roots of the tree represent intrinsic inner assets that provide the tree with the strength to survive, and even thrive, amid the elements. The external forces against the tree represent the everyday adversities within caregiving work. These adversities are largely unnecessary and unproductive and yet exist as stressors in virtually every caregiver's workplace to some extent. In this book, I focus not on the weather, but on the roots. The organizational storms (trauma-laden work areas, heavy workloads, violence, lack of administrative support) in the health care system are explored elsewhere. Suffice it to say that fixing the system producing the weather is a worthy and essential endeavour. However, the focus here is on developing the caregiver's calm in the storm—in part knowing that centred and confident caregivers will both demand and facilitate system change.

The Roots Theory describes how the orientation to the inner and outer world inform one's ability to engage in thriving. Furthermore, it describes how connection to community provides the necessary medicine to heal trauma and to take on more compassionate ways of being. There are two basic concepts, or characteristics, that I use to underpin the calm, quiet, stable, and grounded nature of strong roots. The two primary characteristics of these roots are (1) a **sense of coherence** and (2) **congruence** (see Appendix A). Developing a sense of coherence centres on improving our orientation to life; congruence is about self-compassionately deepening our roots by improving our orientation to self. Together, these two characteristics enable us to self-actualize into our best and most authentic self; they equip us to thrive.

Our sense of coherence includes mindfulness and self-efficacy. It shapes how we relate to the outer world and how confident we are when navigating life's challenges. Developing a sense of coherence improves our ability to manage internal and external stimuli with confidence, knowing we have the resources necessary to resolve potential threats to our well-being. When our sense of coherence is high, meaning drives us into alignment with our desires and a calling that extends beyond ourselves.

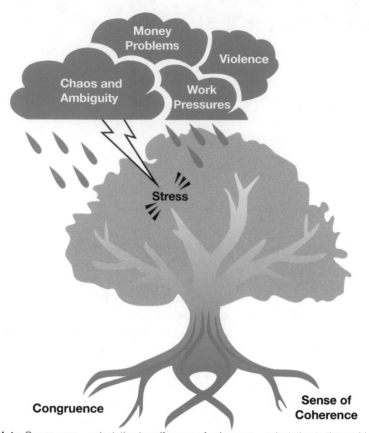

Note. Congruence = orientation to self; sense of coherence = orientation to the world.

Fig. 1.1 The Strength of the Roots. The depth and strength of our roots (personal and collective resources) determines our perception of the "weather" (external stimuli), which can be viewed either as a stimulus we can navigate or as a stressful threat to our basic needs and survival. The "weather" takes many forms and includes racism, discrimination, trauma, and moral injury, which can also activate internal, unresolved trauma and stress from our past, contributing to higher stress levels. When deeply rooted, we are more likely to view challenges optimistically, seeing them as meaningful/synchronistic opportunities for healing and clearing to promote future thriving. When roots are shallow, we cannot distinguish between past and present, and the "weather" seems overwhelming. As a result, the ability to thrive is hampered. Operating from this survival mode quickly depletes our energy.

Congruence includes self-compassion and determines how we relate, respond to, and express the stimuli arising from our inner world. The more congruent we are, the more we freely express our authentic self. If we have unconditional positive regard for ourselves, then we can self-compassionately tend to inner tensions when challenges do arise.

When we are lacking in congruence and a sense of coherence, we are more apt to spiral into stress states, disabling our ability to thrive and leading to a host of mental and physical health issues. Together, congruence and a sense of coherence enable us to thrive in high-stimulus work environments, yet few training programs articulate their importance, and even fewer provide the tools to attain them. This book provides insights and evidence-informed tools that promote congruence and a sense of coherence, which are essential to establish the deep roots necessary to buffer caregivers from many of the stressors endemic in the workplace. While some have had the benefit of garnering these personal resources in their childhood, the research (and my life experience) demonstrates that when we reconnect to the essence of who we are and the innate resources within us, these assets can also be developed in adulthood.

The Conceptual Framework Behind the Roots Theory

Sense of coherence (Antonovsky, 1979): Sense of coherence centres on our orientation to life, our ability to reframe and resource with confidence and optimism. Our degree of sense of coherence informs our sense of agency, meaning making, comprehension, predictability, confidence, and self-efficacy. Presence and mindful reorienting is a core factor in the development of a greater sense of coherence.

Congruence (Rogers, 1959): Congruence centres on our orientation and connection to self and others. It is the aligning of our "real" (actual) self and "ideal" (potential) self. Authentic expression and deepening self-compassion are key for developing congruence.

When combined, congruence and a sense of coherence enable us to thrive. Thriving roots are those deeply rooted in personal authenticity and in connection with the world. From this grounded place, we can mindfully live with purpose, joy, courage, and compassion.

These two concepts are best developed within a relational container that promotes awareness, self-regulation, self-compassion and other compassion and connection, and alignment with one's calling. **Polyvagal theory** provides the theoretical framework that describes the healing capacity of the communities of practice that embody the Roots Theory. Ultimately, when people experience a felt sense of unconditional positive regard, they securely attach to themselves and others, which promotes a greater tolerance for passing stimuli. With a calm nervous system, there is a greater ability to feel into the inner and outer resources that enable humans to thrive.

Vision for a Deep-Rooted World

Cultivate a deep well inside yourself and you will never thirst.

While this book pulls from research focused on professional caregiving, it also applies to the informal caregiving roles we take on, such as parenting children and caring for dependents. In an ideal world—the world we envision for the generations to come after us—we begin life depending on others for soothing and to have our basic needs met.

We then mature into independent, self-soothing adults. In this ideal world, as children, we would experience a sense of unconditional positive regard, empowering us to express ourselves authentically. As a result, we would develop high levels of congruence and self-compassion, enabling us to accept and embrace our popular and not-so-popular features. We would incubate in an environment that promotes the confidence to step into meaningful caregiving roles, trusting that we have the resources to manage whatever challenges may arise and that, in the end, all things will work out reasonably (sense of coherence). With adequate developmental and material resources (congruence and a high sense of coherence), we would soothe ourselves in the face of suffering, knowing our inner world always has just the right medicine in our time of need. We would come to know this inner world as a place of stillness, the eye of the storm when the winds howl around us: these are thriving roots. With intention and alignment, we come to view the world and take action from this empowered way of being. In a deep-rooted world, everyone has the resources they need to cope with the rain, and better yet, to use the rain to spur our growth and inspire service to others.

Navigating Global Threats

Just like trees (see Figure 1.1), we are members of a larger forest with an opportunity to collectively resource, taking what we need in times of need and giving what we can in times of plenty. Global threats to humanity, such as a pandemic, are an opportunity for humans around the world to come together to collectively navigate a common challenge before it becomes a chronic stressor. In areas that were hit hard by the first wave of the COVID-19 pandemic, there was a tremendous mental health impact on professional caregivers and frontline essential service workers (Lai et al., 2020; Tsamakis et al., 2020). Many struggled to find their footing in their work and life roles as the first wave of the outbreak subsided.

Each of us has varying degrees of personal resiliency, reflected in the depth of our "root" systems. As a result, transient "weather" systems will feel more threatening (stressful) to some than others. The "weather" is the events, thoughts, and emotions that circle us, taking many forms, individually and globally. In these rapidly changing and often chaotic situations, a common form of "weather" is ambiguity. When ambiguity is high, it causes many of us to spiral into fear states that fester amid a sea of potentially threatening scenarios. Adding to the ambiguity, collective actions taken to navigate the potential threat can cause even greater insecurity, especially for those whose physiological needs (food, shelter) or sense of safety are threatened. As a result, stress levels are high, which can lead to either chronic anxiety (sympathetic nervous system stuck in the "on" mode) or freeze, leaving us feeling disconnected and depressed (parasympathetic nervous system stuck in the "on" mode). By grounding collectively, as opposed to isolating individually, we are more likely to manage these common human challenges before they evolve into chronic stressors.

At the risk of overcomplicating a complex topic, on a practical level there are three evidence-informed qualities we can cultivate to promote personal and collective resilience in these collectively uncertain times:

1. According to polyvagal theory (Porges, 2011), we are more likely to regulate our stress and confidently manage challenges when *we feel securely connected to others*. For instance, in a pandemic scenario, while physical distance may be a requirement, social distancing is not. In this age of technology, we can stay connected to others despite physical restrictions.

2. To bolster our sense of coherence (Antonovsky, 1979), *we can expand our awareness of the plethora of inner and outer resources at our disposal*. We can ground ourselves by taking an inventory of the structures (family, work, hobbies), assets (a safe place to live, food, warmth), activities (exercise, breathing, hobbies that bring joy), and relationships (people you feel safe being authentic with) that help you feel resourced and secure amid the felt chaos. When we feel out of control and lost in a sea of insecurity, reminding ourselves of our resources is imperative. It is our resources that help us interrupt the stress response and that boost our confidence so that we can creatively navigate the challenges that arise before they turn into chronic stressors.

3. To keep us connected, and thus prevent states of fight, flight, or freeze, *we can use these uncomfortable emotions to cultivate habits that promote self-compassion* (Rogers, 1959). In other words, we can increase our capacity to self-regulate and self-soothe when discomfort comes our way. We do this by showing up authentically with the people with whom we feel safe, those who can acknowledge and normalize our suffering. When we pay attention to what is arising within, we have an opportunity to provide ourselves with the loving-kindness necessary to feel and tend to past and present wounds. This process begins with noticing when difficult thoughts and emotions arise, then stepping back to recognize these stimuli as transient messengers, rather than overly identifying with them. With this stepping back (nonattachment), we are more able to provide loving-kindness to ourselves, much like we would respond to a dear friend.

While global urgencies and emergencies often feel threatening, they are excellent opportunities to brush off our resources, strengthen our sense of belonging in a larger community, and cultivate greater personal and collective resilience.

Spirituality in the Roots

We are not human beings having a spiritual experience, rather we are spiritual beings having a human experience.

Teiylhard de Chardin

There are elements in the writing here that may be interpreted as spiritual. However, I wrote this book with no particular religion or religious lens in mind. Rather,

I encourage readers to relate to the material in a way that works for them, regardless of their religion or lack thereof. The words surrounding spirituality are used philosophically and are not affiliated with any god or religion. The term spirituality acknowledges that there is an "immaterial reality imperceptible to the senses" (Encyclopaedia Britannica, 2020). With this definition, engaging with our spirituality looks different for different people. It may have you communing with the forest or attending Sunday mass or gazing with wonder at a painting. Seminal author Richard Rohr (1999) describes this sacred space as **liminality**, representing the threshold between what is known and the mystery of what is yet to come. It is in this space that most of our significant embodied transformations emerge. Staying embodied in this space is essential to shift from one way of being to another. To do so, we must navigate, not shut down, the felt chaos that arises in the in between.

This text takes you on a journey that is born largely from humanistic (Maslow, 1943; Rogers, 1959), transpersonal (Porges, 2011; Rogers, 1959), and transcendental and integral theories (Wilber, 2001). Spirituality is the essential component that fuels our transpersonal and transcendental capabilities. Neuman (1995) and Watson (1988), both seminal theorists in nursing, incorporated spirituality as a core element of whole-person caregiving. Over a decade of research links spirituality to health outcomes as evidenced in a study by Loeb et al. (2003) showing that a spiritual focus promotes a greater ability for older persons to manage multiple co-morbidities. Similarly, Brady et al.'s (1999) study reported that a spiritual focus was positively correlated with a higher quality of life. Despite substantial evidence for the positive effects of spirituality, we as caregivers often broach the topic with a great deal of trepidation.

Spirituality is woven into the content presented here using terms such as essence, higher power, higher self, or Spirit. If any of these terms is a stumbling block for you, explore others that you are comfortable with. While religious differences can divide us, I believe that we can find common ground in the idea that we are all tethered to an essence or interconnectivity that transcends the limits of our humanity. The development of our roots requires a tethering to this essence, accessed and strengthened by dropping into our inner world. In this way, I discuss spirituality as a doorway to connect to essence—the core of who we really are beneath our cultural conditioning.

> *All meaningful and sustainable behavioural changes emerge from a spiritual reorientation or shift—from those moments when our entire frame of reference changes. Once we shift spiritually, in time and with this new and expanded way of "being," old and unhelpful ways of "doing" naturally fall away.*

Connecting to a spiritual source that provides us with a felt sense of unconditional positive regard cultivates self-compassion, loving-kindness for others, objectivity, meaning, and guidance amid a sea of passing feelings, thoughts, and experiences. Incorporating spirituality, in whatever way that looks to each of us, enhances the mental and physical health benefits of meditation practice (Wachholtz et al., 2017). To develop the key requirements of thriving, I take you beyond cognitive knowing (the "figuring it out" mind), promoting an ability to let it fall into the background of a much larger and spiritually inclusive reality. This common spiritual thread holds each part of the book together.

And now here is my secret, a very simple secret: It is only with the heart that one can see rightly; what is essential is invisible to the eye.
                              Antoine de Saint-Exupéry, The Little Prince

MENTAL ILLNESS OR SPIRITUAL DISTRESS?

Engaging in thriving requires both an intermingling and an evolution of our physical and cognitive frameworks, inspired and fueled by a ground-shifting spiritual awakening.

The body acts as the vessel that enables the spirit to actualize in the physical world, providing a tangible reflection of how individualism and collectivism intertwine. When tuned into one's individual spirit, the indomitable and abundant force within, we expand beyond the vessel it inhabits to align collectively and compassionately with all beings. We are all this glorious combination of spirit and body, whole as individuals, and collectively part of something that is far greater than the limitations of our physical form.

The biology and conditioning of our nervous system developed within a blueprint of scarcity and fear millions of years ago. When we default to this fear, our thoughts, emotions, and resulting behaviours emerge as projections of the old belief systems connected to unhealed wounds. Our spiritual self is the conduit that connect us to a power greater than our physical selves, reminding us of our wholeness and enabling genuine and compassionate connection to each other and to the planet that hosts us.

Without spirit, the efforts of the body lack inspiration. Without buy-in from the body, the spirit becomes trapped, unable to actualize in the physical world.

When immersed in a world fixated on adornments and the appraisal of others, our orientation to spirit shifts. The spontaneous, spirit-filled self feels incongruent with what the external world demands. As a result, the spirit becomes a threat to the body's felt need to gain the approval of the conditioned world. As the spirit grows dimmer with each layer of conditioning, the defensive nervous system becomes our primary concern. Spiritual distress signals become a source of anxiety to the body, reminding us that we have forgotten who we are. As a result, the relentless need to *do* lacks spiritual inspiration, eroding our emotional energy stores and causing dis-*ease*. When separated from and out of tune with spirit, the body cannot navigate the world objectively. This separation leads to spiritual distress that remains until we tune in again. Tuning in is the process of relearning what it means to be a human *be*ing.

Addressing spiritual distress begins with stepping into a new blueprint, moving from fear to abundance. We do this by finding containers that promote spiritual expression, enabling us to feel safe to *be* authentic. In time, we regain the trust necessary to enable the body to come into right relationship with the spirit. With this trust, the conditioning falls away, and the spirit grows brighter. We reach a tipping point, the resistance of the body dissipates, and we are able to see the conditioning for what it is. We set our *be*ing free from the illusive conditions of the physical world, and our orientation shifts from fear to abundance. From this space, the spirit informs the *do*ing of the body, providing the ease, confidence, direction, and inspiration to live this short life abundantly. Finally, it is important to normalize the frustrations along the way. When we experience spiritual insights, embodied shifts (sustained changes in behaviour) often take longer. Rather than allowing shame to fester because of the felt **incongruence**, this is our opportunity to consciously cultivate self-compassion. With self-compassion, the body relaxes. And when the body relaxes, we begin to cultivate the environment necessary to embody the essence of who we are.

The Journey Ahead

This book is divided into 12 chapters. We begin by discussing the actualization of the "real" self and, through exploration of stressors and resiliency development practices, we learn to engage in thriving. By studying this book and engaging with the exercises, you will try a variety of tools, noticing what resonates and setting aside what does not. Part 1 of the book focuses heavily on *coming to know*, explaining why this work is needed, exploring the components of health care culture that are, ironically, unsupportive of health and well-being, and ultimately convincing the mind that the journey is indeed worth our time and attention. Once we feel motivated and ready, Part 2 will take us deeper into experiential practices, promoting the development of congruence and sense of coherence through a variety of attuning, strengthening, clearing, and aligning practices.

Here is a general overview of the topics covered in each chapter:

- Part 1: Coming to Know Through the Research
  - Chapter 1: Root Strength: Sense of Coherence and Congruence: Introduces the core concepts and framework undergirding the experiential nature of this work
  - Chapter 2: Coming to Know How to Thrive: Describes the concept of thriving and the necessary components to engage in it

- Chapter 3: Coming to Know About Stress: Describes the concept and complexities of stress and the common sources that lead to it
- Part 2: Coming to Know Through the Felt Sense
  - Chapter 4: Attuning to Your "Roots": Moves into the realm of felt sense, whereby we begin exploring the strength of our roots
  - Chapter 5: Strengthening Congruence With Self-Compassion: Describes the importance of self-compassion and provides the core components and tools to promote its development
  - Chapter 6: Navigating Stressors: Clearing the "Noise" and Managing the Weather: Provides insight into managing external stressors, all of which draw upon tools that engage our inner resources to feel and release unresolved emotions (trauma) that we were previously not equipped to navigate
  - Chapter 7: Strengthening Sense of Coherence: Mindful Reorientation: Focuses on mindfulness—staying connected to the inner self, building mindful habits, and letting go of our tendencies to ruminate on thoughts of the past and the future. Sense of coherence develops as we mindfully recognize and learn to trust our inner resources, cultivating a greater ability to see the world from this more objective lens.
  - Chapters 8: Strengthening as We Till the Soil of Our Childhoods: We continue clearing areas of incongruence. As such, without getting stuck in narratives that disempower us, we gently feel our way back to our upbringing, tilling the soil of our childhoods.
  - Chapter 9: Strengthening Our Self-Soothing Capacities: Calm at the Roots: We explore the tools and techniques that promote the ability to self-soothe instead of looking to chemicals and activities as a distracting reprieve. Self-soothing is a natural result of coming to know, trust, and take comfort in our inner world.
  - Chapter 10: Clearing Past Trauma: The Unresolved Weather of the Past: Delves deeper into resolving trauma, using mindfulness to reorient ourselves in the face of difficult experiences and connecting, strengthening, and deepening our sense of support and grounding to our spiritual roots.
- Part 3: Aligning With Calling in Community
  - Chapter 11: Aligning With Calling: Roots Over Fruits: Describes how "living our calling" is what it looks like to thrive. We align our choices with our essence (values and desires) and the unique life purpose that flows from that essence.
  - Chapter 12: Aligning in Community: Connecting Root Systems: Turns outward to focus on service and leadership. To sustain any meaningful changes in health care culture, priorities and decision making are rooted in the understanding that lasting change requires a spiritual transformation at every organizational level.

Making the Most of the Journey

While the journey through this life curriculum is informed by science, how we shift goes far beyond coming to know the research. Science helps us come to know by showing us the clues along the way. But deep knowing, the kind that moves us into new ways of being, occurs by coming to know through experiential learning, enabling us to develop our felt sense (Figure 1.2).

The process by which we develop a new trajectory—from coming to know to alignment with calling (Figure 1.3)—reflects the learning methods that promote sense of coherence and congruence (see Figure 1.3). This learning approach follows the principles of adult learning and metacognitive skill development (Stolovitch & Keeps, 2011). As you immerse in the tools and techniques, you will engage in exercises that relate to the five transformative practices—coming to know, attuning, strengthening, clearing, and aligning—each of which further develops our felt sense. In this section, I outline how these

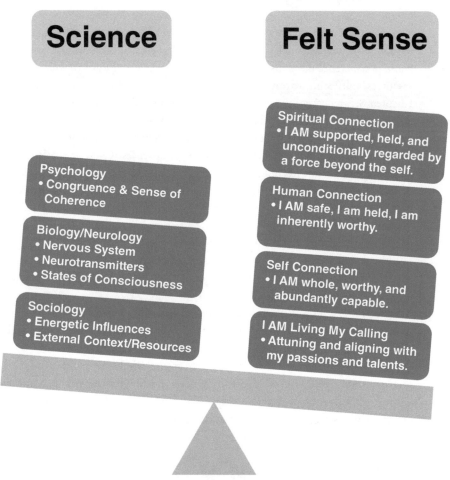

Fig. 1.2 This journey is informed by science, undergirded by widely adopted concepts and principles. The tools provided on the journey correlate with evidence-informed strategies to bolster sense of coherence and congruence. Once we come to know the science, we can surrender to a much deeper knowledge, enabling the inner world to direct our steps as we attune and strengthen our felt sense.

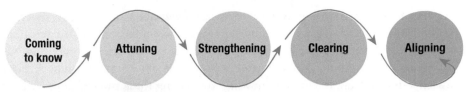

Fig. 1.3   A New Trajectory. From coming to know to alignment with one's calling.

transformative practices have emerged from an evidence-informed framework so that you can make the most of the journey. In doing so, I hope that you will trust the process, moving past scientific knowing to a deeper experiential knowing. The five transformative practices are as follows:

- **Coming to Know**
  - Empowered learning: catering to your learning style
  - The core requirements of stress mitigation and thriving
- **Attuning**
  - Reflecting from the heart
  - Connecting new learning with experiences and context
  - Practising a variety of exercises to integrate learning
  - Noticing what you notice: distinguishing signal from noise
  - Tuning by bringing new learning into focus: pruning the knowledge tree
- **Strengthening**
  - Developing sense of coherence through activities that promote:
    - Meaning making
    - Self-efficacy
    - Mindfulness
  - Developing congruence through activities that promote:
    - Authentic expression
    - Self-compassion
- **Clearing**
  - Identifying old belief systems: pivoting via reorientation
  - Identifying and digesting areas of incongruence and trauma
- **Aligning**
  - Leaning into your "real" self: connecting to authentic values and desires
  - Embracing connectivity beyond your container
  - Living your calling
  - Goal setting that aligns with your calling, propelling you toward your vision
  - Setting out on a new trajectory via new habits and new ways of being
  - Stepping into compassionate leadership

Activities and practices enable shifts in our way of being, challenging old beliefs with evidence-informed tools and techniques and offering new perspectives to reorient ourselves. As illustrated in Figure 1.3, we *come to know* about our biology, psychology, and human tendencies by building awareness and understanding the research. We apply the research to our experiences and unique contexts. By practising, we cultivate habit formation, to *come to be* more whole as we transform superficial knowledge into a deep, integrated knowing. By making these small changes, we set out on a new trajectory. Like an airplane adjusting its orientation by one degree, these changes are barely perceivable in the beginning, but over the course of the flight, these incremental changes lead the plane to its final destination. *New trajectories* are about making small, intentional adjustments to our orientation to the world and our orientation to self, which over time will alter the course of our lives.

Because we are all different, some exercises will resonate and others will not. Keep what you like and let go of the rest, trusting that the tool you need will come to you when you need it. Additionally, if we interpret tools as magic bullets, coming from a "fix me" mentality, we promote further incongruence. However, if we approach the work with curiosity and self-compassion, we strengthen our self-trust, self-integrity, and sense of coherence and congruence in the process.

Knowledge is not what you can remember, but what you cannot forget.

As demonstrated in Figure 1.3 and Appendix B, this book follows a framework where participants "come to know" by remembering the heart of their identity. This coming to know process, outlined earlier, promotes agency, an ability to reframe and reorient, and a deep sense of connection inwardly and outwardly. We cultivate agency, reorientation, and connection by:

- **Attuning** to personal and collective resources. We attune by dropping into our bodies and inner worlds and tuning into our unique values, calling, spirituality, and inner and outer sense capacities (e.g., intuition, insight, physical senses). Attuning promotes agency and helps us distinguish between the imprints of social conditioning and habitual, survival/stress behaviours. This also includes attuning to healthy relationship support: the wisdom, compassion, witnessing, and mirroring of group participants.
- **Strengthening** by cultivating connection and mindfulness: understanding "the weather" of our workplace environments as well as trauma, stress, and the process of recovery; using tools and practices for physical and emotional regulation; and cultivating relationships of unconditional positive regard with ourselves and fellow participants.
- **Clearing** coping strategies that no longer serve us through self-compassion, insight, shadow work, and releasing shame. We regulate the nervous system to clear the stress response. We clear out the old thought systems that are no longer serving us.
- **Aligning** and **reframing/reorienting** our personal and professional identity with our authenticity, our "calling" to live in the most meaningful, joyful, and healthy way possible.

Practices Are Not Prescriptions

There are many suggestions and exercises included in this book; these are not intended as magic bullets, but to enhance self-awareness through exploration, experimentation, and critical reflection on how each practice may or may not resonate with our unique needs and desires. Assuming that the practices will suit everyone only breeds homogenization. Our brain chemistries, our past experiences, our projections, and our vulnerabilities are all different. Given our unique needs and desires, there can be no general prescription that will work for all. Rather, the exercises are tools to try out: you can decide for yourself whether they heartfully resonate and whether they are helpful on your journey toward a greater sense of coherence and congruence.

Respond to every call that excites your spirit.

Rumi (1997)

Attuning is a reflection practice where we filter events, opinions, and practices through the lens of our heart. Using this form of reflection (taking notice of what resonates) as you work through the concepts and after each practice is the most important part. Through reflection we come to know ourselves and what engages our hearts and minds, including our desires or lack of desire to continue with certain practices. Be mindful of what comes up for you with each practice; let go of whatever is not resonating and hold on to what is. When you find you are "attaching" to a practice or tool, remember that they are guideposts on this journey of self-discovery and self-healing. Notice which ones seem to illuminate undigested dissonance from the past that is perhaps ready to heal; notice how they stir your emotions and desires.

Circling With Unconditional Positive Regard: Cultivating a Community of Practice

A **community of practice** describes a group of people who share an intention for something they do and learn how to integrate it into their daily lives, learning to do it better as they interact regularly (Wenger-Trayner & Wenger-Trayner, 2015). In the context of this work, it describes a group of people with a shared intention to cultivate a space of unconditional positive regard, aiming to minimize stress and other barriers to thriving and to maximize one's ability to flourish individually and in community. As a group, the community of practice facilitates the ability to operate from this place in their day-to-day lives through relationships and practices that expand awareness and promote self-regulation and stress mitigation, heartful connectedness, and an ability to live one's calling.

It is within a community of practice that we learn self-compassion, which describes the embodiment of unconditional positive regard, enabling us to mirror the same inwardly. It is important to cultivate your circle of support, those people in your life that you feel unconditionally positively regarded by, that see you as whole and inherently worthy of love and belonging no matter what. I expound upon these relationships later in the book, but it is important to begin this part of the journey sooner rather than later, as much of this work requires a willingness to be vulnerable. To be willing, we need to feel safe. Cultivating a safe inner and outer environment enables us to feel safe, even held, fueling the courage necessary to step out into new territory.

CO-CREATING A CONTAINER THAT PROMOTES HEALING

> *Circle started around the cook-fires of humanity's ancestors and has accompanied us ever since. We remember this space. When we listen, we speak more thoughtfully. We lean in to shared purpose.*
>
> The Circle Way (2019)

Remaining in isolation can take us only so far. Finding our people, those who can remind us of who we are and help us tether more securely, will take us the rest of the way. Healing happens at the pace of trust, and because we are relational beings, trust is built in relationship to self, to others, and to self with others (being witnessed as we express ourselves in the world). As illustrated in Figure 1.4, one way to cultivate trust is by formally circling up with like-intentioned others. It is our

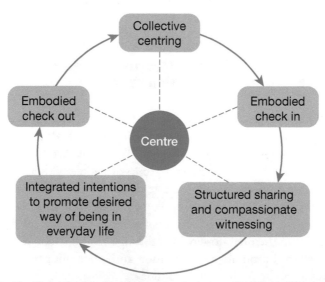

Fig. 1.4   The Circle Way. *The Circle Way: A Leader in Every Chair* (Baldwin et al., 2010).

circle of support that holds us, steadies us on the more difficult parts of the journey. Furthermore, being witnessed as we take on new ways of being expedites our ability to have meaningful shifts, where we can embody new insights and intentions in our day-to-day life. Each time we step out in courage by saying what we think or respond to how we feel in the company of others, our trust in the container and ourselves grows. Those who see us for who we are and who celebrate authenticity help us relax into the healing process. While no *one* circle will feel safe for every person in every moment, we can maximize the felt safety of all by following a predictable structure and developing collective agreements to which every member contributes and with which every member agrees.

One way to encourage individual agency is to explicitly make agreements that promote acceptance of and trust in each other's emotional regulation needs. For instance, some may dislike saying goodbye or hugging, some may need breaks away from intense stimuli to avoid using dissociation as a coping mechanism, and others may need to move around to tend to their physical needs. Enabling members to mindfully manage biological distractions, transitions, and potential activators by doing what feels good and safe is unconditional positive regard in action. Furthermore, celebrating these self-compassionate practices within the circle promotes congruence and sense of coherence. In addition to agreements, having a structure reduces ambiguity (a common stressor) and strengthens the group's shared intentions. The core circling practices promote speaking with intention, listening with attention, and tending to the well-being of the circle.

Reconciliation: Stepping out of the Box

As a third-generation settler in Canada, I have struggled to connect to truth and reconciliation efforts. While I support the cause, it never felt applicable to my day-to day life until recently.

As I have started to awaken to who I am, separate from my conditioning, I am also awakening to the dehumanizing nature of the system we live and work in. This rigid, perfectionistic system is a living and breathing result of colonization (establishing control over people, forcing assimilation to one way of being). And the truth is, I spend a good part of my day reinforcing it.

COLONIZATION HURTS (EVERYONE)

Ironically, I have spent years working on inner reconciliation, making peace with adversities from childhood, making amends with those I have wronged, and updating old and unhelpful belief systems. No matter the inner work, I recognize that I walk around each day forcing myself into the neat little boxes prescribed to me from a young age. I do not enjoy stepping into these boxes. They feel rigid, predictable, and lifeless. To fit inside, I must make myself small, quieting my inner voice so I can assimilate. Once inside the box, I do not feel good. I feel oppressed, held down, ashamed because my real self does not feel welcome there. I must quiet my authentic self, instead taking on the ideal display prescribed to me. Inside this box, my emotions feel threatening because they tell me to get out, that it is not safe, that I do not fit there. I am feeling threatened because I know these emotions are important messengers: they are telling me what needs to be done to heal, to self-actualize into my most authentic and best self. But that box is all I have known for so many years, and I am too afraid to step out. What if I am alone out there? What if I shed the walls around me, revealing my true self, only to face rejection? And then, after ruminating on these thoughts, I freeze, immobilized from acting. And so I stay in the box. I retreat to a feeling of safety, clinging to the familiar walls, finding comfort in the predictability they bring.

In this individualistic culture, we like our boxes. There is the box we work in, which we spend much of our lives serving feverishly, rewarded by extra letters that bolster the power and respect of our birth names. Then there are all the other boxes that we hop in and out of: the church box, the parent box, and the "gotta look socially competent" box.

I spend most of my day moving between boxes, wearing them like a well-insulated jacket and then removing each box when it no longer serves its purpose. And what purpose is that? I want to be accepted and loved; I want to feel like I belong to something bigger than myself. Each box holds a promise of a sense of belonging, and somehow that deep primal need seems to justify putting my "real" self to sleep. Waking up feels dangerous. I have served this colonized system for so long that I am afraid to be free of it. I am afraid that if I step outside of the walls, I ... I ... I don't know. And that not knowing terrifies me.

Then it happened. I found people like me—people that want to step out, be free, be seen, and in that seeing, to love and be loved, sans boxes. Even more exciting is that this box-burning work is infectious, and sure enough, an entire community is emerging all around us.

It is time to open our eyes to the consequences of conforming and colonizing. We all carry trauma from this homogenizing system we live in. To genuinely reconcile with others, we must first face our own truth, reconciling with who we are in this world and how in our sleepiness we continue to contribute to colonization.

I am coming to know that we are more than the boxes we hide in. We are so much more...

Attuning for the Journey Ahead: Cultivating Habits and Centring

Centring is what happens when we stop doing, allowing us to feel and tune into the spirit of our being. When we tune in, in this way, we find stable ground in the essence of who we are.

Imagine each area of self is an essential piece of the whole longing to be authentically expressed. Much like a vessel that exists to be filled, so too are these pieces completed as we recognize, allow, and nurture them to fullness. With each nurturing practice, we add another drop of water to these waiting parts of self, these vessels inside us that long to be filled and fulfilled. Eventually, the vessel's surface tension grows to a point that it can no longer remain bounded by the walls of the cup and an undeniable shift occurs. To this end, try several practices, find what resonates with you. You will cultivate habits that, in time, will fill and fulfill the parts of your self that long to be accepted, allowed, expressed, and loved. Remember to manage your expectations, as these shifts take time; some will require far more drops for the cup to fill up before they finally spill out of the container they are bound by. Trust the process.

Centring is about coming back to your centre, the unchanging essence of who you are. There are several ways to come back to your centre, and I recommend it as a core habit to develop. Here are a few centring techniques to try:

- **Feel your feet on the ground** anytime, anywhere (when able, put your bare feet on the earth).
- **Lift your eyes to the sky**, imagine this sky as your witness, the all-knowing entity that knows *you*, the *you* that exists beyond the conditioning. For some, looking to the sky is a reminder of a loving and all-knowing God or a higher power that makes us feel loved and accepted as we are.
- **Focus on the breath, or better yet, focus on the space between your breaths**. Let your breath anchor you, reminding you that *you* exist outside of the noise of internal and external stimuli. *You* are not the noise; you are the space, the observer of the noise. Each time you focus on the breath, you are stepping back from the noise, cultivating nonattachment and objectivity.
- **Loving-kindness**. Through loving-kindness practice (several practices are available in this book), we learn to lead with the heart—our physical and spiritual centre. So often in the West, we are conditioned to lead with the head, analyzing the most efficient, most socially acceptable plan of action. As a result, we can lose our sense of self and the desires that stir and excite us. By reconnecting to the heart, we access the most powerful part of self, centring via loving-kindness practices directed inwardly and outwardly.

In addition to theory and research, you will be given an opportunity to develop a sense of coherence and congruence by picking and choosing from a variety of experiential and reflective practices presented in Experiential Practice Opportunity sections and Attuning/Reflecting Opportunity sections.

Attuning/Reflecting Opportunity

Tapping into a sense of meaning and joy in this work is necessary to centre and sustain ourselves on the rougher parts of the journey. It is about remembering who we are and what really matters to us. Being mindful to simply take notice (refraining from analyzing or judging good or bad), what is it about taking this journey of remembering that sparks your desire? What do you fear?

Attuning for the Journey Ahead: Coming to Know How to Thrive

As you move forward in the text, I hope you will lean in to develop trust in the process. You can do this by paying attention to the felt sense, noticing when your body expands and when it contracts. Listen to the subtle cues, tuning into your inner wisdom. This is your most trustworthy guide on this journey.

Despite what you might have learned in the culture that you are incubating in, to forge the deep and resilient "roots" necessary to navigate the passing "weather," we must tend to the body and the felt senses within. This embodied form of knowing empowers the healing process. To cultivate this form of knowing, try on the experiential practices in the text. They will guide you away from the "figuring it out" mind so you can move back into your body (the "felt sense"). Aligning with this intention, Chapters 1 through 3 focus on satisfying your "figuring it out mind." Once trust is developed at the level of the mind, we are more likely to invest in the process at the level of the body and spirit (your "felt senses"), which is necessary for healing and the focus of Chapters 4 through 12.

To summarize the process (see Figure 1.3), you will *come to know* about common human needs, the impetus of stress and the core assets of thriving. As a reminder, we then take the knowing deeper by *attuning, strengthening, clearing, and aligning*:

- Come to know by exploring the research, focusing in on the requirements of thriving (Chapters 1 and 2)
- Attune with the inner world, letting the outer world fall into the background. Distinguishing between the "signal" of you versus the "noise" of the conditional world will enable you to tune into your highest purpose (Chapters 3 and 4).
- Strengthen via heart-centred, self-soothing practices that forge connection by improving congruence (including self-compassion—Chapters 5, 8, and 9) and a sense of coherence (including mindfulness—Chapter 7) as the developmental factors that promote thriving.
- Clear out your inner space by developing tools and techniques to reorient old belief systems and resolve areas of incongruence and trauma (Chapters 3, 6, 9, and 10)
- Align with your calling, vision, and leadership potential by engaging in practices that attune and strengthen your ability to connect to and empower the "real" self (Chapters 11 and 12)

Continue to travel in relationship with like-intentioned others—this will provide you with a physical reminder that you are not alone. Every leg of this journey is another opportunity to remember what it means to be human, resolving what has come before to prepare for something new. Now we will *come to know* about the requirements of thriving.

CHAPTER 2

Coming to Know How to Thrive

Root Strength
May you find your balance amid order and chaos.
Enough order to trust in love and enough chaos to freely dance with the mysteries of life.

May you develop the wisdom and compassion to navigate the tensions within, of power and powerlessness, independence and intimacy, contentment and yearning.

May you root deeply in your inner world, enabling all of life to be a meditation, buffering you from the ever-changing landscape of the outer world.

To this end, whatever conditions present on the surface, may you ground deeply in the strength of your roots and may you feel the connectedness and nourishment of the forest that holds you.

We all encounter numerous forks in the road every day. The path we take, impacted by a variety of factors, determines our ability to thrive. The forks in the road represent the everyday moments when we as caregivers give and receive, fill and are filled. Taking the thriving path describes those moments when we are honest about who we are and how we express ourselves in the world. It is the everyday moments when we immerse in meaningful conversation, when we get so lost in the fun of completing our tasks that our workday flies by. As we develop a habit of being in the moment, the experiences of ease, fluidity, and flow compound. As a result, we toil less about what was and what we expect to come. When challenges arise, we engage the practices that ground us, enabling us to reconnect to a sense of meaning and an ability to feel excited (rather than stressed) by the work challenges that we now feel empowered to navigate.

If we encounter a fork in the road and take the other path, ignoring the inner call to satisfy the wants of others, the felt efforts will outweigh the felt rewards. From this eroding place, we begin to wear out, feeling a lack of energy that makes tasks feel obligatory and onerous. From this orientation, time tends to creep by as we do our best to ignore the distress signals lighting up within us. The mysteries of the day feel unpredictable and threatening, filled with the insecurity of what is to come and whether we have the resources to manage it. Challenges that arise threaten our last drops of energy, and as a result we feel tired, emotionally exhausted, irritated by those things and people that require our attention. We fear we are becoming *that* caregiver, the one we always swore we would never be. And so, to prevent such an atrocity, we put on a smiling face and we push down the negative emotions that burn within us. This is a familiar place for many of us. How did we get here?

Thriving, as I see it, is living a self-actualized professional and personal life. It is living life to the fullest, being authentic and present in the moment, and feeling contentment despite the inevitable twists and turns of life. From a place of inner security, when there is suffering or sadness, we recognize that feeling and emoting is a healthy and liberating part of life.

Aligning with Rogers' (1951) work, the act of thriving means "to actualize, maintain, and enhance the experiencing organism" (p. 487). When we are acting out of our inspired and authentic selves, we are engaging in self-actualizing activity. A self-actualized person is one in whose

> ...contact with reality is simply more direct. And along with this unfiltered, unmediated directness of their contact with reality comes also a vastly heightened ability to appreciate, again and again, freshly and naively, the basic goods of life, with awe, pleasure, wonder, and even ecstasy, however stale those experiences may have become for others … For such people, even the casual workaday, moment-to-moment business of living can be thrilling, exciting, and ecstatic. (Maslow, 1968, p. 214–215)

Self-actualized people accept their fallible human nature and are more tolerant of uncertainty and ambiguity in the workplace. These caregivers will have significant interpersonal work relationships and freely accept their colleagues' spontaneous thoughts and behaviours. They have a clear sense of reality and an objective tolerance for the incongruent nature of professional ideals. They take on unpredictable events with creativity and a sense of humour. They continue to feel an appreciation for life, despite its unpredictable nature, and look forward with optimism to the limitless opportunities on the horizon (Maslow, 1954).

The self-actualizing process centres on the ability to engage with life from a congruent place. Being authentic (congruent) is the manifestation of the intertwining connection of our mind, body, and spirit. It involves taking ownership of our life and fully participating in it. Rather than taking marching orders from external authorities, we rely on an internal compass that guides us through our felt senses, enabling us to see the world and actions in the world through our eyes rather than the eyes of others (Rowen, 2015). When we feel safe to express ourselves congruently, we are more likely to feel fulfilled. As a result of our fulfillment, instead of looking solely at our own needs, we begin to gladly tend to the needs of others from this place of abundance (Starcher, 2006). Conversely, when motivated by a role ascribed to us by others, we act from an obligation to gain approval, consumed with meeting our felt need to be loved and accepted by others. From this place of scarcity, our own needs will continue to be overshadowed by the needs of others.

Thriving

Based on the interweaving of terms in the literature, self-actualization and thriving are interchangeable terms. Both share definitions using similar descriptors. For example, those who are thriving feel alive, full of energy, and optimistic about their progress and learning. (Mortier et al., 2016; Porath et al., 2012)

Why do some people thrive while others struggle to survive each day, even though they work and live in similar environments? There are key personal assets that determine whether people can express themselves authentically and whether they will feel threatened by external **stimuli** (events unfolding around us). Because most stimuli in and of themselves do not provoke stress, but rather our interpretation of them, bolstering our confidence in our personal assets improves our likelihood of thriving.

While some people learn these skills in childhood, they can also be learned in adulthood. The "weather" (see Figure 1.1) represents the external factors that can help or harm our ability to thrive. However, internal factors play a just as great, if not greater, role in thriving.

Even though this text is focused on the cultivation of one's personal resilience, it is equally important to also consider what strategies might support changing the parts of the work environment (or our role in it) that continue to distract us from thriving. Put in terms of threatening weather systems, no matter how deep a tree's roots are, when a tornado presents, all trees are at risk of being uprooted. We must acknowledge both, as personal resiliency and environmental factors are not mutually exclusive.

Both our personal resilience (roots) and external factors (weather) contribute to our ability to thrive. However, when we engage in thriving, we are less likely to experience the weather as a threat. For instance, we are less vulnerable to role ambiguity (unclear expectations), interpersonal tensions, and the unpredictable nature of our personal and work environments. When work environments have less extreme weather conditions, such as less co-worker hostility, manageable workloads, less ambiguity, and more order and predictability, they promote thriving. The two are interdependent. While having strong roots buffers us from stressors, they are impactful and intertwining parts of the equation. To regularly live in a thriving state, there must be a balance between systemic environments that provide us with a sense of confidence that our basic human needs will be met *and* we must engage in the deep inner work required to self-actualize into our best and most authentic self.

In this section, I cover three core intrinsic factors that we all encounter: (1) The *basic human requirements to thrive*; (2) *congruence* (orientation to self), which enables us to reconcile our "real" world and "ideal" world; and (3) *sense of coherence* (orientation to the external world), which determines our ability to understand and

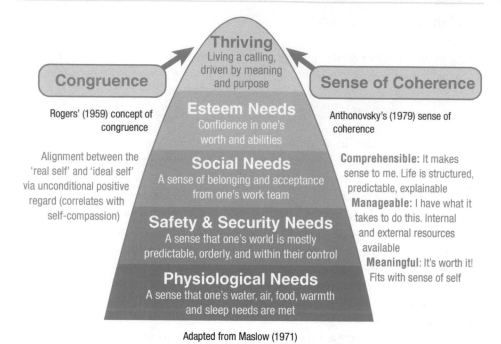

Fig. 2.1   Formula for Thriving. Maslow's hierarchy of needs (adapted) is interwoven with the concepts of thriving, congruence, and sense of coherence. All three concepts suggest that basic requirements must be met in order for us to engage in thriving. Whether in a professional or personal context, these basic needs apply. For instance, we long to feel a sense of belonging with and acceptance from our work team.

confidently manage external stimuli. Finally, we look at how the three concepts compound and interweave. Figure 2.1 illustrates the relationship between our basic needs, congruence, and sense of coherence. Assuming we all have common requirements and that humans, and thus caregivers, are ultimately motivated to thrive/self-actualize, we can then also assume that if a primary need goes unmet, we will experience stress that distracts and often disables us from thriving, until the need is satisfied. Congruence and sense of coherence determine whether we interpret internal (emotions) and external (thoughts and unexpected events) stimuli as obstacles to navigate or as threatening stressors.

The Meeting of Human Needs as a Precursor to Thriving

When unable to transcend towards self-actualization due to an unmet need, one will experience stress until the unmet need is satisfied. (Maslow, 1943)

Recognizing that thriving is a complex topic influenced by a variety of cultural factors, most of us can agree that there are certain human requirements that must be met before we can engage in self-actualization/thriving. When we cannot get these basic needs met, the stressor (threatening stimulus) will distract, if not completely derail, us from thriving (Maslow, 1943). As Maslow continued to develop his theories, he recognized that traditional humanism, whereby self-actualization is the end goal, is incomplete. Extending beyond humanism, transpersonal psychology acknowledges mystical or spiritual states. This process describes how we cross the threshold from one way of being to another—moving through liminal spaces—whereby we leave what we once knew, transcending beyond the self to embody a more collective sense of security in who we are and our place in the larger human mosaic. Psychologist Ken Wilber describes this integrative approach as a need for development and transcendence, or the need to "grow up and wake up," which provides a more complete picture of the requirements and experience of thriving (Macdonald & Friedman, 2020).

While Maslow's (1943) hierarchy of needs has garnered plenty of criticism for its linear nature and shortcomings related to spirituality and cultural influences, most of us can agree that we have basic human needs and that these needs must be met. If they are not met, we will at least be distracted and potentially disabled from thriving. Despite the theory's shortcomings, for the purpose of describing the impetus for stress, Maslow's hierarchy fits. Maslow describes the core human needs in five categories arranged in order of priority. These needs are physiological survival, security, belonging, esteem, and thriving. Because there are cultural factors take into consideration, I do not focus on the hierarchical nature of the pyramid, as it is not empirically supported nor helpful in understanding the nature of stress. Furthermore, in later years, Maslow added transcendence as an additional level, recognizing spirituality as an impactful factor and also showing that as we self-actualize, we will often naturally transcend to be more outwardly focused (Maslow, 1968). The theory of unmet needs is an adequate framework to understand that we are motivated to satisfy our basic human needs, and that our more primal survival needs such as hunger, thirst, warmth, and sleep are highly distracting/disabling if not addressed. For caregivers, these needs include adequate work breaks to hydrate, eat, and rest, away from workplace stimuli. Caregivers also require adequate food, sleep, and shelter outside of work. If workplace stimuli (i.e., stormy weather in Figure 1.1) threaten the ability to meet our needs, leaving them unsatisfied, caregivers will struggle to thrive, distracted by the primal need to fulfill their unmet needs.

Once one set of basic needs is met, such as physiological needs (no physical threats to our survival are present), it becomes easier to turn our focus to our need for emotional safety, security, belonging, and esteem. If we as caregivers cannot attain emotional security, a sense of belonging, and esteem, including confidence to navigate challenges at work, we are unlikely to engage in thriving. When we start something new, we tend to feel like we have shallower root systems (low sense of coherence and congruence). As a result, novice caregivers are more likely to report having one or more unmet needs in the workplace (Rhéaume et al., 2011).

As a result of this lack of grounding and related confidence in their resources, novice caregivers are more likely to perceive events/stimuli as a threat to their primary needs. For example, Janice, a new graduate nurse, shared her experience as she entered her professional practice:

> *[In the beginning], I was so stressed from work, I would just come home and cry. I would go right to bed … I couldn't add one more thing [to my life apart from work], even if it may have helped. I was too overwhelmed. I wasn't taking breaks. It was just too busy. I was so stressed … we were all just drowning … You are so overwhelmed by the need to feel like you needed to prove yourself that I … missed a lot of breaks. There is this feeling that if you are asking for help too much or bringing things up that you will be viewed like, 'Hey, what's not working here, what's wrong with you?' (Dames, 2018)*

According to Maslow's theory, if we continue to endure *threatening weather* such as missed food and rest breaks, endure hostility from more senior members, or feel too emotionally unsafe to use our voice, it can result in moral injury. If left unresolved, it will continue to distract us from thriving. As a result, we are at higher risk of burnout. Conversely, with deeper roots, established by high levels of congruence and sense of coherence, we are equally vulnerable to physiological threats, but we will have a higher stress threshold in the realms of emotional security, belonging, and esteem needs.

A HIERARCHY OR A TIPI? INDIVIDUALISM VERSUS COLLECTIVISM

While the individualist culture this book emerges from largely informs the lens from which it is written, it should be noted that a core component of thriving requires a shift toward a more collectivist way of being. The Maslow/Blackfoot controversy illustrates the foundational difference between two frameworks that look similar, but in principle are quite different. Some historical researchers, such as Ryan Heavy Head, speculate that Maslow's hierarchy of needs is largely informed by the Blackfoot (Siksika) Nation he visited in 1938 while developing his theories (Feigenbaum & Smith, 2019). While his hierarchy of needs originally represented the collectivist Blackfoot way, Maslow misrepresented the foundational cultural framework from his individualist lens (Heavy Head, 2018). Maslow's potential adaptation of the Blackfoot way reflects an attempt to adapt a collectivist model (tipi) to an individualist power structure (hierarchy). While hierarchical power structures are a dominant characteristic of Western individualist cultures, with self-actualization placed at the top, this does not appear to have been the original intention. In the original pyramid, now known as Maslow's hierarchy of unmet needs, the Blackfoot way embodied collectivism, with self-actualization placed at the bottom, providing the foundation for community actualization (see Figure 2.2).

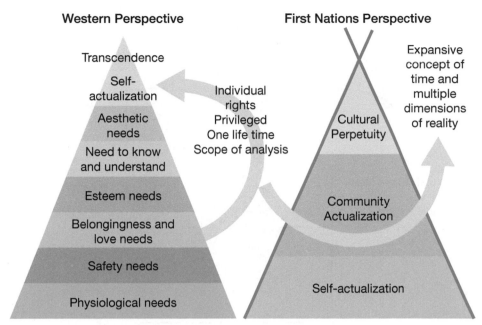

Western Perspective

First Nations Perspective

Transcendence

Self-actualization

Aesthetic needs

Need to know and understand

Esteem needs

Belongingness and love needs

Safety needs

Physiological needs

Individual rights
Privileged
One life time
Scope of analysis

Expansive concept of time and multiple dimensions of reality

Cultural Perpetuity

Community Actualization

Self-actualization

Fig. 2.2 Maslow's hierarchy of needs informed by the Blackfoot Nation, Alberta, Canada. (Used with permission of Cindy Blackstock, PhD.)

Polyvagal Theory and Perceived Unmet Needs

Through the lens of polyvagal theory (Porges, 2011), illustrated in Figure 2.3 and described in more depth in Chapter 3, the nervous system is constantly scanning for threats. This scanning happens outside of our thinking mind and often dictates how we react based on how we interpret the events happening around us and how secure we feel in our resources in a given moment. When threatened, our nervous system becomes activated, distracting or even disabling our ability to stay embodied in the present moment (a requirement of thriving). However, according to polyvagal theory, when we experience a felt sense of unconditional positive regard from others, we gain a greater ability in that moment to ground ourselves securely, which promotes a greater tolerance for passing stimuli. With a calm nervous system, we have a greater ability to feel into the inner and outer resources that help us navigate challenges, enabling us to quickly get back to thriving in the moment.

Cultivating Choice: Drop by Drop Until the Cup Overflows

Viewed through the lens of trauma-informed practice principles, choice is a luxury for many. When we come to a challenge with confidence, enthusiasm, and optimism (high sense of coherence), we have a greater ability to view stimuli objectively

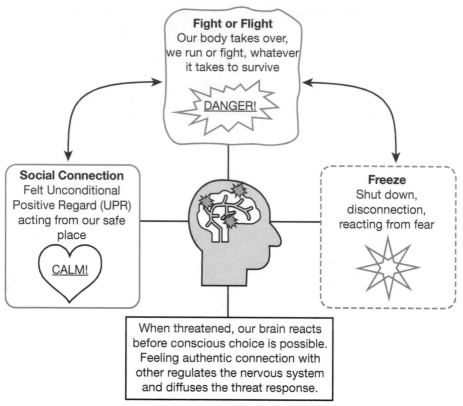

Fig. 2.3 Polyvagal Theory. We can retrain our neural pathways through social interactions that feel safe. When we feel safe, we can show up authentically, trusting that we will be met with unconditional positive regard. Grounding more securely in relationships characterized by unconditional positive regard regulates our nervous system, enabling us stay connected to the sensations in our body (embodied) and expanding our window of tolerance for stress.

and are more likely to act in ways that are congruent with our values and goals. When we come to a challenge with a low sense of coherence, often because of unresolved wounds (trauma) and old belief systems, we are prone to perceiving the stimuli as threatening. When threats feel intense, the nervous system becomes activated, causing us to react with fight, flight, or freeze, limiting if not completely disabling choice. When this happens, we are far more prone to reacting subconsciously, doing or saying things that don't feel congruent with our values and goals.

To cultivate choice, imagine each effort to come to know, attune, strengthen, clear, and align as one more drop into our resourcing cup. The fuller the cup gets, the more our sense of coherence and congruence develops, with every drop representing an investment in the cultivation of more choice in our day-to-day perceptions and resulting actions. We may not feel like the individual drops we add to the cup make a difference, but in time the surface tension builds to a point that it can no longer remain as it is. Eventually, one of those individual drops will cause an undeniable shift, moving us beyond the walls we have felt confined by. There are many old stories that we will evolve beyond, each story with its own cup, slowly filling drop by drop. As we intentionally invest in ourselves, we add another drop. We can trust that in time, emancipation will come, providing us with a newfound sense of awareness and freedom. When these overflows occur, perhaps more familiar to us as an "Aha!" moment, it means that old belief systems have evolved and we will awaken to a new way of knowing that deeply and completely changes our perceptions and resulting trajectory.

When we understand this ability and inability to choose, we can offer compassion and forgiveness to ourselves and others. Because we all share in this human experience, we can at some level relate to the sense of powerlessness and **shame** that comes when we react from fear. In this way, we all experience this form of **emotional transference**, where an experience reveals an old wound from the past and it suddenly feels fresh. Even seemingly small challenges can pull us back to the intensity of the feelings associated with that first core wound, underscoring old and often misguided belief systems and resulting in spontaneous projections that emerge in a variety of harmful ways. What if we could look beyond the shame of our reactions, self-compassionately and curiously tending to the wound that lies beneath? What if we saw the experience as a gift, an opportunity for healing? As we heal the wounds beneath, we promote a greater ability to respond with a different orientation in the future. In these ways, drop by drop, we cultivate choice.

Congruence as a Requirement for Thriving: Reconciling Our "Real" Versus "Ideal" Self

> *Our deepest calling is to grow into our own authentic selfhood, whether or not it conforms to some image of who we ought to be. As we do so, we will not only find the joy that every human being seeks—we will also find our path of authentic service in the world. (Palmer, 2000)*

Thriving requires authenticity (congruence), which is the gatekeeper to fulfillment of our desires and higher states of consciousness; this is where transpersonal and spiritual ways of being are accessed. The concept of **self-integrity**, which is interchangeable with congruence, comes from living honestly, when our words and actions align with our values, beliefs, and preferences. If life experiences and the work environment provide feelings of emotional security and acceptance, enabling caregivers to feel safe to be authentic, then they would be more likely to thrive. Self-integrity, our ability to be authentic and feel whole, is priceless. Doing or saying anything that erodes your sense of self, stripping you of inner peace, is too expensive.

Self-compassion and congruence intertwine. To attain congruence, we must have a high degree of self-compassion, which enables us to act authentically despite the risk of disapproval from others. When we are self-compassionate, we are more likely to act congruently, expressing our "real" self by allowing spontaneous emotion, accepting and owning our shortcomings along the way.

Congruence describes our orientation to self, an alignment with heart and spirit that results in an ability to express ourselves authentically. Most of us can point out some differences between who we are and who we believe we ought to be. Influential psychologist and researcher Carl Rogers (1959) developed his theories on congruence, thriving, and personality concurrently with his endeavours in empirical research. The concept of congruence between the "real" self and "ideal" self provides insights into the basic belonging and esteem needs required to engage in thriving.

When you accept your flaws, you are free of the fear of shame. When you are free of shame, scrutiny from others loses its sting.

Rogers suggested that for a person to achieve congruence, they require an environment that provides them with unconditional positive regard. Unconditional positive regard, which is further described in Chapter 8, emerges from grace, enabling us to value and accept one another despite our failings. When we believe we are unconditionally and positively regarded, we become willing and able to act authentically without, or despite, a fear of rejection. Within this safe, accepting, and empathic space comes the willingness to be open and to self-disclose.

Unconditional positive regard reminds us that we are enough as we are, separate from cultural conditions, past behaviours, and achievements. From this nurturing and regulating space we begin to heal.

To better understand how we assimilate to view ourselves and other humans in terms of conditions, imagine a newborn baby. See its very essence and innate sense of worth, its precious spirit, apart from any conditions. We can easily attach a sense of unconditional positive regard to this newborn. Now, imagine attaching conditions to this baby's innate worth and value. This baby must achieve several goals, maintain a certain body type, attain the right degrees, live in a certain dwelling, and drive a certain car to be acceptable and loved. As ludicrous as this may seem to apply conditions of worth to a baby, we lose sight of this sense of inherent worth as we assimilate, and we often expect others to assimilate in the same fashion. These enculturated conditions often shroud our ability to accept others' innate essence apart from societal ideals. When one believes that others are worthy of unconditional positive regard, they can then mirror the same inwardly; this is **self-compassion**. It acts as a buffer against these feelings of threat that emerge when we feel insecure about our basic needs getting met. When we respond with self-compassion, we interrupt the stress response by providing the unconditional positive regard to ourselves that we are longing for from others. Self-compassion meets this need. We are therefore more likely to keep the potential threat in perspective, act to resolve it, and as a result, prevent stimuli from becoming stressful. Within this context, self-compassion intertwines with congruence in its acceptance of the "real" self, despite immersion in a culture that focuses heavily on the "ideal" self. Acceptance of one's self enables us to base our decisions on what we believe is best for us, despite the differing, and often distracting opinions of others. With this sense of inner security, self-compassion serves our self-esteem needs, promoting a greater ability to engage in thriving.

> **Self-compassion** enables us to hold awareness from a place of abundance, as we provide unconditional positive regard inwardly. From this place, we believe we are good enough. **Awareness without self-compassion** leads to perfectionism, which is fueled by shame. From this place, we grapple with the insecurity of not feeling good enough.

Similar to Maslow (1943), Rogers argued that there are contextual requirements needed before a person can develop fully. Rather than illustrating these needs via a hierarchy, he compared it to a tree that will not flourish without sunlight and water (Rogers, 1959). Flourishing requires that we grow up in nurturing environments that cultivate authenticity and promote a sense of belonging, where we feel known and accepted. These nurturing spaces result in our ability to engage in thriving. This same premise applies to the ability for caregivers to thrive in their role(s).

To further describe congruence, a person's level of congruence between their "real" self and "ideal" self is a primary indicator of their likelihood to engage in thriving (Rogers, 1986). Professional incongruence (illustrated in Figure 2.4) is the misalignment between actual experiences and the "ideal" picture (Rogers, 1986). For example, if the caregiving ideals we learn in our training cannot be actualized

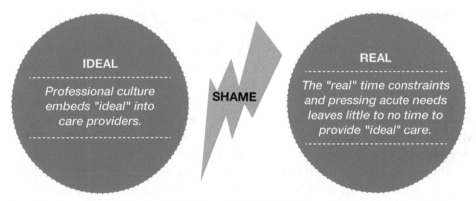

Fig. 2.4 Incongruence Between the "Ideal" Self and the "Real" Self. The more incongruence we feel between the "ideal" self and the "real" self, the further apart these two circles are and the more shame we will carry for not being who we believe we should be. A felt sense of *unconditional positive regard* for self and others promotes our ability to live with the vulnerability necessary to act congruently.

in the field, shame often results. If we cannot resolve this incongruence, we will experience chronic shame, which is often felt as a chronic sense of anxiety or stress in our work role. Our degree of incongruence depends on how far apart the perceived "real" self is from the "ideal" self. These incongruences affect decision making because we are likely to do things to please others rather than satisfying our own needs. Those who have a greater discrepancy between the "real" and the "ideal" will be at greater risk for maladjustment, resulting in feelings of shame and dissatisfaction (Rogers, 1959). Furthermore, those with unresolved **trauma** and/or resentments toward themselves or others are likely to feel and act incongruently because of the resulting unconscious projections that we deny in ourselves will eventually spill over on to others.

As for the workplace context, congruence between the "real" self and "ideal" self relates to the perceived unconditional positive regard we experienced in childhood, an experience that enables deep roots to grow. From this place of grounded security as adults, we can express ourselves authentically in the workplace. Additionally, a felt sense of unconditional positive regard from at least one colleague further encourages us to express our "real" selves (rather than a prescribed "ideal"), even when it differs from the status quo. This concept is underscored in the research on caregivers, where those who had strong, trusting relationships with colleagues are more empowered and have higher quality of life and work scores (Casole, 2016). Conversely, when self-worth and sense of value at work feel conditional, it erodes our confidence, our ability to trust our emotions, and our decision-making capacity. When we work in environments that feel conditional, we are more likely to prioritize the opinions and values of others above our own, leading to further incongruence. As a result, the stress that emerges from this less secure orientation distracts us from being in the present moment, hampering our ability to thrive.

Congruence Between the Heart and the Mind

Ground-breaking researchers Beatrice Lacey and John Lacey (1974) found that the heart is in constant communication with the brain, a connection that has powerful psychological and physiological effects. While we often rely on our cognitive ability to analyze and reorient our thoughts as a way to cope with stress, it is actually through the heart that we truly orient ourselves in the world. The heart is the centre from which we learn to authentically respond to the world around us. Furthermore, psychophysiologist Rollin McCraty (2015) has described how the heart's magnetic field is 100 times stronger than that of the brain and that this field can be felt from 3 feet away. Energetically, the heart is 60 times more powerful than the brain! The science is clear: mindfully engaging the heart as we move through our day has a powerful impact on all aspects of our health. By doing so, we also can also positively impact the world around us.

Strengthening Practice: Cultivating Heartful Social Coherence

Because we humans are always in connection and communication with the complexities of our inner workings, and also to each other and to the natural world, social coherence influences our ability to thrive. Like many important topics, there are several coined terms used to describe similar concepts and the terms sense of coherence (Antonovosky, 1979), our orientation to life, and social coherence, our degree of harmonious relational alignment, are both related but different concepts.

Rollin McCraty (2010), head of the research team for the Institute of HeartMath, describes social coherence as a harmonious alignment with others that enables the optimal flow of energy and communication to facilitate cooperative and synchronized action. This form of coherence includes physiological synchronization, emotional connection, and cooperation with others, all of which impacts our capacity for coordinated action.

◎ Experiential Practice Opportunity

By cultivating appreciation and compassion individually, we engage the heart, shifting into a more coherent physiological and energetic state (McCraty, 2017). Because the electromagnetic field of the heart extends beyond our physical body, we inherently influence the energetic state of those around us. When groups intentionally work to be more heartfully engaged, there is an enormous opportunity to gain greater capacity for synchronized action. There are several heart-engaging activities throughout this book. For instance, you can focus on breathing in and out of the heart, immersing in a felt unconditional positive regard for yourself and/or others. Or you can engage in any other loving-kindness practice that cultivates heartfelt compassion and appreciation.

We generate greater social coherence as a group or in pairs. To do so, begin with cultivating loving-kindness internally by immersing in feelings of unconditional positive regard, either by imagining a loved one providing it to us or by directing it inwardly to ourselves, and then radiating it out to others in the group.

These heart-engaging techniques (see Experiential Practice Opportunity) can also be used to shift from incoherent to coherent states during times of relational stress. For instance, when we feel threatened or frustrated with someone, it often lands us in a physiologically and socially incoherent state (McCraty, 2017). By intentionally engaging our heart to generate appreciation and compassion, we can often reorient ourselves to a more coherent (and often more objective) state.

Thriving in the Mind: Working With Our Neurology

Thriving brains navigate challenges before they become stressors. They self-regulate and make conscious choices that promote wellness. We frequently carry unhealed past adversities and live and work in overstimulating and often energetically toxic environments, all of which takes an immense toll on our neurology. To work objectively and creatively with our neurology, we may need to explore and accept vulnerabilities that may not be immediately changeable so that we can focus on what we *can* change. From this place of acceptance, we can spring into action in a new empowered way.

Our brain cells communicate through electrical patterns called brain waves, which are categorized as alpha, beta, delta, gamma, and theta. Each of these patterns represents different states of consciousness that depend on whether we are relaxed, sleeping, meditating, concentrating, alert, frightened, and so on. We frequently measure these waves via noninvasive electroencephalography (EEG). When we are in states of stress and anxiety, the brain tends to operate using high-frequency beta waves. When relaxed, the brain operates using lower frequency brain waves. The good news is that we can transition between these states with mindfulness, meditation practices, and binaural beats. Training our brains in this way has many benefits such as promoting relaxation, enhancing performance, and reducing stress, pain, migraines, and a host of mental health issues (Cruceanu & Rotarescu, 2019; Lee et al., 2019; Rebadomia et al., 2019). By training our brains using meditation, neurofeedback, binaural beats, or other brain entrainment tools, we learn to recognize when we enter lower frequency brain wave states. With practice, we can mindfully shift into more productive states. We spend most of our day operating predominantly in beta wave states, which is often fitting because it keeps us alert and focused as we move throughout our day. However, when beta waves are dominant, especially at higher frequencies, they limit creativity and can cause hyper-alertness, which fuels stress and anxiety and burns up our energy. In this high-alert state, our nervous system is more likely to get activated, pushing us into fight, flight, or freeze and reducing our ability to act objectively.

Depending on our neurology, mindfulness/meditation history, and unique preferences, what works for one individual to shift out of beta wave states— enabling us to relax and gain important insights—may not work for another. For instance, those who regularly practice meditation will have a greater ability to maintain the concentration needed to experience a shift with traditional sitting meditation methods. Some need a physical ritual such as running, walking, yoga, sweeping, and so on to shift to lower frequencies. Others prefer repetition and vibration using chants such as "Om" to transition to other states (Anand, 2014; Harne & Hiwale, 2018). From beta waves, we can move to these other states:

- **Alpha waves**, commonly accessed via mindfulness, promote a relaxed state of alertness that enables reflection, relaxation, and improved cognitive performance (Cruceanu & Rotarescu, 2013; Rebadomia et al., 2019). With practice, we can sink deeper into the lower frequencies.

- **Theta waves** promote memory consolidation (Reiner et al., 2014) and a greater ability to recognize unwanted prejudices toward others. This state enables us to act counter to our ingrained instincts, whereby we can recognize the difference between the rational course of action and the ingrained instinct (Cavanagh et al., 2013). In theta, we are more likely to practice nonattachment, enabling us to objectively navigate challenges and reorient ourselves via renaming and reframing.
- **Gamma waves** are the subtlest of the brain wave frequencies. They require a quiet mind. Yet when we are in this state, we are highly active, with enhanced focus; heightened senses, consciousness, and compassion; and a greater felt sense of inner and outer connection. We can access and sustain gamma waves by practising loving-kindness (Berkovich-Ohana et al., 2012; Lutz et al., 2004). When our brains are at this frequency, which promotes open heartedness, we are likely to feel more connected and a greater sense of well-being. Because gamma waves promote feelings of well-being and connection to self and others, those who lack sufficient time in gamma states are more likely to feel disconnected and depressed (Khalid et al., 2016).
- **Delta waves** promote deep relaxation and sleep modes. It makes sense that those who operate at high-frequency beta states, rapidly burning energy stores, may subconsciously gravitate to rituals to shift to a more relaxing state.

Our mental health and related behaviours and rituals are closely linked to brain wave states (Newson & Thiagarajan, 2019). Some conditions, such as attention deficit hyperactivity disorder and obsessive–compulsive disorder, typically occur in individuals who tend to have more lower frequency brain waves, delta and theta, with decreases in alpha, beta, and gamma (Newson & Thiagarajan, 2019; Travis, 2019). In terms of addictions fueled by high-frequency beta states, the addictive behaviour is likely shifting the brain in a helpful way. Our behaviours and rituals span a variety of culturally acceptable and not-so-acceptable activities and mind-altering substances. Whether labelled bad or good, if we objectively explore our behaviours, we may find they are indeed shifting us into the more focused or restful state we are craving. These shifts may be described as "zoning out" or "switching gears," but in neurological terms, we are transitioning between brain wave states (Newson & Thiagarajan, 2019). Given that these behaviours or rituals may be serving us in this way, if we want to make changes, and thus reduce harm, we will be far more successful if we can replace them with new rituals that serve us in this same way. Furthermore, to interrupt unwanted habits, we often need to reorient ourselves, relating to the behaviour in a new, nonthreatening way. Genuine and lasting reorientation typically happens in lower frequency brain wave states, when our sense of threat is low and we are relaxed and open hearted; this is why hypnosis can be so effective in interrupting habits (Li et al., 2017). Essentially, if we hope to change behaviours, it is important to consider how we can self-compassionately and creatively work with our neurology to set ourselves up for success.

> ### Attuning/Reflecting Opportunity
>
> Think of an activity that helps you relax. Quite likely, the activity and behaviours you are immersed in are promoting lower frequency brain wave states, enabling you to relax. From this relaxed state, you can feel into the abundance of your inner resources, allowing you to practise *being* instead of *doing*—or, to put it more accurately, to *do* from a more connected and empowered state of *being*. At times, the behaviours that promote states of rest may actually be harmful to us. When this is the case, even though we see the harm, because we are experiencing a reward despite the harm, we may feel resistance if we try to break the habit without a healthy substitute. For example, if you want to change the habit of turning to food for comfort, you will need to find a replacement that provides a similar reward to reduce reliance on the old unwanted behaviour. This is where we get to try out several tools, play with them, and see what works to help us transition into more helpful brain wave states. From there, we can cultivate a new habit. With this knowledge in mind, what habit is helping you to relax these days?

The Dance: Navigating Obstacles to Congruence

Dancing involves surrender to the music of the moment, enabling spontaneous and authentic expression. Incongruence between personal values/desires and professional obligations is a barrier to thriving because it inhibits authentic expression. We become self-conscious, which pulls us into our mind and out of our body. Our ability to make meaning is limited when we craft our actions out a felt sense of obligation, which strips us of the inspiration that emerges from a thriving state of mind. An example of how this might emerge in the workplace is demonstrated by a Canadian study involving 23 new graduate nurses. The strongest motivators for the new graduates to leave their place of work was a lack of empowerment, measured as an inability to internalize goals and feel safe to express their authentic selves in the workplace (Rhéaume et al., 2011). Based on Rogers' (1986) theory, this common scenario reflects incongruence between the learned "ideals" of our profession and the "real(ity)" of the work in the field. The further apart the "real" and "ideal" are, the more incongruence and resulting shame we will feel (Rogers, 1986). Figure 2.4 illustrates the incongruence between the ideals of the profession and the reality of the work, with the incongruence hampering our ability to engage in thriving (Rogers, 1986). We all strive to be our best, most inspired selves at work, which then enables us to naturally encourage others to do the same. If we become blocked from transcending in this way, we will feel too self-conscious to engage in the dance, producing a felt incongruence, which leads to shame and ultimately chronic stress. This stress can motivate us to make a change, doing whatever we can to remove the block. If the stressors are unchangeable, there are two potential scenarios: one, we will look for another work role or environment that will enable us to thrive; or, because there are many situations that make leaving a well-paying job infeasible, we will bide our time and often succumb to frequent moments of emotional exhaustion and hostility. Most of us who have been in the field long enough can relate to both scenarios.

THRIVING IN ROLE TRANSITIONS

Another core aspect of thriving is the intertwining of our personal and professional journey, which requires multiple role transitions. It is difficult to balance our energy as we take off one hat and put on another. For those of us who have or had small children, you may be familiar with the guilt you feel when you get home and are too exhausted to engage with your children. Or for those who are more introverted, it can be a challenge to maintain friendships outside of high-stimulus work environments when being at home alone is what you need to recharge outside of work.

Taylor and Dell'Oro (2006) liken the balance of roles to a dance: we learn new and varying rhythms as we tak e off one hat and put on another. This book focuses on developing the core assets required to find our rhythm by engaging in thriving while navigating personal and workplace stimuli/stressors:

> *Having and displaying integrity is more a matter of being able to move in ways that are consistent with the originating and developing themes of our lives. Teachers, guides, and practice make us better dancers because they help us listen more carefully and follow the music we hear more confidently. We learn which movements fit the rhythms and which do not. There is rarely just one way to enact an excellent dance to fit a particular melody—and sometimes, when we have learned to hear the music more clearly, to understand it more deeply, we find that we have to change our steps. (Taylor & Dell'Oro, 2006, p. 95)*

On a similar note, Desmond (2012) described this artful process as a living intelligence that is "open, attentive, mindful, and attuned to the occasion in all its elusiveness and subtlety" (p. 192). It is an experience that contributes to the situation and receives fulfillment in the same moment.

Thriving requires a constant balance of filling and being filled, implying a certain degree of flexibility and a sense of security within caregiving work cultures. Flourishing cultures produce a graceful environment where caregivers can find their footing in the face of a rapidly changing work environment. There is room to learn from mistakes and opportunities to adjust our steps to attune to our unique rhythm.

THRIVING IN RIGID SYSTEMS: HOW HEALTH CARE SYSTEMS CAN PROMOTE INCONGRUENCE

Another element of congruence relates to the ability of caregivers to be authentic in the workplace. O'Callaghan (2013) described a hidden curriculum in medical cultures, where cognitive expression is praised and emotional expression is largely suppressed, fueling incongruence. This hidden curriculum is rampant in postsecondary settings, which then informs professional habits, co-worker relationships, and patient/client care. The implicit message delivered in this hidden curriculum is that our "real" (emotional) self is not welcome in the practice setting, which is instilled by shame and intimidation and ultimately results in incongruent practitioners. When students incubate in an environment of intimidation and shame during their training, they enter the workforce with well-engrained habits, pushing their "real" self into the shadows and perpetuating the same expectations onto their colleagues, mentees, and clients (O'Callaghan, 2013). Conversely, role-modeling emotional congruence promotes reciprocal behaviours, which encourages authentic displays of emotion and perpetuates nurturing and respectful behaviours to co-workers and clients. The element of being "real" occurs via transparency, undergirded by compassion and reliability (Rogers, 1968; Venise et al., 2015). These same implicitly learned behaviours promote congruent workplaces and identify formation.

The socialization and embedding of professional "ideals" begin in the postsecondary setting (Benner et al., 2010). Our degree of congruence between our "real" self (roots) and professional "ideals" depends on the alignment between our personal and professional values. When we do not feel emotionally safe to express our "real" selves, we often act in ways that result in further incongruence. This incongruence, a state in which we are less connected to our roots, further creates a constant state of ambiguity (threatening weather) with who we really are. This in turn produces high emotional labour.

Arlie Hochschild, a sociologist and feminist thought leader, coined the term emotional labour, describing it as the practice of emoting states of being incongruent with our genuine feelings. (Hochschild, 2012)

In the workplace, our degree of incongruence between our "real" emotions and the "ideal" we are expected to display correlates with the rate at which we burn our emotional energy. Those who tend toward incongruent displays, causing a form of moral injury, are more prone to emotional exhaustion and burnout. This understanding centres on our ability, or inability, to be authentic, which is a primary characteristic of thriving (Maslow, 1987).

A BARRIER TO THRIVING: NOT KNOWING OUR SELF

When the practice of being who we should be rather than whom we are becomes a well-established way of life, we can no longer rely on our emotions to accurately guide us. Our genuine values and feelings about events and other people become muddled to the point where they become generally inaccessible. "They have learned how to con themselves, and no longer know who they really are" (Bergquist, 1993, p. 73).

Based on Rogers' (1959) work, feeling ambiguous about our self, how we feel, and the values that drive us prevents us from resolving emotional dissonance. This ambiguousness, resulting in incongruence, is echoed in these novice caregiver statements (Dames, 2018):

> *Whatever happened was my fault in some way.*
> *[Mary]*

> *I don't like to confront tension, I guess I'm worried for being called out for being wrong or bad or whatever.*
> *[Rhonda]*

> *If something goes wrong in the room ... I automatically think it is my fault somehow ... I was terrified of not being what others expected of me, or even what I expected of me ... terrified of failing. It felt like it would destroy me.*
> *[Tabitha]*

Conversely, in workplaces that promote and celebrate diverse ways of being, thinking, and doing, it is likely that individuals will exercise their personality traits and personal values in their professional role. This book focuses on improving congruence through the development of authentic expression, self-compassion, and forgiveness practices. To promote congruent decision making, you will work to align your goals, actions, and life roles with your values and desires.

Attuning for the Journey Ahead: Digging Deeper Into Sense of Coherence and Thriving

> *While we can't always change what we are doing, we can change how we do it. It is not external events that produce stress; rather, it is our orientation to the stimuli (threat versus a challenge we can confidently navigate) that determines whether it feels stressful.*

Adding to congruence (our orientation to self), sense of coherence (Antonovsky, 1979) describes the cognitive components of thriving, which impacts our orientation to our thoughts and our external world and the ability to navigate stimuli before they become stressors. When we interpret stimuli as a threat, it activates the body's stress response, which distracts us from thriving. Aaron Antonovsky developed the concept of sense of coherence over 40 years ago while working with Holocaust survivors. He aimed to understand why some people appeared resilient to "dis-ease" when faced with stressful events, while others were more likely to succumb to illness. His work contrasted the status quo theories held by researchers, where common medical culture perceived stress as negative and a threat to health (Eriksson & Lindström, 2007).

Conversely, Antonovsky viewed stress as a natural part of life. As such, while congruence reflects our orientation to self (our ability to authentically express ourselves), sense of coherence reflects our orientation to the external world. Aaron Antonovsky's (1979) sense of coherence predicts our ability to engage in thriving as reflected in its correlations with health outcomes and whether or not stimuli are interpreted as stressful. Sense of coherence is widely accepted as significant and reliable across cultures (Eriksson & Lindström, 2005).

THE COMPONENTS OF SENSE OF COHERENCE

Sense of coherence is a descriptor of orientation to life and a predictive tool for health outcomes. It describes a person's confidence to manage life's stressors and feelings of **optimism** that events will work out reasonably well (Antonovsky, 1979). Sense of coherence includes three components:

- Comprehensibility
- Manageability, and
- Meaningfulness (Antonovsky, 1987).

First, comprehensibility describes the extent to which we can make logical sense of the events taking place in our life and whether these events feel consistent and structured. Second, manageability is determined by the confidence we have in our ability to cope with stimuli, which may or may not be stressful. Third, meaningfulness describes sense-making and gratitude, which makes difficult events feel worthy of their commitment.

Antonovsky (1987) found that individuals differed in their sense of coherence and that these differences have immediate and long-term effects on our mental and physical health. Those who have high sense of coherence scores are less likely to view a stimulus as a stressor. The stressor is seen as comprehensible and solvable, resulting in feelings of being grounded and in control (Pallant & Lae, 2002). When a stimulus produces stress, these individuals are more likely to choose coping mechanisms that promote health and deal with tensions (Antonovsky, 1979).

In a study of 51 fourth-year nursing students in Western Canada, those with lower sense of coherence scores were less satisfied with nursing as a career choice and more likely to use substances to cope (Dames & Javorski, 2018). The impact of sense of coherence has been documented in many studies: individuals with low sense of coherence scores are more likely to experience higher levels of stress from workplace stimuli (Eriksson & Lindström, 2006; Erim et al., 2010; Nahlen & Saboonchi, 2009; Streb et al., 2014) and are more likely to engage in substance use to cope (Dames & Javorski, 2018; Larm et al., 2016). Conversely, those who have higher sense of coherence scores are more likely to engage in thriving, make healthier coping choices, exercise more, choose healthier foods, have stronger feelings of optimism, resilience, hardiness, and control, and live with an overall higher quality of life (Andersen & Berg, 2001; Bergh, et al., 2006; Eriksson & Lindström, 2007; Hassmén et al., 2000; Myrin & Lagerstrom, 2006; Wijk & Waters, 2008).

Based on a 21-year longitudinal study of 1 265 children in New Zealand, other qualities that trended with the higher sense of coherence scores were a positive temperament, higher intellectual skills, and a positive view of the self (Fergusson & Horwood, 2003). In a recent qualitative study (Dames, 2018), participants who had a high degree of confidence (a component of sense of coherence) and who could easily find meaning (also a component of sense of coherence) from other life roles felt buffered from some of the ambiguity they felt as a novice caregiver. For example, Tabitha's confidence in another life role had a positive impact on her work role:

> *Because I'm so new, I don't know everything and have questions all the time, it easy to wonder if you will ever get it, but then you have to remind yourself that outside of nursing I know that I am really good at this and this, and in terms of my identity I am first and foremost a mother and an [athlete]. It feels okay to feel crappy at work when I know that I'm really awesome over here! (Dames, 2018)*

Antonovsky (1979) described how developmental and material assets promote flourishing, which is similar to Maslow's (1971) requirements of thriving. The more assets we have, the higher our sense of coherence and the better our ability to engage in thriving. These assets include self-esteem and social supports outside of work, which impact our ability to tolerate and manage socially unsupportive work environments. These assets can also be material assets such as our financial picture, empowering us to leave a work environment that is causing us chronic stress. Our ability to attain developmental, social, and material assets maximizes our personal resources and positively correlates with our level of sense of coherence. High sense of coherence promotes an ability to manage stimuli before they feel stressful. Therefore, we as caregivers can bolster our ability to manage stress and to thrive by developing these resources.

Finally, sense of coherence intertwines with development of **self-efficacy** and **mindfulness**. Self-efficacy describes our level of confidence and motivation to manage life events (passing weather). Mindfulness is defined in depth later in the text, but as an overview, it is the process of stepping back from passing thoughts and emotions to cultivate nonattachment. From this place, we can investigate stimuli objectively, which prevents them from feeling stressful or threatening. If we cannot view them objectively (nonattachment), we are more likely to avoid and resist our emotions, disabling our ability to resolve or at least manage them. A high sense of coherence often prevents stimuli from feeling stressful, and as a result, it is a protective factor against stressful work environments (Gillespie et al., 2007). This book focusses on the development of mindfulness because it is the doorway to reorientation. How we orient ourselves in the world determines our ability to engage in thriving. For example, cultivating gratitude and optimism improves sense of coherence, buffering us from stress by improving our ability to creatively manage stimuli before they evolve into stressors.

To summarize the requirements of thriving, we cultivate a greater ability to thrive by developing congruence (alignment between the "real" self and "ideal" self) and sense of coherence (a more confident, meaningful, and predictable orientation to life). Congruence relates to how grounded we are in the inner world. Sense of coherence describes our ability to navigate the external world confidently and creatively. Calling enables us to lift our eyes toward a north star, immersing us in our vision and propelling us forward. When we develop these three characteristics of self, we minimize stress and maximize our ability to thrive.

As we deepen our roots through congruence and sense of coherence, we draw on the resources needed to work with our emotions and navigate external stimuli before they become stressors.

 Attuning/Reflecting Opportunity

Consider your felt confidence to manage challenges, your understanding of events occurring around you, your ability to predict many of life's events, and the degree to which life's tasks feel meaningful. How would you describe your sense of coherence?

Attuning for the Journey Ahead: Coming to Know About Stress

Moving forward in the text, I hope you will lean in to develop trust in the process. You can do this by paying attention to the felt sense, noticing when your body expands and when it contracts. Listen to these subtle cues, tuning into your inner wisdom. This is your most trustworthy guide on this journey.

Despite what you may have learned in the culture that you are incubating in, we must tend to the body and the felt senses within in order to forge the deep and resilient "roots" necessary to navigate the passing "weather." This embodied form of knowing empowers the healing process. To cultivate this form of knowing, try on the experiential practices in the text. They will guide you away from the "figuring it out" mind so you can move back into your body (the "felt sense"). Aligning with this intention, Chapters 1 through 3 focus on satisfying your "figuring it out" mind. Once trust is developed at the level of the mind, we are more likely to invest in the process at the level of the body and spirit (your "felt senses"), which is necessary for healing and is the focus of Chapters 4 through 12.

To summarize the process (Figure 1.3), you will come to know about common human needs, the impetus of stress, and the core assets of thriving. We then take the knowing deeper by attuning, strengthening, clearing, and aligning:

- Come to know by exploring the research, focusing in on the requirements of thriving (Chapters 1 and 2)
- Attune with the inner world, letting the outer world fall into the background. Distinguishing between the "signal" of who you are versus the "noise" of the conditional world will enable you to tune into your highest purpose (Chapters 3 and 4).
- Strengthen via heart-centred, self-soothing practices that forge a connection by improving congruence (including self-compassion—Chapters 5, 8, and 9) and sense of coherence (including mindfulness—Chapter 7) as the developmental factors that promote thriving
- Clear out your inner space by developing tools and techniques to reorient old belief systems and resolve areas of incongruence and trauma (Chapters 3, 6, 9, and 10)
- Align with your calling, vision, and leadership potential by engaging in practices that attune and strengthen your ability to connect to and empower your "real" self (Chapters 11 and 12)

Now that we've reflected on our sense of coherence, the core factor that determines whether an event feels stressful, we are ready to move into Chapter 3, where we *come to know* the concept of stress and the common activating factors that emerge in caregiving work environments.

Coming to Know About Stress

We now have enough science to confirm that our emotions are an integral part of maintaining biological equilibrium. When we repress our emotions, not allowing them to surface, they become a biological stressor, compromising our immune system and activating our nervous system, putting us at risk for a host of acute and chronic ailments.

So far, we have explored the requirements for thriving and the challenges that we individually and collectively must navigate on our way back to wholeness. To cultivate this wholeness, we need to welcome and partner with the nervous system as part of our collective ecosystem.

We cannot heal at the level of the mind while being split off from the body. Since psychic anxiety is often somaticized, we must stay connected to the sensations in our body to embody healing. To embody healing, we express or manifest the healing in a tangible way. However, when we feel threatened (stress), we often disconnect from the body as we cling to security in the outer world. This is the coping or defence mechanism known as dissociation. When stress is unmanaged, it derails our ability to thrive. The stress response is ubiquitous—23% of Canadian adults report that most of their days are highly stressful (Statistics Canada, 2014). While we often think of stress as a mental construct that only affects the mind, when unaddressed, stress has profound effects on the body that lead to a host of chronic mental and physical symptoms (O'Malley et al., 2015). These symptoms often defy any specific medical diagnosis and are described in the DSM-5 under the new heading of *Somatic Symptom and Related Disorders*.

Moving through this section, we will walk through the common stressors that together create a perfect storm for caregiver burnout. We will then move into the theory of stress mitigation and thriving and the practices that will help you find the eye of the storms.

Stress

Storm Watching

By Crosbie Watler, MD, FRCPC, a Canadian thought leader and seasoned psychiatrist

Challenges are objective events that occur to us externally. The outcomes of many challenges are outside of our ability to directly predict or control. We imagine that we have control when we create a "problem" for ourselves to manage, our mind churning on possible outcomes, when in reality all we control is the process. A student can either worry about the outcome of an exam or commit to the process of studying. Many of life's challenges are process related—health, relationships, financial planning. For each challenge, we need to identify whether we control the outcome directly or only the process. We can then commit fully to the steps involved in the process, detaching from outcomes we cannot directly control. This is sports psychology 101. It pays to approach life's challenges in this way. Think of the elite athlete who commits to the process of training and preparation. On game day, she must show up from a place of calm detachment from the outcome. In doing so, she preserves her finite powers of attention to actually perform better.

External challenges will come and go like the weather, but you are not the weather. You are the *witness* of the weather. You are metaphorically sitting in the chair, watching the storm from a safe and secure place. The weather does not touch you. There is space between you and the weather. Whatever happens in the weather of your life, at your essence *you* are neither elevated nor diminished. This is the practice of mindfulness.

Mindfulness is more than just paying purposeful attention to the present moment. It also means being aware of *who is paying attention* to this moment. The silent witness attends to the moment with nonjudgement and nonattachment. This is the domain of "I can handle whatever happens," where challenges become opportunities for the development of self-awareness and resilience.

WHERE DOES STRESS COME FROM?

Until recently, Western science had little understanding of how an external challenge triggers a stress response. Life is by definition challenging. As Dr. Watler illustrates (see the box Storm Watching), stress is a *response* to the challenge. Challenges are real and objective, while stress is subjective—stress is merely a possibility. We do not *have* stress in our lives; we create it when we use maladaptive coping tools—patterns of reactivity that do not serve us.

As the Western scientific community has come to better understand the mind and the brain, and more specifically how neurotransmitters respond to threatening thought patterns (Figure 3.1), we have developed tools that allow us to think more critically about the stress response and can often regulate the response by mindfully shifting our perceptions. This new understanding of stress empowers us to use our attention with intention and to bolster our tools and techniques to manage the stress response.

Stress can be deconstructed as follows: after we encounter an objective external challenge, we can either use an adaptive coping response or our stress response gets triggered. In this book, we distinguish the challenge from the experience of the stress response. A combination of extrinsic and intrinsic factors activates the perception of threat. Extrinsic factors are things that happen outside our immediate or direct control—metaphorically, the *weather* of our lives. Common examples include relationships, roles, finances, successes, and failures.

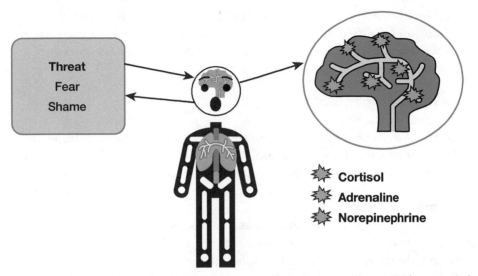

Fig. 3.1 Stress Response. Beneath our conscious awareness, the brain is constantly scanning (neuroception) for threats. When a potential threat is sensed, chemicals are released, leading to a cascade of biological and emotional events. When intensely activated in the body, we are typically feeling fear or shame concurrently.

Stress can be defined in two ways: as the stressor (external source of "bad weather") or as the experience of **distress**. We can distinguish the *source* of stress from the *experience* of stress. A combination of extrinsic and intrinsic factors activates the perception of threat. Extrinsic factors are things that happen outside our inner workings (the "weather"), such as secure relationships, financial security, physical safety, and so on. Intrinsic factors describe how securely grounded we are in ourselves (our "roots"), which is reflected in our congruence and sense of coherence. We often have little control over extrinsic factors, but those with well-developed intrinsic factors are less likely to feel intimidated and threatened by unpredictable and often challenging "weather" patterns. When extrinsic factors feel threatening, those with strong roots will have more confidence to resolve the threat before it becomes a chronic stressor.

To illustrate a perception of threat, consider this example. Rhonda was a research participant in her mid-twenties. She was new to nursing and struggling to thrive in her novice role. In her account, Rhonda captures the epitome of stress on the job, describing the need to face disturbing events at work without the confidence or resources to operate effectively:

> It [safety] feels at risk on pretty much every shift. Last set a patient charged me with a med cart … The day before that a patient took a sheet and put it over my head … We had a patient's family member shoot himself outside the hospital, and the hospital did not do anything, like no debriefing or anything, which made me feel really unsafe and unsupported. Pretty much every shift people are threatening us, saying that they are going to come back with a gun … I would come off a night

and have two days to turn around and go back for a day. I was a wreck. I was so exhausted. By the third night shift, every time I would turn into a crazy nurse by the third night. I was so emotional, I couldn't function, and I couldn't sleep. (Dames, 2018a)

HOW DOES STRESS WORK?

Cognitively, stress works like this: If we believe that a primary need is being unmet or feels threatened, we will experience stress until the unmet need is satisfied or until the stimulus that threatens it dissipates. The experience of stress among care-givers signals an unmet need or a threat to our needs. Persistently unmet needs undermine our ability to thrive.

Biologically, the stress response works like this: When we feel threatened, our amygdala taps the hypothalamus, which then sends a signal to our nervous system, activating the release of the stress hormones epinephrine, norepinephrine, and cortisol. Stress hormones are designed to get our attention in a big way, making sure we take action to resolve the perceived threat. As a result, an automatic biological response ensues, engaging our sympathetic nervous system. We experience an increased metabolic rate and muscle tension; elevated heart rate, blood pressure, and respirations; increased blood sugar; and arousal of the immune system. These physiological changes, collectively referred to as the **fight–flight–freeze–fawn** responses, have evolved to help us identify and escape from danger. However, as we well know, the fight–flight–freeze responses are often activated at times when we would be better off staying calm and relaxed; for example, when speaking in public. In addition, the more sensitive we are to stress, the more likely our nervous system is likely to be triggered when there is no true danger to us.

As an example of the fight response, consider this situation: You honestly, and perhaps a little too bluntly, communicate how frustrated you are with the workload inequities between individuals on your team. In response, one of your co-workers reacts in a sharp and defensive tone. Both parties have now taken on a "fighting" posture with the following characteristics:

- Flexed/tight jaw, teeth grinding
- Fighting eyes and tone of voice
- Desire to slam, stomp, kick
- Feelings of anger or rage
- Homicidal or suicidal feelings
- Twisted stomach or nausea, and
- Crying.

Here is an example of the flight response: You are intimidated by an administrator who seems to look down on you. When they are around, you tend to talk nervously, which further fuels your insecurity. As a result, when the administrator is around, you tend to quickly look for an opportunity to escape. The flight response is characterized by:

- Restlessness
- Anxiety
- Shallow breathing
- Sense of chaos in life with little space for grounding between events, and
- Excessive exercise.

The **freeze** response might look like this: It is a busy day at work and there is far more need than there are bodies to meet the demand. Between the background noise and the felt chaos, you've been on the edge of overwhelm for a good part of the day. A client approaches you, wagging their finger and yelling accusations. What was manageable anxiety has now become a numb heaviness in the body and a blank mind. The freeze response manifests as follows:

- Feeling cold and numb
- Sense of heaviness and rigidity
- Holding the breath
- Sense of dread
- Decreased heart rate and/or pounding heart
- Constantly scanning for threats, and
- A sense of "stuckness" in the body.

Finally, here is an example of the fawn response: The work environment has been an emotional battlefield for a while now, where shaming remarks are more the norm than the exception. You're noticing that no matter how poorly you're treated, you spend all of your energy trying to appease others rather than tending to your own emotional needs in the moment.

The fawn response could be characterized by:

- Saying "yes" when you want to say "no"
- Changing your values based on who your with
- more awareness of the emotions of others than your own
- putting more weight in the opinions of others than your own
- feeling guilt and fear of rejection when you authentically express yourself.

We can measure stress by tracking cortisol levels in the body. Often referred to as the "stress hormone," cortisol is produced by the adrenal cortex in response to physical and psychological stress. Cortisol impacts numerous metabolic processes as well as the immune system, both of which are significant contributors to a variety of acute and chronic diseases. The release of cortisol occurs when we think threatening thoughts, which then activate the sympathetic nervous system to flood the bloodstream with cortisol. Researchers use cortisol measurements to quantify an individual's experience of acute and chronic stressors. There are many ways to interrupt the activation of the sympathetic nervous system and instead activate the parasympathetic system, which enables the body to relax. Throughout the book, I refer to cortisol as the single best biological indicator of the experience of stress, and I highlight practices that activate the parasympathetic nervous system to counteract its effects.

DISTRESS

The stress response is not always negative. The experience of stress can alert us to situations that demand our attention and motivate us to resolve them. However, when the stress response extends beyond the threatening event or exceeds our capacity to cope, it becomes distress. When distress goes unchecked, it becomes chronic and we quickly lose perspective. While some types of stress can enhance our ability to resolve stressors, distress undermines this ability. Chronic stress, when it becomes distress, leads to numerous negative mental, physical, and spiritual consequences.

Workplace factors that interplay to compound stress include past trauma, **vicarious trauma**, unmanaged emotional labour, effort–reward imbalances, workplace hostility, physical violence, and heavy workloads. In terms of developmental assets, our sense of coherence (our orientation to the stimuli) and congruence (or ability to express ourselves authentically) impact whether a stimulus feels threatening. If so, we experience the stimulus as a stressor. If not, the stimulus is simply a challenge to navigate. The intensity of our experience of stressors and our felt confidence to resolve them interplays with our likelihood of using substances or distracting activities to cope, as well as our capacity to be objective and creative and to relate to others from a place of wholeness. All these factors produce ripple effects in our personal and work relations and the larger system in which we live and work (Dames, 2018b; Schwabe & Wolf, 2013).

Diffusing: Stepping Back From the Stress Response (Nonattachment)

NONATTACHMENT

When we get fused or attached to the feelings that result when our nervous system becomes activated, we are likely to react, limiting our ability to choose the most beneficial action (for ourselves and others) in that moment. **Nonattachment** is the quality of having a sense of coherence and describes an ability to step back and maintain perspective. From this more objective place, we can consciously work with the emotions that result from potential and often passing threats. Our body is designed to protect us from these potential threats. It is doing exactly what it is supposed to do, alerting us and helping us to tend to potential threats before they become actual threats. Before we can even form a thought, our well-intentioned body responds to these potential threats, getting us ready to fight, flee, or, if too overwhelmed, freeze. The stress response was never our enemy; quite the opposite, it is a protector, an ally on our journey. However, this ally often gets confused, conflating the past with the present, causing a form of emotional transference that can feel quite threatening. For example, someone in our current life may remind us of someone who hurt us in the past. As a result, we react to this person as though it is the person from our past rather than the present, which keeps us from seeing both the person in front of us and the situation for what they really are. In this way, if we overly identify with the physiological reactions created by the nervous system, we become confused; rather than working with the nervous system, we begin to feel enslaved by it.

Another form of nonattachment in relation to others is **rational detachment**. This form of nonattachment is characterized by an ability to not take the behaviours of others personally. It enables us to recognize that the hostile behaviours of others are less about us and more about unresolved hurts from the past being projected onto the current situation. From this vantage point, we can keep things in perspective without getting stuck in our own assumptions and fears. Because we don't view another's behaviour as personal, it also isn't threatening to the nervous system. When we are grounded in this nonattached position, we can shift our focus from what is wrong to what can be done about it. On a related note, and as elaborated on in Chapter 10, rational detachment can also be applied to situations where we project our past hurts onto the present day. If we confuse one with the other, we are apt to spiral into stress states, simply because the mind is conflating a past event with the present.

The stress response pulls our attention to perceived threats that need tending to. We do not consciously choose whether we will position ourselves to go into fight, flight, or freeze; it happens before thoughts even form. Some will start in fight or flight and then quickly move into freeze. Others remain in fight or flight, not moving into freeze at all. Ideally, we can stay in fight or flight, as we still have access to our inner and outer resources, enabling us to manage the felt threat so we can return to a state of equilibrium. Once we get into freeze, our ability to connect to our inner resources and creatively tap into our outer resources is extremely limited.

Our stress response tendencies are related to our past experiences and related assumptions. These assumptions come from our brain's ability to organize past insights and learnings into patterns, enabling us to intuitively and spontaneously react before we can form conscious thought; this is **brain chunking** (Neath & Surprenant, 2003).

BRAIN CHUNKING: OUR INTUITIVE ASSUMPTIONS

As a reminder, an event is not what typically causes stress. How we interpret the event is the source of our stress. A stressor develops when we consider an event a threat to our primary human needs. Brain chunking is a helpful way to understand how we form our assumptions outside of conscious choice. It represents our intuitive intelligence, the compilation of our lived experience and how we have come to know and understand the world. It is brain chunking that explains how we can rationally act before we have an opportunity to consciously think. This intuitive knowing is helpful when we need to respond quickly in emergencies, but not so helpful when we are trying to break habitual stress reactions. If the intuitive stress response sends us into a fight, flight, or freeze response, our ability to maintain an objective perspective is hampered, if not eliminated. In this way, when we feel threatened, our biology and neurology compel us to react from a fear-based framework. To reorient ourselves, we must cultivate a space between ourselves and the sense of threat. This space represents nonattachment. From this more objective vantage point, cultivated through nonattachment, we have an opportunity to rewire old patterns and consciously engage with our intuitive intelligence. By doing so, we can interrupt the involuntary impulse to react from a place of fear. As a result, we cultivate choice and can therefore act from a different, more creative, and optimistic framework. Brain chunking is explored further in Chapter 5.

Dissociation Versus Nonattachment

Dissociation is a subconscious reaction to fear. Nonattachment occurs when we step back from emotions to objectively work with them. One occurs subconsciously and leads to impulsive and involuntary reactions. The other is conscious, enabling mindful action; the latter cultivates choice. Mindful action enables the emotions to come and go as needed, without making us feel attached or threatened by them.

NONATTACHMENT CULTIVATES CHOICE

Confidence in our choices and resources bolsters sense of coherence. The ability to step back occurs when we disidentify with the event in addition to our thoughts and emotions about the event. We become the curious observer. We identify more from the space from which we are observing, rather than identifying with the thing or sensation we are investigating. We can notice the thoughts and emotions, welcome them as biased guests (informed through brain chunking), consider their message, and then let them fall into the background. When we step back, creating a space between us, the stimuli, and the noise that arises from the stimuli, we attain a state of nonattachment. *I am not that—I am the witness of that.* Again, we become like the detached observer of stormy weather. Without the capacity to create this space or grounding in response to a threatening event, we are left at the mercy of our thoughts and emotions, surrendering to the stress response, and reacting from fear. This lack of space disables conscious choice. Attaining nonattachment is what enables us to consciously act from choice and prevents us from involuntarily reacting to passing stimuli.

POST-TRAUMATIC STRESS DISORDER

Post-traumatic stress disorder (PTSD) is a common condition, especially among caregivers who work in high-stimulus and trauma-laden work environments. For example, in an emergency, the first people on the scene, such as firefighters, police, paramedics, and a variety of others tend to the most chaotic and often frightening moments in other people's lives.

The diagnosis criteria for PTSD include symptoms that reflect reexperiencing, avoidance, reactivity, and cognitive and mood impacts (National Institute of Mental Health, 2019b). Unlike PTSD, which is related to a specific event, **complex PTSD** stems from the feeling of being unable to escape ongoing traumatic events such as chronic abuse and negligence (National Health Service, 2018). The symptoms are similar to those listed for PTSD but may also include feelings of shame or guilt, difficulty controlling emotions, dissociation, isolation, relationship difficulties, risky behaviour and self-harm, and suicidal thoughts.

Post-traumatic stress occurs when a threat from the past informs our perception of present-day events, disabling our ability to maintain perspective. The current event may not be an actual threat, but it subconsciously reminds us of a time from the past, when a need went unmet, wounding us to the point that it continues to inform (out of self-protection) our current experience. Viewed through this lens, when unmanaged, PTSD limits our ability to step back, making nonattachment and objective decision making difficult if not impossible. When the nervous system is intensely threatened or activated, a common symptom of PTSD, the intense physiological attachment to the stress response often leads to involuntary reactions. Once the cascade begins, we may not recognize what has happened until it plays out. However, we can work with the experience, investigate what activated us, and come up with a self-compassionate plan that can help us prevent or notice the activation earlier the next time around.

Despite what individualistic Western cultures teach us, sharing the road with others facilitates and expedites our healing. Healing requires the development of trust, and the quickest way to develop greater trust in ourselves and others is through vulnerability in relationship. When we come to believe we are unconditionally positively regarded by others, we are far more likely to release the shame that keeps us fused to the stress response. By expanding our awareness of how stress works, we are more apt to recognize the event, which provides an opportunity to step back from it. We have then cultivated a space between *it* and *us*. In this space, we can see the event for what it is, investigating it more objectively, enabling us to keep it in perspective. We see the experience for what it is, a pattern or assumption based on a past adversity. From here, we can nonjudgementally work with the assumption, which was developed from subconscious brain chunking, and investigate how fitting or true it is in the moment. Most times, we will find that we are not actually threatened in the here and now. When we feel less attached to the passing threat, we discover a newfound sense of choice. Empowered by confidence in our research, we can now consciously and self-compassionately recognize and tend to the past wound as both separate and intertwined with what is happening in the current moment. This is a demonstration of congruence and sense of coherence.

Finding Our Way Home in Community: Polyvagal Theory

We all need people. Let's be each other's people…

As illustrated in Chapter 2 and in Figure 2.3, polyvagal theory (Porges, 2011) interweaves with Maslow's theory of unmet needs (Maslow, 1943) and attachment theory (more in Chapter 8; Bowlby, 2012), impacting how we perceive stimuli and our ability to emotionally regulate, be in authentic relationships, and mitigate or interrupt the stress response. Polyvagal theory shifts us away from the idea that compulsive behaviours reflect a lack of willpower. Quite the opposite—the nervous system directs our behaviour before our thinking mind can intercede. Behaviours reflect the state of our autonomic nervous system (Flores & Porges, 2017). Relating this process to what is known as PTSD, the nervous system is reacting to a past threat before the conscious mind can objectively evaluate the situation. Once the brain floods with chemicals, we are often unable to make objective decisions, causing us to react before conscious choice can occur. In this way, when the nervous system is activated, depending on the intensity of the felt threat, conscious choice or willpower is not a part of the equation.

We can retrain our neural pathways through social interactions that feel safe. When we feel safe, we can show up authentically, trusting that we will be met with unconditional positive regard. Grounding more securely in relationships characterized by unconditional positive regard regulates our nervous system, enabling us stay connected to the sensations in our body (embodied) and expanding our window of tolerance for stress.

In terms of how the body attains homeostasis, according to polyvagal theory, we can retrain our neural pathways through social interactions that feel safe. When we as a community understand polyvagal theory, we have a great opportunity to rewire our neural pathways through relationships of unconditional positive regard. Rewiring neural pathways in a community characterized by unconditional positive regard improves our ability to form secure attachments and reduces anxious or avoidant reactions. When we practise this new way of being with others, being witnessed and celebrated with unconditional positive regard, we are more apt to then integrate the same felt sense in our relationships to ourselves and others. Embodying this secure way of being empowers us to keep authentically showing up, allowing us to consciously express what is happening inside of us to the rest of the world.

When we show up authentically in community with others with whom our body feels safe, we work in tandem with (rather than at odds with) our brain (**neuroception**), which inhibits the stress response and promotes a greater ability to thrive (Flores & Porges, 2017). Because connection through relationship is at the heart of healing and reorienting, we must shift away from our individualistic—and often disconnected—ways of being. We heal in community with others. While we may have come to believe that we are safer alone, the flaws imbedded in this orientation are becoming clear as we work our way through an international mental health crisis. Relationships characterized by unconditional positive regard remind us of who we are, separate from our cultural conditioning. As we remember, the veil of our confusion lifts, enabling us to rediscover our wholeness.

> *In times of stress, the best thing we can do for each other is to listen with our ears and our hearts and to be assured that our questions are just as important as our answers.*
>
> Fred Rogers

FINDING COMMON GROUND AND CELEBRATING DIVERSITY

A sense of trust develops when we *believe* there is common ground between us and others, where we feel a sense of belonging. With this relational common ground, we take ownership in the agreements and expectations between parties. In this way, we develop a more predictable and secure relational container, one that can be understood and relied upon. When planted securely in this environment, we can relax into the relationship, enabling us to put a greater focus on *be*ing embodied together rather than the transactional form of *do*ing that comes from fear and obligation.

In terms of diversity, all too often it can be interpreted as a threat to our need to belong. When we lack a sense of unconditional positive regard, we are more prone to contribute to homogenization, which is reflected in how we attach to the conditions on the surface (skin colour, language, belief systems, gender, etc.). From this insecure orientation, we tend to subtly (or not so subtly) force common ground, snuffing out diversity wherever we can. Health care culture is known for having workers who exert control through homogenizing tactics, such as scrutinizing those who challenge the status quo and shaming those who threaten the unwritten cultural rules (Cho et al., 2006; Jackson et al., 2002; Jacobs & Kyzer, 2010; Laschinger et al., 2010; Lively, 2000; Porath & Pearson, 2012).

We regain balance when we come back to compassion. Doing so enables us to find the common ground in our shared humanity, the inner signal that connects us despite the noisy conditions on the surface. For example, we all long to be fed, sheltered, and accepted, to love and be loved, and ultimately to be seen and celebrated for who we really are. In these ways, we find common ground. From this abundant place, our differences are a reason to lean into the mysteries between us. With curiosity, we can delight in and learn from the varying ways of *being* and *doing*, an artful blend of nature and nurture. We can celebrate diversity as a beautiful mosaic to behold, with immense opportunities to learn and grow together.

Empathy and Vicarious Trauma: Hurt Too Close to Home

Empathy describes the ability to put oneself in another's shoes, especially in times of suffering. According to a recent study by Buffone et al. (2017), there are two ways to cultivate empathy. You can imagine what the other is feeling or you can imagine yourself feeling what they are feeling, taking on the feelings as if they were your own. While the two approaches may seem similar, the long-term impact each of them can have on us is notably different. The first provides a degree of nonattachment that buffers us from overidentifying with the situation and more closely aligns with compassion.

Blatchford's (2019) description of her experience walking alongside a loved one with Parkinson's disease illustrates empathetic engagement:

> ...*when your heart is being broken open by life, there can be moments when you may feel your breaking merging with the breaking others are experiencing. It's as when waves, from various directions, created by different disturbances, meet and become one within a river or on the surface of a body of water. One glance at the face of another, or others, and you know what they are feeling. Their feeling washes over and into you, becoming yours, too. (Blatchford, 2019)*

Caregivers are often expected to be selflessly empathetic, often engaging in this second form of empathy without an awareness of the long-term impact. When these unwritten cultural "ideals" are prescribed to caregivers, despite potential harms, they contribute to high rates of moral injury, emotional exhaustion, and burnout. While we praise caregivers for empathetically listening to their clients, it is important to also cultivate an awareness of the risks of overly identifying with clients, as it can result in vicarious trauma. Vicarious trauma occurs when the traumatic experience of another negatively impacts the provider's identity and beliefs, which when unresolved can lead to cynicism and despair (Saakvitne & Pearlman, 1998).

For example, in my line of work, empathizing with another can play out for me as follows:

I work as a forensic nurse examiner, which includes tending to adults and children who have recently experienced a traumatic event. When I work with children who are similar in age to my own children, I am prone to overly identifying with them and their distraught parent. The more the parent and/or the child reminds me of myself or my children, the more difficult it is to separate my emotions from theirs, resulting in emotional transference. Adding to this emotionally activated state, there is often moral or ethical dissonance that results when we feel that the traumatic situation is not fully resolved. For instance, this may occur when we feel as though we are sending a client back into a situation where they clearly have an unmet need. When the compounding feelings overwhelm me, and I cannot resolve them in those moments because my job is to tend to the client's emotions, I am at risk of subconsciously freezing (*dissociating*). While this state may appear similar to nonattachment, when it comes to these cases, it is more often a subconscious fear-based reaction whereby my body compartmentalizes the emotions because I don't feel safe expressing them. As a result, there have been a few cases that still come to mind even a year or two later, unearthing the emotions I felt at the time of working through the case. I have learned over the years that if I overly identify with the client—as if I or a loved one were the victim instead—and dissociate from the resulting emotions, they get pent up as trauma until I resolve them. When the emotions well up, even years later, I need to take the time to feel and digest them in order to release them.

When we connect with others through empathy, we are vulnerable and open, often resulting in an inner change that can shift how we relate to the world; this effect can be cumulative and permanent, impacting us personally and professionally. Empathy enables us to deeply connect with the experience of others, which has both upsides and downsides. The research shows that when we feel connected to another, it can mitigate suffering (Sturgeon & Zautra, 2015). Sharing our pain or sharing in the pain of another has two benefits: it increases our sense of connection, reducing felt isolation, and it promotes an ability to put the situation in perspective, assuming that the person with whom we are sharing our story can provide some objectivity. Furthermore, the person providing empathy benefits by gaining a greater sense of purpose, happiness (Steger et al., 2008), and overall psychological well-being (Manczak et al., 2016). However, by sharing in another's suffering, we are also vulnerable to the stressful aspects of suffering, including a cortisol spike and heightened inflammatory profiles (Manczak et al., 2016).

Compounding the stress-related impact of sharing in another's suffering is that those who are more sensitive (able to read and feel other's emotions) also tend to have more of a **negativity bias** (Chikovani et al., 2015). A negativity bias means that negative events have a far greater emotional impact on us than positive ones, with the effect of negative events lingering longer than that of positive ones. People with a negativity bias are more likely to pick up on fear and sadness than on pleasant emotions; as a result, they are likely prone to compassion fatigue and vicarious trauma.

As a protective factor against vicarious trauma, those who can separate their emotions from those of another by focusing on compassion—*imagining* how another feels rather than imagining ourselves in their shoes—are less likely to suffer the ill effects of overidentifying through empathetic engagement (Electris, 2013). However, depending on our emotional management skills, our tendency toward having a negativity bias, and whether another's situation reminds us of our own, we may be unable to separate our emotions from another's. As a result, we will be more likely to overly attach, feeling the trauma as if it is our own and dissociating from the emotions out of a felt necessity to stay focused on our client's needs. Finding our unique balance between when we engage in empathy, compassion, or dissociation takes awareness, practice, and self-compassion as we work with our unique tendencies and make adjustments as we go.

Attuning Practice: Empathy and Me—Harmful or Helpful?

Is there a way to feel empathy in caregiving work when people are suffering and dying without experiencing vicarious trauma? In short, yes. Depending on the situation, how much we identify with the other person's narrative, and whether there is a related unhealed wound in us, engaging in empathy is not always best. However, if we can mindfully manage empathy, the benefits will outweigh the risks, and in most cases, will buffer caregivers from burnout (Wilkinson et al., 2017). There are a few important points to be aware of though. First, it is not helpful to put on an obligatory empathetic display if it doesn't feel authentic. Faking it contributes to emotional labour (discussed later in this chapter). Second, if it feels authentic and you can separate your process from the other person's, mindfully managed empathy will allow you to be present with the person without (figuratively) carrying them home with you or experiencing suffering so deeply that it feels like your own. Through mindfulness, a component of sense of coherence, we can step back from the situation, which promotes objectivity, and then determine which path is best for us on a case-by-case basis. If you notice that your pattern of coping means that you cannot step back far enough to be objective, it can be helpful to get that objective perspective from a professional counsellor, trusted colleague, or friend.

Attuning/Reflecting Opportunity

Reflect on a situation at work involving another's suffering that continues to activate difficult emotions for you. If you haven't encountered any of these situations, this may be a sign that empathy is more helpful than harmful. If you can pull up a case or two, reflect on what made those cases different from the others in terms of how the person's suffering impacted you. Can you recall whether there were similarities in your lives, perhaps putting you at risk of overidentification? Reflect on how you might engage differently the next time: What would it look like for you to engage compassionately (setting a clear boundary between their pain and your emotions) rather than empathetically (feeling as they feel)? Can you see and feel a difference?

Sometimes, other people's experiences are too close to home, making it impossible to erect an emotional boundary. In these cases, we can have an emotional safety plan at work. The plan doesn't have to be formally established, but it is helpful to know how we can reach out for help. For instance, perhaps you can plan to switch patients or clients with a co-worker. If removing yourself from the situation isn't an option, are there a few colleagues you can debrief with? Having an emotional safety plan in place will help to prevent your own experience of trauma from evolving into unresolved trauma or PTSD.

Strengthening Practice: Escaping the Empathy Trap

In caregiving professions, we often spend large parts of our workday focused on other people's needs, which can lead to emotional exhaustion if left unchecked. By developing greater awareness of what is ours and what is our client's, we increase our **emotional intelligence** and ultimately engage empathy from a place of wholeness.

Empathy is a combination of our natural human desire to connect with others and a byproduct of our social conditioning. Tuning into another via empathy enables us to draw closer to others and to feel truly heard and understood by another. When we choose to feel empathy for another, the connection is empowering; however, when the emotions of another feel involuntarily pushed onto us, these feelings of connection can feel violating, which can fuel relational resentment.

Striking the balance between others' emotional needs while also honouring our own requires emotional intelligence. We develop this emotional intelligence with practice as we consciously attune to our own emotions, learning to distinguish them from the feelings of whomever we are connected to, then stepping back when we lose our balance. Relying on others to hold their emotions back in order to gain reprieve is not a realistic nor fair expectation. That means the onus is on us to first take notice when we begin to feel trapped and then make the choice to emotionally withdraw, to a degree, until we can regain our balance.

You can transition from feeling trapped by an obligation to embodying empathy by choosing to step into it. To engage from this more empowered place requires the ability to step back (nonattachment), a skill that we gain through awareness and practice (Stern & Divecha, 2015). In this way, we consciously notice our emotional state while we are empathizing with another. Expanding our awareness of the source and message of our emotional felt sense enables us to distinguish the subtleties of someone else's emotions from our own. We learn to distinguish our "signal" (essence) from the external "noise" (thoughts, conditioning, others' emotional energy) by coming to know the tune of our inner world, which hums at its own unique frequency. As we receive emotions, welcoming them as important guests, we can tune into their message. Pendulating between the inner and outer work, tuning into the signal amid the noise, prevents us from feeling involuntarily held hostage by another's emotional experience. This awareness enables us to choose to continue feeling with people; but the moment it feels harmful, as an act of self-compassion, we can also choose to step back.

Stepping back does not necessarily mean physically removing ourselves, although it can! Rather, it creates a subtle space that enables us to transition from feeling *with* someone, as if another's emotions were our own, to feeling *for* them, with a clear distinction between their emotional experience and ours. On a more practical front, especially in the beginning, we may need to create a distinct physical or verbal boundary. For example, slipping out for a bathroom break can be a great way to physically separate ourselves without raising social alarm bells. We can set a boundary by verbally acknowledging other people's suffering while also honouring where we are at. For instance, one could say, "Wow, that sounds so difficult! I'd really love to hear more about it, but I'm exhausted right now. Can we meet up tomorrow?" Or, if our loved one is coming to us with an urgent emotional need that we feel we need to attend to in that moment, we can practise transitioning from empathy to compassion, whereby we take a grounding moment (a heart breath or two is a great strategy to quickly ground ourselves), and then verbally honour what is theirs and what is ours. For example, we can acknowledge their suffering by saying, "Wow, that sounds difficult," and then ask how we can help by saying, "Is there something that I can do to help?" While the move is subtle, we are compassionately responding, and yet it is clear that this is their experience, not ours.

Setting these boundaries may feel like we are inconveniencing others, but the relational benefits are enormous. By setting boundaries and thus taking care of ourselves, we are letting our loved ones know that they too can set boundaries and take care of themselves. Setting these boundaries is an essential part of cultivating relationships where we can provide and receive unconditional positive regard. This takes practice and vulnerability, and may require us to communicate what we are working on, especially when others receive these boundaries as rejection. Letting others know that we sometimes struggle with distinguishing our emotions from others' and that we are working on managing our emotions in a healthier way reassures them that the boundary setting is about us, not them. Expressing ourselves in this way can elicit empathy in others, deepening relational connection and cultivating relationships that encourage authentic expression.

Speaking of unconditional positive regard, cultivating relationships in which we feel cared for and where we can receive empathy is a great way to help us attain a balance of giving and receiving. However, just as we are learning to set boundaries, it is important that we can also honour others' boundaries, recognizing that someone else needing some emotional space is not personal; this too takes practice!

Those of us who spend much of our day more focused on the emotions of others than our own often have super-sensitive emotional antennas that pick up on the emotional energy around us. In addition to developing a greater awareness of what is ours and what is others' and setting boundaries when we lose our balance, we can reorient ourselves when we fall prey to assuming we know what others are feeling and why. This skill is an asset when we are caring for others from a place of wholeness, whereby we are our most objective self, but not so helpful when we falsely assume we know what is happening and act or react accordingly. We can check our assumptions by first taking notice when an assumption has hatched, and then asking for more information or simply stating what we think we are hearing and asking whether our understanding is accurate.

As we build our emotional muscles, we become more able to embody unconditional positive regard. Just like practising compassion and self-compassion are skills we can develop, so too is expressing empathy and self-empathy. Emotionally managing and rebalancing when we feel off-kilter enables us to relate from a place of wholeness, a requirement for us to be fully present with others. We can attain homeostasis through social interactions that feel safe. As described in polyvagal theory, when we authentically show up in community with others who feel safe to us, we are working in tandem with our brain (neuroception), inhibiting the stress response, and promoting an ability to thrive as our authentic self (Flores & Porges, 2017).

Emotional Labour in the Workplace: Fake It Till You Can't Take It?

Emotional labour, a term coined by Hochschild (2012), occurs when we make an effort to act differently from the way we feel. It is putting on the cheery face that others expect even when we are feeling lousy. In the workplace, excessive emotional labour dampens our ability to thrive because thriving requires authenticity. Authenticity is also a core feature of Maslow's (1987) theory and Rogers' (1959) concept of congruence between the "real" self and "ideal" self.

A meta-analysis of 109 studies made it clear that incongruent emotional states (surface acting) have a range of negative consequences related to burnout, job satisfaction, the ability to effectively complete work tasks, and caregiver retention rates. Conversely, those who maintain emotional congruence did not incur these same negative consequences (Mesmer-Magnus et al., 2012).

Hochschild (2012) articulated three ways of being and acting that determine the amount of emotional energy used during interactions. The first is surface acting, which burns the greatest amount of energy stores and represents a disconnection from authentic emotion. Surface acting is a complete detachment from emotion, which may be done subconsciously as a fear-based coping habit or consciously, knowing that we must display an emotion that is not authentic to how we really feel. The second option, which is more in line with a mindful stepping back, is deep acting, whereby we attune to an authentic emotion while we are having to put on a certain prescribed display.

In a study by Brotheridge and Grandey (2002), surface acting resulted in a diminished sense of personal accomplishment, but when deep acting was employed, employees felt a greater sense of efficacy at work. Deep acting mitigates emotional exhaustion by enabling us to stay connected to authentic emotion while displaying the emotions that our work role demands of us. For example, Cherie, a new graduate nurse and research participant, explains how she handles mistakes, which she ties to her ability to connect to her feelings of unconditional acceptance from her mother. In her account, Cherie shares how those positive feelings buffer her from feeling personally threatened when she makes mistakes at work and enable her to act from a grounded, objective space:

> My mom and I have always been very close, and she has always been a sort of bedrock. My self-acceptance started there … I mean I make mistakes at work, but I don't really feel bad about it. There is usually something in the environment that enables the mistake to happen, so it is more important to look at what is happening to cause that to happen in the first place. It isn't all about me. (Dames, 2018a)

In a similar situation, where self-esteem may feel threatened, rather than dissociating out of fear, Janice finds strength and authentically connects through her faith, drawing on this strength during difficult work moments:

> My faith helps me feel that you know it's okay, I've done what I can to make it right, I've changed what I can change, I know I am forgiven, and I can move on. (Dames, 2018a)

In addition to surface acting and deep acting, the third option is to express ourselves authentically, without filtering or crafting a particular display for another. When we are authentic, we are not wrestling with self-consciousness, which enables us to maintain our emotional energy stores. The more we have to emote positive emotions while we are experiencing negative ones, the greater the surface acting, which leads to incongruence and ultimately emotional exhaustion. When surface acting becomes an ingrained work habit, we are at greater risk of burning out. To address the issue, you can learn to use deep acting skills, which mitigate the consequences of incongruence. This ability to deeply act allows for connection to "real" emotions while adhering to the "ideal" cultural display rules. An example of deep acting is cultivating cheerfulness by thinking about something in your life that you are excited about or for which you are feeling grateful even while you are feeling tired. Employers that require emotional displays can train employees to deeply act, which reduces emotional exhaustion and burnout in the workplace (Tracy, 2005).

Attuning Practice: Deep Acting With That Thing That Makes Your Heart Sing

Deep acting is helpful when we must display an emotion that is incongruent with our authentic emotion. This tool applies to all areas of our lives, as emotional display expectations are plentiful at work and at home. Deep acting is an alternative to emotional dissociation, where we push our genuine emotions down, disconnecting from our inner world, which can lead to unresolved trauma and subconscious projections. To deeply act, we attempt to connect to something or someone that elicits a positive emotion, immersing in and savouring it so that we can view the situation through a more loving and flexible lens.

> ### Attuning/Reflecting Opportunity
>
> Think about something(s) in your life that makes your heart sing. Perhaps a loved one comes to mind, a pleasant memory, or an event that you are looking forward to. Can you write down a few that will be easy for you to recall in your time of need? This is how you engage in deep acting. It takes practice. With intention, you can develop a habit of this form of embodiment, interrupting a tendency to surface act.

At the organizational level, making sure that caregivers' "real" selves are welcome will reduce the need for us to surface act (taking on a prescribed ideal) and minimize the unnecessary emotional effort required to maintain artificial displays. This skill can be learned in the education setting. In many cases, as educators, we train students to emulate professional comportment standards, but when emotions arise that are incongruent with the prescribed image, many students are not prepared to manage the unresolved dissonance that results (Gray, 2009). While maintaining professional standards requires some consistency among how members uphold the collective image, we must strike a better balance to limit surface acting and emotional dissociation and protect emotional our energy stores.

Holding space for emotions, despite perceived social pressures, is an important emotional management skill (Russ, 1998; Taylor & Cranton, 2012). For instance, when I work with children who have experienced trauma, I often feel the need to push my emotions side in order to tend to the child. If I cannot hold space for my emotional messengers, I risk adding a layer of unresolved trauma that will quite likely project itself into a future moment. If left unresolved, it may continue to haunt me, coming to mind at unpredictable times, adding to my emotional labour until I tend to it. Ultimately, when the burden of emotional labour overshadows workplace rewards, it causes an effort–reward imbalance (Lewig & Dollard, 2003)—the next stressor I discuss here.

Projections and the emotions they provoke are our greatest teachers.

Effort–Reward Imbalance: Not Worth the Effort

Caregivers who are consistently experiencing an effort–reward imbalance may be at a higher risk for adverse physical and mental health impacts and eventual burnout (Bakker et al., 2000; Eriksson & Lindström, 2006; Jesse et al., 2015). According to an international systematic review of effort–reward imbalance among caregivers (Nguyen Van et al., 2018), there continues to be a high effort–reward imbalance, especially among caregivers with less power in the workplace. For instance, care aides may have a higher effort–reward imbalance than registered nurses, and, in turn, registered nurses are likely to have a higher imbalance than physicians. The effort–reward imbalance continues to be a major contributing factor to a caregiver's intent to leave their position (Boamah & Laschinger, 2016). Those with an imbalance toward the effort end of the spectrum will rarely thrive, and many may leave the profession altogether (Currie & Carr Hill, 2012). There are many types of rewards, including but not limited to compensation, and different people value different types of rewards. Some common examples of rewards mentioned in the literature include taking on satisfying work, establishing a professional identity, feeling a sense of place, and feeling empowered and in control during the workday. These rewards result in greater job satisfaction and retention rates (Zurmehly et al., 2009). A sense of control and empowerment are often lacking in caregiving. As these nurse research participants illustrate, their need for a certain degree of control and predictability (sense of coherence) is threatened:

> *They can pull us wherever and it doesn't matter. I don't feel heard, and I have no control. I feel like we are pawns that they just toss around however they want. (Sarah)*

> *I don't feel supported because I don't know the people. I haven't gotten a good orientation to the places I'm floated to … I just feel flustered and stressed, and then that impacts how I nurse and how I come across to my co-workers. I feel like I look like this terrible nurse, but I know I'm not. I'm just out of my comfort zone. I just don't know how they function; I don't know their routine. (Janice)*

> *Staffing is huge, not enough and being redeployed into areas where they don't have experience. (Mary)*

> *[On floors I'm redeployed to] the care aids were totally different; there was no communication, they weren't answering call bells … there is no floor organization, no flow, no consistency, no senior nurses, lots of new graduates, high turnover, it's super stressful. (Sarah) (Dames, 2018a)*

A felt sense of commitment to the organizational vision and perceived opportunities for promotion also reduce attrition rates (Beecroft et al., 2008; Kovner et al., 2009). While some caregivers may leave, many remain in the profession in a burned-out condition, resulting in workplace hostility (Schaufeli & Buunk, 2003).

Workplace Hostility: Eating Our Young

Workplace hostility is a result of the shame that emerges from individual incongruence. Influential psychiatrist and psychoanalyst Carl Jung called shame the "soul-eating emotion." If we dig deep enough, under every enduring emotional discomfort, we will often find shame at its roots. As research participant Tabitha told me:

> *I've had a senior nurse literally say, "We always eat our young, I don't know why we do it, but we do, so get over it." The younger nurses were … afraid of being targeted. There is a lot of talking behind people's backs. I've heard on a few occasions that you can't speak up because you will be busted for bullying … people are afraid to say anything; they bully behind the scenes now … It's not a safe space at all. (Dames, 2018a)*

The saying that "nurses eat their young" reflects the way our individual shame spills over onto others. As a result, **horizontal violence** emerges in the workplace. There are several common forms of horizontal violence such as criticizing, belittling or making hurtful gestures or comments to or about a co-worker in front of others, or intentionally excluding a colleague (Mitchell et al., 2014). These expressions of co-worker hostility produce stress, resulting from a felt threat to our need for esteem and belonging. Caregivers will find it difficult to thrive in environments where co-workers are hostile to one another. These novice caregiver statements from my recent research (Dames, 2018a) illustrate the reality that co-worker hostility is still "alive and well" in the workplace.

Cherie expressed hesitation among new nurses who felt "bullied" to come forward. They were afraid to challenge the status quo, which would have her stay quiet. She worried that if she did speak up and no one stepped in to protect her, she could be penalized by the senior nurses who uphold the cultural status quo.

Over-reporting is another form of co-worker hostility. Scrutiny from more senior caregivers can erode self-esteem (a primary need). As Candice shared, "There is one nurse that follows me all the time, and every little thing that she thinks I missed or did wrong gets reported. I don't think she was doing it to personally attack me, but it is just who she is as a nurse."

Enculturation in the ways of being of a particular culture begin during our caregiver training. We learn the norms and we learn to play the game if we want to be accepted into that culture (primary need to belong). As Mary shared, "… Even the senior nurses on the floor, watching them as a student, they would get shamed for speaking up or saying something … When you're a student, you just don't have the right to stand up for yourself. You just … learn it by being around it … I fear being publicly shamed. I experienced it as a student; I was publicly shamed in the hallway by two nurses … One lit into me, and the other stood there, watched, and didn't say anything. It was because I didn't chart in a timely manner."

The determining factor between whether a stimulus is a mere distraction that we can quickly recover from versus something that completely derails us is our sense of coherence. When we know we have the necessary resources to manage a challenging stimulus, it is less likely to feel threatening. When we do not perceive the stimulus as a threat, we can confidently and objectively navigate the challenge without feeling paralyzed by it. Conversely, those with a lower sense of coherence often lack confidence in their ability to manage stimuli, making them more prone to perceiving a stimulus as a threat; this perceived threat is fueled by shame, discussed later in this chapter. Conversely, a high sense of coherence enables objectivity, promoting a greater capacity to resolve or at least manage feelings of dissonance and the ability to engage or quickly reengage in thriving (Dames, 2018a).

Madeleine Leininger (1994), a prominent theorist in the field of health care and nursing culture, defined culture as the dominant values, patterns, and normative practices that are transmitted by those who identify with the professional role. Nursing culture has become known for putting nurses at risk for horizontal violence, demonstrated by the fact that 85% of nurses have reported being the victims of incivility (Jacobs & Kyzer, 2010). In a Canadian longitudinal study of 415 novice nurses, one-third reported feeling bullied at least twice per week (Laschinger et al., 2010). Another Canadian study surveying 226 novice nurses found that nearly 70% of them experienced severe burnout related to negative workplace environments (Cho et al., 2006). Lively (2000) found that senior caregivers who held a higher status had more social support in expressing emotion than those of a lower status. Individuals with a higher status set emotional display rules and determine when these displays are appropriate (Lively, 2000; Porath & Pearson, 2012). Individuals who question these power imbalances, disturbing the status quo, may become targets themselves. This pattern is subtly supported by management, who discredit the disturbers in a variety of ways. For example, they scrutinize an employee's work or publicly ridicule them, which eventually silences them (Jackson et al., 2002). The pressure to maintain the status quo, which gets threatened by those who do not conform to the implicit cultural rules, is a homogenizing force within health care providers.

There are three underlying phenomena worth diving into when it comes to workplace hostility: shame, perfectionism, and homogenization. While homogenization is a process, perfectionism is a disorder, and shame is a weapon of choice for those driven by unconscious and maladaptive needs to control the behaviours and identities of others.

Shame: When We Don't Measure Up

Everything that irritates us about others can lead to an understanding of ourselves.
                                                                    Carl G. Jung

According to Carl Jung, nearly every enduring irritation we feel about others is a **projection** of our shadow self and thus can be traced back to an unaccepted and therefore unintegrated part of our "real" self. These unintegrated parts of our "real" self are those parts that we began hiding as children to ensure that we were loved and accepted by others—this was not a choice, but a primal survival need. The more of our "real" self that remains hidden in the shadow, the more incongruent we are. When we see a reflection of this hidden part of ourselves in others, it reminds us of our incongruence, which results in shame (Jung, 1970).

Shame is one of the most powerful motivators and disablers in the human experience (Bond, 2009). It represents the painful feelings that occur when we become conscious of behaviours of ours that are incongruent with our core beliefs and values.

"In shame, perfection is sought; one is either perfect or a total failure, one does not experience anything in between" (Bond, 2009, p. 134). Among many caregivers, shame occurs when the socially prescribed "ideal" is incongruent with our "real" self, resulting in moral injury. The socially prescribed "ideal" is the display rules of how to professionally "know, be, and do," and in caregiving professions, they often become entwined and confused with our "real" values. For example, caregivers such as paramedics, dentists, firemen, veterinarians, counsellors, nurses, and physicians wear their professional identities in and out of the workplace. Among their friends, family, and community groups, they are caregivers, even when they aren't formally wearing that hat. Caregivers rarely get to take their professional hat off. Because of the enmeshing of our professional and personal lives, if we are expected to put on a cheerful and stoic display at work, even when we feel grumpy and uneasy inside, we are likely to mirror these same incongruent displays in our personal life. The enmeshing of professional display rules and personal values corresponds with Rogers' (1986) concept of congruence and provides insight into why feelings of not measuring up to professional ideals may correspond with intense feelings of personal shame.

Toward solutions to shame, Brené Brown (2006), a prominent shame researcher, describes the cores skills need to recognize and accept vulnerability and to build shame resilience by (1) validating ourselves and practicing self-compassion, (2) maintaining critical awareness of socially prescribed "ideals," and (3) attaining relationships that promote an ability to talk about shame, enabling the shame to surface, be processed, and be released. Workplaces that provide an opportunity to reflect on shaming when it occurs are more likely to expose the socially prescribed "ideals" at their roots (Jahromi et al., 2012).

Anything that's human is mentionable, and anything that is mentionable can be more manageable. When we can talk about our feelings, they become less overwhelming, less upsetting, and less scary.

Fred Rogers

Perfectionism: The Pressure to Perform

A recent meta-analysis involving over 40,000 college students in North America and the United Kingdom found that perfectionism—be it self, socially, or other prescribed—is on the rise, especially among our younger generations (Curran & Hill, 2019).

Put simply, **perfectionism** is the dogged pursuit of absolute flawlessness (Frost et al., 1990) and the driving force behind co-worker hostility. Maladaptive perfectionism and particularly socially prescribed perfectionism can create toxically stressful environments for those who do not fit neatly into the status quo (Jahromi et al., 2012). Current health care culture often promotes tendencies toward perfectionism; as a result, high levels of anxiety and depression are commonplace (Jahromi et al., 2012).

Most of us will have experiences with perfectionism. Some may slip in and out of it in milder and more adaptive forms, while others will spend every waking hour driven by a compulsion to attain a standard that is unreasonably high. In the more adaptive form, striving for perfection can be beneficial, as it motivates us to complete work and produce the best product possible (Harari et al., 2018). In its more adaptive form, perfectionism leads us to keep our high standards to ourselves as opposed to socially prescribing our ideals onto others. We are more likely to be self-motivated, be goal oriented, adapt to obstacles that may delay achievements, and find satisfaction from our accomplishments (Ellis, 2002). The downside of perfectionism, evident in its maladaptive forms, is the natural inclination to hold others to the same idealistic standards, which can cause unreasonably high expectations (Melrose, 2011). If we cannot meet these idealistic standards, detrimental mental health effects often result (Melrose, 2011). These health effects often correlate with fears of criticism and failure and when left unaddressed can lead to moral injury, emotional exhaustion, and eventual burnout (Chang, 2012; Gould et al., 1996; Sevlever & Rice, 2010).

TWO PERFECT DOORS

There are two dimensions of perfectionism: "excellence-seeking," whereby we are driven to achieve high standards, and "failure-avoiding," whereby we are driven to avoid shortcomings. Both versions are ultimately driven by the same core factors such as black and white thinking, a compulsive need to attain lofty standards, and self-worth evaluations that are contingent on one's achievement of their idealized standard (Harari et al., 2018; Hewitt & Flett, 1993).

PERFECTIONISM SPILLING INTO THE WORKPLACE

When mired in perfectionism, we are likely to be threatened by our internal alert system (i.e., our emotions), often ignoring and internalizing feelings of worthlessness, shame, and failure (Petersson et al., 2014; Shafran et al., 2002). Over time, this habitually defensive way of being will cause an overall lower tolerance to stress (Ellis, 2002; Petersson et al., 2014). These maladaptive forms of perfectionism lead to self-destructive behaviours, which extend into prescribing the same unrealistic expectations onto others (a phenomenon called socially prescribed perfectionism). Socially prescribed perfectionism uses shaming tactics to pressure others to live up to unrealistically high standards; when culturally reinforced, it has toxic effects on workplace morale, resulting in perfectionism being a chronic workplace stressor.

Perfectionism and sense of coherence inversely link; those who have a low sense of coherence score have higher perfectionism scores; therefore, improving sense of coherence buffers us from extreme forms of perfectionism. (Rennemark & Hagberg, 1997)

Homogenization: A Black and White World

While we can all resonate with the idea that there is indeed beauty in our individuality and how our differences can contribute to a rich and diverse workforce, when we are enculturated in homogenizing environments, we develop a fear of otherness. The fear and the homogenizing tendencies that follow are a natural outcome of our professional upbringing. We homogenize the workplace by shaming those who threaten the established culture (Adamson & Clark, 1999). Refusing to acknowledge otherness is the fuel that sustains cultural homogenization (Palmer et al., 2010). **Homogenization** is a "lose–lose" process: those who advocate for diversity become vulnerable to scrutiny, but those who comply with assimilation often feel unsettled and ambiguous (incongruent). Chronic denial or suppression of our "real" self in order to assimilate produces incongruence and is a barrier to thriving (Rogers, 1959). Palmer et al. (2010) suggested that, in homogenizing cultures, diversity produces implicit fears of conflict, which further pushes differences into the shadows and makes them even more divisive. High expectations (perfectionism) in nursing fuel homogenization. In a way, this form of hostility is the dark side of perfectionism in the profession.

Peer approval and acceptance plays a fundamental role in our psychological well-being and long-term physical health (Baumeister & Leary, 1995; Dickerson et al., 2009). In health care, garnering the approval of our work team, and especially senior members who implicitly set the cultural tone, is often a matter of career survival; as a result, the more vulnerable members (those who fall outside of the status quo) rarely challenge homogenization.

Physical Violence: A Disturbing New Normal

Physical violence is a common concern in many health care environments (Gates et al., 2011; Roche et al., 2010). Cherie, a novice caregiver and research participant, was surprised and disempowered by how common it is for patients to physically hurt nurses at work:

> *The amount of violence I see is so much more than I was expecting. Also thinking of reporting it, what are they going to do? The report will go back to my [manager], and they will say, "well he has dementia," and then it is normalized. It just seems pointless to report it … nothing is going to change. (Dames, 2018a)*

SAFETY IS A HUMAN NEED

The unmet need for safety in caregiving occupations is a major issue. Research shows that many caregivers working in acute care areas experience violence in the workplace, which has detrimental effects on their mental health and their ability to care for their clients (Gates et al., 2011; Roche et al., 2010). Frequent experiences of violence lead to a normalization of violence, where staff feel unable to resolve the threat and therefore accept it as "a part of the job." The normalization of physical violence prevents many health care providers from feeling safe in the work environment (Gates et al., 2011; Roche et al., 2010). These feelings of threat will at least the very distract and may even disable workers from thriving. Typically, the first one or two violent events activate an acute stress response, which then commonly evolves into similar events being dismissed as normal, often cloaked in humor. While the normalization of this threat may resolve the intensity of the stress, it does not resolve its lingering effects. Stress elicited by frequent violent events precipitates long-term mental and physical health consequences.

In order for a caregiver to reflect on their experience, process their emotions, and articulate themselves, they need time and space away from the high-stimulus health care environment as well as the awareness and tools to facilitate these activities. Unfortunately, heavy workloads and the normalization of violence may prevent caregivers from finding the time or recognizing their need to resolve this common stressor.

Heavy Workloads: Too Busy to Breathe

In an era of insufficient funding and limited resources, many practitioners try to do more with less. These larger systemic forces are a stressor that often weighs heaviest on frontline providers, who stand in the gap between systemic shortages and growing health care demands. A 2004 study of 393 nurses representing many work sites in the United States found that less than half of them could take any uninterrupted breaks during a typical 12-hour shift (Rogers et al., 2004). For new nurses, it is common practice to miss breaks and stay late to keep up with the caregiving workloads in health care, where the work volume for newer providers is the same as it is for their more experienced colleagues (Lea & Cruickshank, 2017; Rhéaume et al., 2011). Because they lack experience, these new caregivers often need to double-check their decisions, a necessary safeguard against mistakes. However, the employer may not acknowledge the workload associated with these extra steps. In my own career, I've observed that employers often do not take learning curves into account when assigning workload to novice caregivers, expecting them to carry workloads equal to those of more experienced employees. As a result, new caregivers become even less likely to take breaks and often fear scrutiny (shame) if they fail to carry the same workload as their more experienced colleagues.

Heavy workloads contribute to unmet needs because caregivers are missing breaks, working long hours, and unable to find space away from external stimuli to address mental and physical requirements. Caregivers are unlikely to thrive in the workplace as long as these needs go unmet.

IMPACTS OF CHRONIC STRESS

Even when the many stressors mentioned earlier in this chapter are absent, and the workplace is generally happy and healthy, working in high-stakes (life or death), high-stimulus environments can cause sensory overwhelm, activating the stress response. Events that compound to make an environment high stimulus include long to-do lists combined with interruptions, constant alarms and call bells ringing, patients and family members calling out for help, multiple people moving around, and fast paced and rapidly changing activities. It is no wonder that these work environments often produce a felt sense of threat and activate the stress response. For example, a nurse may question their decision—which, if wrong, could have life or death consequences—but not feel they have the time to double-check it, as other patients in peril are in need of immediate care.

As described earlier, those with a higher sense of coherence will be more likely to experience stressors as momentary distractors from thriving rather than feeling completely derailed by them. However, there are certain weather conditions (external stressors) that must be managed. For instance, in a study comparing general ward nurses and neonatal intensive care nurses, the higher the stakes in the work environment, the higher the levels of cortisol and stress felt among workers (Fujimaru et al., 2012). Another study by Vessey et al. (2010) found that the frequency and rates of co-worker hostility had detrimental effects on the psychological and physical health of nurses. As a result, it negatively affected job satisfaction, retention rates, quality of care, and patient outcomes.

Most of us can relate to the mental impacts that stress has on our ability to think and cope; however, we may be less aware of the long-term mental and physical risks we may face if stress goes unaddressed. High stress levels correlate with endocrine and immune dysfunction, lower vaccine responses, cardiovascular disease, rheumatoid arthritis, delayed wound healing, and rapid disease progression (Baum et al., 1993; Castle et al., 1995; Dickerson et al., 2004, 2009; Kiecolt-Glaser et al., 2002; Smith & Zautra, 2002). These sustained feelings of stress are a significant health issue, leading to burnout if left unaddressed (Cowin & Hengstberger-Sims, 2006; Deary et al., 2003; Garrosa et al., 2011; Luthans & Jensen, 2005).

BURNOUT

Burnout is a state of chronic occupational emotional overload (Thunman, 2012) or a "state of exhaustion in which one is cynical about the value of one's occupation and doubtful of one's ability to perform" (Maslach et al., 1996, p. 20). The pathological components of burnout overlap with those of clinical depression (Bianchi et al., 2015). Burnout is considered the single most common occupational health hazard second only to musculoskeletal injuries. Furthermore, burnout is estimated to have doubled in incidence in the last 10 years (Thunman, 2012).

When our *doing* in the world lacks meaning or runs counter to our belief system, it results in incongruence and ultimately moral injury, which is a primary contributor to burnout. The less caregivers can authentically express themselves and their emotions, the more they experience shame. The more emotional dissociation and dissonance they experience, the more likely it will manifest as anxiety or depression. Depressed and anxious caregivers are less able to manage their emotions, making their risk of burnout exponentially higher.

Novice caregivers who leave the profession commonly report that they left because of burnout (Suzuki et al., 2010), and research suggests that the stressors leading to burnout begin during the undergraduate years. Nurses who experience it at school are at significantly higher risk of leaving their position after only 10 to 15 months (Rudman & Gustavsson, 2012). According to the World Health Organization, caregiver burnout is a global issue (Perry et al., 2012) that will require a widespread effort (aiming at both the roots and the weather) to address. One person's burnout has a ripple effect, extending to the surrounding staff, who have to cope with diminished workplace morale and often take on extra work because of high rates of attrition and absenteeism.

DEFLATED MORALE

Many caregivers who suffer from emotional exhaustion and burnout remain in the field but develop chronic feelings of hostility (Schaufeli and Buunk, 2003). When employees continue to work in a burned-out condition, it causes ripple effects of adverse consequences for themselves, work teams, and clients (Schaufeli & Buunk, 2003). This scenario circles back to co-worker hostility, referred to earlier, with caregivers hurting each other and perpetuating the cycle of violence in the workplace. A homogenizing culture, as described previously, further diminishes morale because it prevents employees from feeling safe to express their "real" self when it does not align with the prescribed "ideals." As a result, employees often repress personality qualities that stand out from the status quo, leading to further shame and diminished morale.

Taking Personality Into Account

Caregivers that work in an environment of their choosing, one that it is congruent with their personality, are at a lower risk of leaving their job (Beecroft et al., 2008). Personality traits influence our ability to navigate workplace stimuli, which makes personality a significant factor in our risk for burnout (Geuens et al., 2015; Hakanen & Bakker, 2016; Swider & Zimmerman, 2010). For example, Geuens et al. (2015) found that caregivers with a certain personality type are five times more likely to burn out, even when taking job-related factors into account. The more vulnerable personality, which shares the same traits as those who have low sense of coherence scores, tends toward pessimism, emotional suppression, and often assuming that the worst-case scenario will unfold. Keeping in mind that we all have days with those tendencies, for the type D personality, this is the norm. Perhaps related to their high degree of emotional suppression is the degree of emotional labour (Hochschild, 2012) that they are managing inside and outside of work. Those with low sense of coherence, the most vulnerable to workplace stimuli, are likely to spend more time surface acting, which is the practice of putting on an emotional display incongruent with authentic emotions; as a result, they rapidly use up their energy stores. If in addition they have a more vulnerable personality type, they are at a disadvantage compared to their peers. Those who are vulnerable because of specific personality traits are more sensitive to stress, more prone to negative self-talk, and more likely to engage in maladaptive coping behaviours. Conversely, those with less trait vulnerability can endure more workplace stimuli before their nervous system activates a stress response (Geuens et al., 2015). Another example of the influence of personality is that of extroverted personality types, who gain energy from social interactions. Because of this trait, they have a greater tendency to thrive in highly stimulating environments, which buffers them from negative workplace events (Clark & Watson, 1999). While our personality type influences how we respond to stress, it is not set in stone and is not an excuse to label or limit ourselves. Our personality is the sum total of various factors related to both nature and nurture (root development) and can change over time as well as through the personal development work described in this book. In this journey back home, it is also good to remember that the essence of who we are is not always well reflected in the personality type we have been conditioned to take on.

 Attuning/Reflecting Opportunity

After reading about the common workplace stressors, think about which ones you experience at work. Digging deeper, when you experience a sense of danger, what primary need of yours feels threatened?

Stress is caused by being "here," but wanting to be "there."

Eckhart Tolle

Attuning for the Journey Ahead: Moving Into Felt Sense

The factors outlined in this chapter align with Antonovsky's (1979) concept of sense of coherence and the ability to develop assets that improve our confidence and ability to manage stimuli before they become stressors. These factors, both the "weather" and the state of our "roots," interplay and compound to enable or disable our ability to thrive at work. Chronically stressful work environments, where external stimuli are extreme and unrelenting (unmanaged "weather") leads to moral injury, emotional exhaustion, burnout, and high attrition rates (Beecroft et al., 2001).

Developing assets that enable caregivers to establish deeper roots (Figure 1.1), where they feel less threatened by the external stimuli (weather) promotes the ability to thrive as individuals, which then contributes to a collective flow that promotes relational trust and uplifts morale. Many stimuli and stressors are not changeable, such as a certain degree of ambiguity or unpredictability that comes with the work in acute care environments. However, by cultivating and deepening our roots, we are more likely to be able to confidently change what can be changed, accept what cannot be changed, and mitigate challenges before they become stressors.

In Chapter 4, we focus on **attuning** to "felt sense." To do so, we move from *coming to know* from the level of the mind to cultivate the embodied awareness that will guide you on this journey home.

PART 2

Coming to Know Through the Felt Sense

Thriving roots are deeply grounded in personal authenticity and in connection and coherence with each other and the entire natural world. From this deeply rooted place, we courageously embody a way of being, empowered and sustained by a felt sense of purpose, compassion, gratitude, optimism, and joy.

Alexa's Journey

I have worked as a registered health care professional for 6 months now. I work in home and community care. Fresh out of the 4-year tornado of post secondary, I am trying to get my feet underneath me. There are days I feel completely incompetent. I feel like I have no business calling myself a professional. I walk into people's homes hoping that they cannot sense my ineptitude. I feel nervous, unqualified, and incompetent. There are also days I feel as though I am getting it. Days where things click into place. I have answers for people's questions and I skillfully perform care. My training did the best it could to prepare me, but nothing can prepare you for the reality of the work. So, every day I wake up and must tell myself that I am enough, I know enough, and I have the resources and supports I need available to me. This is not easy, and I do not always believe it. I find myself scheming up different career paths. Ones that appear to be more cut-and-dry. I am learning that being a health care professional is not an easy path.

In addition to the struggle for confidence and competence, there is also the part of the job that requires me to witness incredible suffering. A man slowly rotting away in his bed. Women and men living in isolation, with us as professional caregivers their only human connection.

I watched a man die, literally take his last breaths, in my final month of training. School does not prepare us, novice caregivers, for this. How can it? So, on top of the self-doubt and anxiety, we must learn to cope with the emotional labour of this work. We are busy. We are tired. It seems easier to simply stuff it all down and move onto the next thing. Down it goes where it begins to fester. I work hard at allowing myself space to process. Am I doing enough? Time will tell.

The other day at work I was sitting in my car, reading over the chart of my next patient. He was medically complex. Ever the planner, I sat there reviewing procedures and troubleshooting potential complications. I had already done this with my colleagues in the office an hour before. Now I was anxious and alone. Something came over me and I said out loud, "Just get in there." Not to be mistaken for a cavalier attitude, in that moment I had somehow found a place where I trusted myself to be able to handle whatever I may be faced with. I momentarily escaped from the mental torment I wash myself in daily. I know that this was possible because of the work I have done over the last year as part of the Roots Program.

Alexa's Journey—*cont'd*

For me what is most notable is that I have never in fact participated in the full curriculum. I have reviewed and edited the work. I have attended a smattering of in-person and online sessions. I have conversed with my peers about the content. But even so, I have unwittingly adopted the practices the program encourages. I am not immune to the insidious effects of shaming and bullying, but I can now recognize these behaviours even in their subtle forms. I still have maladaptive coping mechanisms, but I find myself sitting with uncomfortable feelings for longer. I forgive myself more for mistakes I make, which allows me to forgive others more readily as well. Being a part of this journey has most certainly made this vulnerable time a little more peaceful for me. To be able to bring this work to more health care workers is an honour that I am grateful to be a part of.

CHAPTER 4

Attuning to Your "Roots"

Wholeness does not mean perfection; it means embracing brokenness as an integral part of life. (Palmer, 2004)

This book aims to underscore the basic requirements of thriving and to promote a greater sense of order and understanding as we collectively find our way home. In this home, we remember who we are, our common humanity, our inherent worth, and a sense of belonging in the world. We do not need to learn how to be human. We know how to be human. Many of us in the West have incubated in an environment that has caused us confusion. We have lost our way. Together, with a good deal of grace and patience, we can begin to separate the signal of who we are from the noise of the conditions of an incongruent culture. We are growing up emotionally as we refriend our bodies and waking up spiritually as we reconnect to the indomitable life force within and around us.

In this chapter, we transition from coming to know at the level of the mind to coming to *be* at the level of the body. Reflective activities, experiential practices, and future direction activities are meant to encourage embodiment, integration, and beneficial habit changes. Actively stepping into the process requires vulnerability. As a result, you might feel some resistance at first. The journey is not linear. When we get too vulnerable too fast, we frequently react by contracting, quickly moving back into our comfort zone. This dance is normal and very much a part of the healing process. Each felt setback is a learning opportunity as we come to know our body's sensitivities. In response, we have an opportunity to listen, learn, and respond with self-compassion. With this compassionate approach, practice is for progress, not perfection. Through intentional and embodied practices, we restore our trust in the intuitive intelligence of the body, remaining connected to the body's sensations and promptings rather than working primarily from the mind. Practice enables us to choose our habits more consciously. Habits enable intuitive routines, which then enable new ways of being to transition from effort to ease.

You will come to see that strong reactions are like a weather system that swoops in, stays for a while, and eventually dissipates. Embodied presence cultivates a wise and compassionate relationship with the reactions rather than judging, rejections, or drowning in the experience. (Brach, 2016)

The Challenge: Orientation

By considering someone else's challenge, or working with another to consider ours, we cultivate nonattachment. We can often find comfort knowing we are not alone and that we can learn from and with each other. Working from this more objective space, we mitigate the stress response. We can then reorient from this position of strength, thus improving our ability to use all our biological, intellectual, and spiritual capacities. With this benevolent orientation, we can face adversities with confidence, knowing we have the resources and support necessary to navigate life's challenges.

To better orient ourselves, consider Tim's challenge. Tim is in his late twenties and has just crossed the threshold into professional practice as a veterinarian. As for his personal journey getting there, Tim lived in his parents' home until he graduated from his veterinarian training. He was hoping that graduation and moving out on his own would provide some sort of emancipation from his looming anxiety and his felt "stuckness." Now that he is living on this own and wearing the professional hat that he's spent so much effort acquiring, he is disappointed to realize he is struggling more than ever. He spends most of his workdays feeling like an imposter, afraid of being exposed or labelled as not ready, competent, not good enough or worthy of his new role and title. As a result of his looming fears, most of his thoughts emerge from a sense of scarcity, fueling a need to hypervigilantly attend to an idealized display and to plan and be prepared for any and all worst-case scenarios. This hypervigilant state is driven by a need to survive, doing whatever is necessary to ensure primary needs are met by managing potential (not actual) threats.

Tim often finds himself unable to think and lost for words when others question his work, which only leaves him feeling more inadequate. He goes home feeling emotionally exhausted, with no energy to interact with others. As a result, he spends his evenings alone, often turning to alcohol, which provides some temporary reprieve from his chronic anxiety. Tim always dreamed of being a veterinarian, and while he accomplished his dream, he can't remember the last time he felt a sense of joy and contentment in his new role.

Using Figure 1.1 from Chapter 1, consider Tim's roots. Consider the state of his roots and how they impact his perception of the weather. Think about where he is now in terms of congruence (how aligned the "real" self and "idea" self are), and sense of coherence (meaningfulness, a sense of understanding and predictability, and the ability to manage stressors and emotions). How does the state of his roots relate to the anxiety he is feeling? Coming from a strengths-based approach, how is Tim resourcing? Consider these same questions for yourself.

Moving From a Focus on the Mind to a Holistic Way of Being

As we move into exercises that encourage embodied knowing through the "felt sense," we begin by expanding awareness of our "real" self, and when ready, we begin to manifest this self in the world. With expanded awareness, we have a greater ability to recognize the outdated belief system that is out of step with our values and calling. By bringing our conscious attention to the resources and barriers that impact our ability to thrive, we have an opportunity to reorient ourselves and take a closer look at the root of the looming threat. With a curious and self-compassionate approach, we can gently uncover the unmet need beneath the felt insecurity. If we are not aware and connected to our core values, we will likely lack the sense of meaning necessary to overcome our fears. If we are not aware of our internal and external resources, we will lack the confidence necessary to enact change. Similarly, if we cannot articulate our vulnerabilities, we cannot manage them. By cultivating self-awareness, we our strengthen sense of coherence, promoting a more empowering orientation to life.

Attuning and Strengthening Practices
Attuning Practices

Cultivate Congruence: Attuning to Desire

As you try on new practices, it is important, imperative even, to note that we are all different. As such, we must pay attention to how our bodies respond. Our brain chemistries, our past experiences, our projections, our vulnerabilities—they are all vastly different! Prompts to reflect and to practise are not prescriptions but are optional tools. You can think of them as an objective experiment. You try an intervention and lean in to observe how the body responds. Is it helpful? Is it serving you? Great, hold on to it while it does. When it is no longer helpful, don't be afraid to let it go. This is how we rebuild trust with our bodies. For this reason, reflection after each practice is the most important part. It is here that we come to know ourselves and what engages our hearts and minds, including our desires to continue with the practices (or not). Be mindful of what comes up for you with practice, deferring to cues from the body as opposed to the obligations of the mind.

After you practice, sit for a moment. You might choose a word or phrase that describes how you feel. What does it look like when a practice resonates? Generally, when a practice grounds us in who we are, it promotes heartful connection and the ability to rest in the inner world. Hold the tool lightly, as in time another tool may call to you. When you need it most, the right practice occurs to you and you can simply say "yes" in that moment. Your job as your body's steward is to take notice when it whispers, answer the call, and trust the process as you respond and tend to the felt desire. You are building awareness of and trust in the body and the messages it is trying to deliver.

Cultivating a sense of desire and choice is imperative. With a focus on meaning and desire rather than obligation and achievement, we are far more likely to want to lean into practices that make us feel more secure and grounded. Rather than holding tightly to individual practices, think of them more like various tools in your tool belt. When your inner signals prompt you, you can choose just the right one for that unique moment.

This practice is about awareness building, enabling us to connect feelings of anxiety and/or depression with moments of incongruity. In American poet Robert Bly's *The Long Bag We Drag Behind Us*, he describes how incongruences develop, often in childhood, and then on into our adult years:

> *When we were one or two years old, we had what we might visualize as a 360-degree personality. Energy radiated out from all parts of our body and all parts of our psyche. A child running is a living globe of energy. We had a ball of energy, all right; but one day we noticed that our parents didn't like certain parts of that ball. They said things like: "Can't you be still?" Or "It isn't nice to try and kill your brother." Behind us we have an invisible bag, and the part of us our parents don't like, we, to keep our parents' love, put in the bag. By the time we go to school our bag is quite large. Then our teachers have their say: "Good children don't get angry over such little things." So, we take our anger and put it in the bag. ... Our bags were already a mile long. Then we do a lot of bag-stuffing in high school. This time it's no longer the evil grownups that pressure us, but people our own age ... Different cultures fill the bag with different contents.*
>
> *We spend our life until we're twenty deciding what parts of ourself to put into the bag, and we spend the rest of our lives trying to get them out again. (Bly, 1989)*

Take a look at your own "long bag." What parts of yourself are still in the bag?

We all experience incongruence from time to time, the result of living in a highly conditioned (and colonized) world. The goal is not to expect perfect congruence between who we are and how we manifest in the world, but rather to be more aware of the "signal" of who we are so we do not get confused by the "noise" of the conditions we have felt the need to adapt to. When we develop a greater ability to reorient ourselves, it enables us to spend more time acting from a place of desire, or "want to," as opposed to a felt obligation, or "have to." This *mindful* awareness cultivates choice, enabling us to live in the joy of *being* exactly where we are. When coming from desire, our *doing* flows from inspired *being*, which produces all sorts of positive ripple effects within us and in the world around us.

> *Mindfulness has two primary components: (1) bringing attention to the moment by moving from the thinking mind to the sensing mind and (2) cultivating curiosity and openness. These components enable objectivity as we step back (nonattachment) and accept whatever arises.*

Congruence requires a willingness to trust our inner promptings, to act in ways true to who we are, despite our fears of being rejected by others. We are able to act with courage when our sense of meaning overshadows our sense of fear. With repetition, trust develops and fear lessens as we come to believe that our internal prompts (sensations, emotions, desires, contractions) are important messengers. What was uncomfortable becomes familiar, even comforting. The emotions that arise no longer threaten us; instead, they become our guideposts, connecting us to our desires and alerting us when incongruence creeps in. As we retrieve those parts of ourselves that were once in the shadows, we feel whole—this is congruence.

In the moments when we have the strength to choose love over fear, we are rewarded not only with the knowledge and confidence that we have done something incredibly challenging and beautiful, but also with the gift of experiencing ourselves as love, and something infinitely more than just the small, fragile ego we thought we were and so desperately needed to protect. We are rewarded with a freedom that surpasses all other freedoms. Ultimately, it is through our willingness to stop defending our idea of ourselves that we discover our true and indestructible self. (Colier, 2018)

Experiential Practice
Working With Our Incongruent Tendencies

This exercise provides an opportunity to take stock in our tendencies toward congruence/incongruence. With awareness comes choice, and with choice comes the doorway to congruence. Using the chart below, adapted from Higgins et al. (1985), list up to 10 qualities of your "ideal" self, those ideal qualities that represent what you feel would represent your best self (your ultimate goals). For example, my "ideal" self is smart, kind, generous.

Then list up to another 10 qualities that represent what you and/or others think are qualities you should possess. For example, I often think others think I "should" be selfless, kind, slow to speak, composed, classy.

Finally, list up to 10 qualities (positive and negative) that you actually possess. For example, I am actually kind, spontaneous, quick to speak.

	"Ideal" Self	"Should/Ought" Self	"Real"/Actual Self
Write down ~10 qualities in each column			

(a) Count how many matches there are in the "real" and "ideal" columns and then count those that mismatch (opposites). Subtract the number of matches from the number of mismatches.

(b) Now, in the "real" and "should" columns, do the same as in the previous step.

This exercise illuminates our inner conflicts between our "real" self compared with the "ideal" self that we or others think we should be. The more discrepancies between the "ideal" self and "real" self, represented by a higher score, the more vulnerable you are to feelings of depression. The more discrepancies between the "should/ought" and "real" columns, the higher your score will be and the more vulnerable you are to feelings of anxiety.

When we recognize the connection between our emotional states and our incongruent thought patterns, we have an opportunity to reframe our thinking. Use the exercise to help make this connection visible.

The next time you notice anxiety or discontentment bubble up, consider the root causes of your incongruence. Ask yourself, what's behind these feelings of incongruence? What quality of my real self am I afraid to express in the world? Consider what might happen if you chose to manifest the "Real" qualities over the "Ideal" or "Should/Ought" qualities that you might typically display. You might even take it one step further by having a conversation with someone who can support you as you practice embracing and expressing qualities that feel more "real"/congruent to you.

Strengthening Practice
Developing Awareness Through Mindfulness

> *Fear not the man who has practiced 10 000 kicks; but fear the man who has practiced the same kick 10 000 times.*
>
> *Bruce Lee*

We dive into mindfulness later in the text, but starting now, through small and frequent efforts, we can begin developing new habits that remind us of who we are, of our resources (internally and externally), and of the security found when we ground ourselves in our life force. These habits are the rituals that provide a bridge between our *being* and our *doing*.

To practise, there is no need to create a ceremony. Simple is best. You don't even need to close your eyes or to find a special place to do the practice. We can engage in mindfulness as part of our busy lives by using reminders within our daily routines that cue us to attend to the present moment.

Mindfulness is achieved by transitioning from our thinking mode, where we are lost in past and future thoughts, to the sensing mode, where we are taking in the world in and around us.

If you forget or your mind wanders during this mindfulness exercise, this is a great opportunity to practise self-compassion. In whatever way feels most natural for you, remind yourself that everyone struggles with focus and mental "noise." These frustrating moments are exactly the time to reorient, putting the focus back on progress not perfection.

When it comes to working with our body and especially our brain in order to cultivate mindful moments—where we transition from *do*ing (checking boxes that no longer feel meaningful) to *be*ing (all activity is infused with meaning)—we need to prioritize the process of getting there over the end result. Distractions are part of the practice as we continue to notice what is happening in the thinking mind and then come back to sensing mode, noting what is actually happening in the moment (outside of the mind's narrative). When sessions are difficult, pat yourself on the back for choosing a great time to help your brain relax—clearly you needed it! The act of consistently bringing our attention back to the practice of *be*ing is exactly how we train our brains to sustain longer periods of mindfulness.

Let's try a few strategies to get you started.

Bring your attention to your environment. Pick one reoccurring event you see or do each day (e.g., brushing your teeth, feeding your cat, eating breakfast, drinking afternoon coffee, entering or exiting your house or office). This will serve as an environmental cue that will remind you to practise mindfulness each time the events occurs.

Bring your attention to a new detail. While you are doing your chosen activity, notice something new that you have never noticed before. Take the experience in through your senses, cultivating curiosity.

Bring your attention to your senses. Feel the touch points, where your body comes into contact with itself or external objects, such as the floor connecting to the bottoms of your feet. Relax those parts that feel the tension, such as relaxing your shoulders away from your ears or letting go of the tension that you may be holding in your belly. Now, feel your spine lengthen: beginning at the soles of your feet, feel yourself lift and lengthen.

Bring your attention to your breath. Take a breath in, imagining the fresh air moving deeply into your chest and throughout your body. As you exhale, imagine the stale air moving out, carrying out the old thought patterns and along with the old areas storing stress. Continue to take a few deeper and longer breaths (4–5 seconds), focusing on fully expanding the lungs, bringing in the new air, letting it cleanse all of the nooks and crannies of your body and mind, paying special attention to moving it into areas of tension; fully exhale, letting your breath carry out old areas of stress and ways of being that are no longer serving you.

Bring your attention to how you feel. Take notice of how you feel physically, spiritually, and emotionally. Practise accepting what *is*, letting go of the need to resist uncomfortable emotions and any need to control or change things. By accepting without conditions, we can step into the here and now, free of subjective judgements (nonattachment). As a result, when we begin to experience the rewards (a more relaxed mind and inspired state of *being*), we can learn to enjoy mindfulness. Once we come to enjoy something, we naturally fall into *being* states, which transform effort to ease.

Intense emotions can deter us from mindfully being with whatever is happening in the moment if they feel too dangerous to sit with. As a result, it is normal for the mind to cling to external distractions in an effort to avoid the uncomfortable feelings in the body. Chapter 6 provides helpful strategies that can help you manage (and de-escalate) intense emotions. Ultimately, these are opportunities to recognize and address unresolved areas of trauma that often bubble up when we bring presence to our senses and emotions, especially in the beginning of the practice.

Viewing Human Needs and Stress Through a Different Lens: Chakras

In the West, the consideration that chakras impact mental, emotional, spiritual, and physical health is relatively new, lacking in familiarity and research. However, a few studies have shown a significant connection between spiritual connection, as reflected in chakra theory, and the expression of physical and mental health conditions (Curtis et al., 2004; Drapkin et al., 2016). In Sanskrit, the term *chakra* means wheel, representing the symbiotic and holistic nature of the energy centres in our body. The chakra system referred to in this chapter originated in India between 1500 and 500 BCE in texts known as the Vedas. In many parts of the East, chakras are viewed as a significant contributor to spiritual, emotional, and physical well-being. They are considered portals to the human energy field.

While there are many chakra models, a commonly adopted model in the West describes seven core energy centres, each of which has its own vibrational frequency and function that contributes to wellness. Much like a river that becomes stagnant when unable to flow, when energy blockages occur, diseases can fester. Even if you do not resonate with the idea of chakras, guided meditations are a great way to develop concentration, enabling you to sustain mindfulness. Furthermore, the loving-kindness component in many of these practices are an excellent way to cultivate self-compassion. There are several online resources with a wealth of guided mediations. If you aren't finding what you like here or you prefer audio versions, try others out until you find something that resonates with you (this is attuning work).

Relating chakras to Maslow's (1943) theory of unmet needs, each of the chakra centres correlates with a basic human need. When we avoid or ignore our inner "signals," which are often drowned out by the "noise" of thoughts and external stimuli, energy gets trapped in the body. Returning to the river analogy, this can cause blockages that impact our emotional, physical, and spiritual homeostasis. When these blockages occur, held up by an unmet need, our body feels threatened, triggering the nervous system to mount a stress response. When the intensity of the felt threat is high, which it often is for those with PTSD, it is common for our interpretation of the current moment to get fused with an unresolved wound from the past.

To illustrate how unmet needs correlate with the different chakras (connecting Western and Eastern perspectives), whatever our income, social status, or theoretical and political beliefs, we all long to feel secure in having the following needs met:

- Our physical needs (root chakra)
- Our need to feel safe (sacral chakra)
- Our need to be loved and to belong (solar plexus chakra)
- Our need to feel unconditional positive regard/esteem for self and others (heart chakra)
- Our need to express our "real" self in the world (throat chakra)
- Our need to self-actualize into our most connected, meaning-filled, and empowered self (third eye chakra), and
- Our need to feel held by benevolent forces greater than ourselves (crown chakra).

Attuning and Clearing Practice: Working With Chakras

As a Westerner, I touch on the concept of chakras in this section and recognize the risk of cultural appropriation in doing so. To mitigate any distortions that can occur as a result of plucking practices from one context and dropping them into another, I encourage you to research the principles and history from which the practices emerge. When you share practices that come from other cultures, please consider referring back to and honoring their origin.

The following meditation script provides an example of how chakra meditations can be used to clear energy blockages that can result from self-destructive belief systems and accumulated stress and trauma. Out of respect to the culture from which chakra practices emerged, it is important to note that a great deal will be lost in translation as we attempt to transplant the practice into our Western context. To honour the Indian cultural origins of this practice, I encourage readers to explore the concept of chakras, their history, and the spiritual intentions behind the practice. To enable your body to change gears from a *doing* (thinking) state to a *being* (embodied) state, it is best to listen to guided mediations rather than read them. Recording yourself as you read a meditation like the one below is a fantastic way to encourage a compassionate dialogue with yourself. Give it a try!

The following guided meditation is used with the permission of Linda Hall (2019), a well-established integrative health practitioner, meditation teacher, and creator of this chakra meditation script. Adapted from the Chakra Healing Guided Meditation Script © Linda Hall. Originally published by www.The-Guided-Meditation-Site.com.

- Allow your eyes to comfortably close, and come down into your breath, into your body, relaxing your belly, softening your mind.
- Feel the support beneath you, connect with the ground below. And let it take your weight.
- Become aware of the sounds around you. Let them be there.
- Notice the light and shade, the air touching the surface of your body.
- Sense the sky above and the horizons stretching all the way round you, the earth below supporting you.
- Allow your mind to empty what it no longer needs to hold on to. Let it go, flow out and away. Allow your body to release what it no longer needs to hold on to, let it go, flow out and away.
- Draw yourself back from where you've been in your day. Draw your energies back home to your centre. Ground yourself in this moment, here.
- Begin to sense the space around you. Breathe with the space and become aware of the rise and fall of your breath, its coming and going, the sensation, sound, temperature.
- Breathe down to where the weight of your body rests, below the base of your spine—to your root—your chakra of belonging. Breathe into your root. Let it soften and gently expand on your breath, taking in nourishment and life force energy.
- Allow your root to connect down, down to the ground below, deep into the earth. And invite in the colour red—the colour of the earth. Bathe your root with red: empowering, embodying, grounding you in the here and now. Let your root take what it needs. And say the words "I am here," "I have a right to be here, as I am," "The earth supports me." While you focus on flooding your root chakra with red, repeat to yourself, "I am safe."
- When you are ready, allow your awareness to move up to your abdomen, just below your navel, to your chakra of emotional intelligence, choice, creativity, movement, and pleasure.
- Breathe into the soft part of your abdomen. Let it gently soften and expand on your breath, taking in nourishment and life force energy. And invite in orange—the colour of the setting sun. Bathe your abdomen with orange, balancing, empowering, motivating. Let your abdomen be fed and say the words "I honour my needs," "I allow myself to be nourished." As you flood your abdomen with orange, repeat the mantra "I am worthy."
- And when you are ready, move your awareness up to the soft area below your breastbone—to your solar plexus—your chakra of personal power.
- Breathe into here, allowing your solar plexus to soften and expand on your breath. And invite in the colour yellow—the colour of sunshine. Bathe your solar plexus with sunshine, replenishing, restoring, nurturing. Let your solar plexus take what it needs and say the words "I value myself," "I am enough."

As you flood your solar plexus with yellow, repeat the mantra "I am more than enough."

- Bring your awareness up to the centre of your chest—to your heart—your chakra of self-development and unconditional love.
- Breathe into your heart, letting it soften and expand on your breath. Invite in green—the colour of spring—or rose pink—whichever feels right. Bathe your heart centre with nourishment, renewal, healing. Let your heart take what it needs and say the words "I am greatly loved," "I allow myself to give and receive love freely," "I am nourished by the power of love." As you flood your heart chakra with the colour green, feel it fill with love and repeat the mantra "I am love."
- In your own time, move up to your neck—to your throat—your chakra of self-expression and personal will.
- Allow your throat centre to soften, expand and b-r-e-a-t-h-e. Invite in blue—the colour of the sky. Breathe the sky into your throat centre, clearing, opening, softening the need for control, freeing self-expression and creativity. Let your throat take what it needs. And say the words "I hear and speak my truth," "I express myself freely," "I allow myself to go with the flow of life." As you fill your throat chakra with the colour of the sky, repeat the mantra "My truth is worthy of expression."
- When you are ready, take your focus up to your forehead—between your eyebrows—to your third eye—your chakra of wisdom and intuition. Gently allow it to soften, expand, and breathe.
- Invite in indigo—the velvety colour of night sky. Bathe your third eye with indigo, soothing, balancing, bringing clarity, insight, and understanding. Let your third eye take what it needs. And say the words "Everything is unfolding as it should." As you connect to your inner wisdom, flood your third eye with indigo, repeating the mantra "I am light."
- Move up, in your own time, to the top of your head—to your crown, your chakra of "oneness," allowing your crown to breathe.
- And gently invite in a light violet, softly bathing your crown, balancing, restoring, harmonizing. Let your crown take what it needs. And say the words "I am one with the Universe," "I am one with the Whole."
- When you are ready, come back to yourself as a whole, back to the ebb and flow of your breath, back to your centre. Breathe into your core. And say the words "I am whole," "I am perfect just as I am." As you connect with the Divine (or your higher self, if you prefer), fill your crown chakra with a soft violet colour, repeating the mantra "I am."
- Allow the energy of the words to bathe your body, mind, emotions, spirit. And take what you need.
- And, in your own time, become aware of the air on the surface of your body. The sounds around you, nearby and in the distance.
- Close your chakras down a little. Just having the intention is enough. Become aware of the support beneath you. Notice how you feel. And hold yourself with loving-kindness, for the beautiful, unique being that you are.
- When you are ready, you can draw this meditation to a close and gently open your eyes.

EXPLORING THE MOST PRIMARY NEED(S): RECOGNIZING CORE BLOCKAGES

When a need goes unmet that feels primary compared to what may feel less pressing, we will often fixate on that one need, neglecting others until we can resolve the issue. These primary needs are not always linear, depending on cultural conditioning, core wounds that need tending to, and a variety of other seen and unseen complexities. For instance, we quite likely will prioritize needs such as food, shelter, warmth, and safety, paying less attention to esteem and connection. Or perhaps we have a long-held belief system that we are somehow not good enough, causing us to prioritize the approval of others, ensuring we please them at the expense of ourselves.

To cultivate curiosity, we can consciously take note of the thoughts that continue to take up space in our day. By doing so, we can welcome them and allow enough time to receive the message, leaning in to explore the correlating felt sense in the body. Recognizing, allowing, and then letting go of judgemental thoughts enables us to look deeper (with an open heart) into what lies beneath our sticky points. By simply noticing, we cultivate space between us and the threatening thought and sensation. With space, we lift the veil, revealing the source of the needs that tend to drive our less desirable impulses.

Reflection Practice: Exploring the Primary Need(s)

Can you recall an area in your life that that brings you frustration, where you feel and see an obvious area that needs tending to (i.e., it could use some serious self-care), but you have little to no desire to develop the necessary habits required to resolve it? Consider what other primary unmet need or haunting belief system may be crying out for tending, subconsciously blocking desires to tend to other needs.

Aligning Practice: Dropping in to Set an Intention

Setting intentions is like consciously choosing the most nutrient-rich soil in which to plant our seeds of change. It involves preparing the soil and taking care of the tender seed to give it the best chance of flourishing. As mentioned earlier in the text, for changes to stick, we must embody them (take on a bodily knowing). In order to embody something, we must move from the thinking mind (*doing*) to sensing (*being*). Art is a great way to help us change gears, as it helps us move from the head to the heart. For example, get lost in a painting, listen to music, or reflect on a piece of writing that inspires you. This short passage by well-known Ojibwe writer Richard Wagamese is a heartful reminder of who we are, enabling us to tune back into "signal" despite the distracting "noises" of life:

> *I am my silence. I am not the busyness of my thoughts or the daily rhythm of my actions. I am not the stuff that constitutes my world. I am not my talk. I am not my actions. I am my silence. I am the consciousness that perceives all*

these things. When I go to my consciousness, to that great pool of silence that observes the intricacies of my life, I am aware that I am me. I take a little time each day to sit in silence so that I can move outward in balance into the great clamour of living. (Wagamese, 2016)

Now that you have dropped in by engaging your heart, try setting an intention that sparks your desire. You might choose one or two intentions that inspire you, but I recommend you keep it so simple that you can easily recall it. Keeping dropping into your inner world to ask whether this intention is coming from *want* ("signal") rather than *should* ("noise"). This requires you to ask your body what it desires, and then leaning in to listen to the inner prompts. When we prioritize our own desires over the desires of others, we are developing agency (a core factor in sense of coherence) and congruence as we allow our inner world to manifest in the outer world.

INTENTION: _____

TIP: By feeling a sense of desire and ownership for your goals and by writing them down, you are more likely to achieve them. As soon as a goal feels obligatory, subconscious resistance will creep in. It is unnecessary to effort greatly or force results. In fact, gentleness is an important quality of self-compassion. It means trusting that when we are ready, the answers to our questions will bubble up from inside of us. No need to force anything. Releasing the need to control and trusting the inner voice will help you craft goals that bring you more meaning and that you are more likely to achieve. We cultivate our ability to hear the inner voice by leaning into it with our awareness and our breath and by immersing deeply by directing loving-kindness inwardly.

Loving-kindness emerges from grace and is characterized by gentleness, consideration, and kindness to ourselves and others.

If the answers do not come right away, or if you are having difficulty dropping into your inner world, that is normal! Focus takes practise, and every practice session is an investment in your progress. If frustration arises, take the opportunity to practise self-kindness much like you would coach a friend or young child who is learning something for the first time. As you continue to refriend yourself, trust will develop, and in time, a yearning to connect will call you in. Hold your intentions and questions lightly, trusting that the answers will come at the right time and in the right way. This process takes patience, it takes self-kindness, and it takes courage.

The Challenge: Navigation

Let's circle back to Tim's challenge. As a novice professional caregiver, Tim spends a great deal of his time assimilating to a prescribed way of being. As a result of the divide between his "ideal" self and "real" self, he experiences shame (a result of

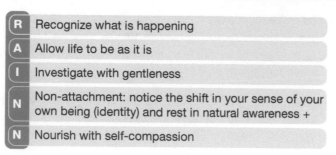

R	Recognize what is happening
A	Allow life to be as it is
I	Investigate with gentleness
N	Non-attachment: notice the shift in your sense of your own being (identity) and rest in natural awareness +
N	Nourish with self-compassion

Fig. 4.1   The R.A.I.N.N. Acronym (Brach, 2013).

incongruence), which is likely connected to his chronic anxiety. By cultivating relational spaces where he feels unconditionally positively regarded for who he "really" is, he is learning that he is enough and is beginning to believe that maybe he is worthy of expressing himself in the world. Because he still feels insecurity knocking at his door, he is intentionally surrounding himself with people he feels safe with, enabling him to fuel his inner pilot light. The more he shows up authentically with people who show him unconditional positive regard, the less shame and anxiety he feels.

In terms of sense of coherence, Tim's orientation to life is characterized by fear and a general feeling of being out of control. This is evident in how he frequently views life's challenges as intensely threatening to his well-being as opposed to events that he feels confident navigating. One of Tim's intentions is to engage the R.A.I.N.N. framework (Brach, 2013) when he notices that his body is activated (see Figure 4.1). He now *recognizes* when fear or anxiety arise. As he recognizes his emotion as a sensation that represents an important message for him to consider, the threat and associated discomfort softens. From this less attached space, Tim is able to see emotion as an important ally, giving him the capacity to *allow* instead of resist. Expanding his awareness in this way promotes a sense of curiosity that fuels a desire to *investigate* the belief system and the perceived unmet need beneath. With this investigation, perceiving the felt senses as messengers rather than feelings lost inside them, he cultivates **nonattachment**. If he cannot attain nonattachment on his own, he can reach out to a trusted other to attain a more objective perspective. From this vantage point, he can *nurture* the wound at the root of his suffering. Finally, if appropriate, he has an opportunity to identify old belief systems that may no longer be true. For the first time in a long time, Tim feels hopeful.

The acronym R.A.I.N.N. is helpful to anchor you as uncomfortable emotions or sensations present themselves (Brach, 2013). The framework provides a process to help us receive and respond to emotions, preventing chronic stress and hostility (and related subconscious projections), both of which emerge when we feel insecure and out of control. Once we tend to the emotional message we are receiving, we are more likely to objectively and confidently enact the changes necessary to reorient ourselves to the felt threat. We can do so by either changing our environment or reorienting ourselves to stressors so that we can successfully resolve them. Resolution does not always mean the stressors go away. Instead, by tending to old wounds and upgrading old belief systems, the stressors no longer feel threatening. Once we tend to the emotion on the personal level, we are far more likely to feel empowered to enact the changes necessary on the contextual, cultural, and systemic levels.

> ### Attuning/Reflecting Opportunity
> Cultivating awareness and confidence in your resources will help to stabilize your "roots" when the "weather" gets rough. What are your resources? These can be any activity, person, or practice in your life that promotes connection and a confidence that all things will work out reasonably well.

Attuning for the Journey Ahead: Strengthening Congruence With Self-Compassion

Taking this journey into the inner world to learn how to manage the outer world is exactly how we collectively remember how to walk this common human path. As caregivers, as humans who have been incubated in a relatively disconnected culture, we are transitioning from the thinking mind to the felt sense in order to heal ourselves.

We have come to know about congruence and self-compassion, attuning and applying the concepts to our inner world. Developing congruence and self-compassion cultivates a safe inner space, one in which we can find comfort and reprieve. As you develop more trust with your body, old wounds that were previously too threatening to feel will come up for healing. This is normal and something to celebrate! It is a sign of your progress. The wound that was too unsafe to feel is now feelable. Reorienting in this way will help you find the meaning within the suffering, to feel the release amid the tension.

Now that we are *attuning* to the felt sense realm, we will *strengthen* congruence by practising self-compassion.

CHAPTER 5

Strengthening Congruence With Self-Compassion

Your task is not to seek love, but merely to seek and find all the barriers within yourself that you have built against it.

Rumi

A congruent life is a thriving life. This section describes the intertwining nature of self-compassion and congruence. By developing self-compassion, congruence naturally follows. To understand the power of congruence, consider an acorn, which is born with all the intelligence necessary to become an oak. It already holds within it the DNA of a full-grown tree. External environmental factors may be more favourable to the growth of a pine tree, but no amount of pressure or preference will change the destiny of the acorn to be an oak. The conditions of the soil and weather will impact the acorn's ability to develop the deep roots required for it to thrive. Trees that develop deep roots are more stable, resilient, and empowered to bring their predestined foliage and fruits into the world. Similar to the acorn, when we work and play in environments that promote congruence (an ability to express ourselves authentically), our ability to reach our full potential grows. When our ability to passionately live out the calling for which we are destined outgrows our fears, we can courageously and authentically blossom in the world. Courage naturally develops parallel to congruence as we align our reality with our unique desires and values.

We need self-compassion to develop congruence between our "real" and "ideal" selves. We learn the felt sense of self-compassion by having unconditional positive regard mirrored to us. In time, as we develop trust in those doing the mirroring, we learn to embody self-compassion, becoming less reliant on external validation; this is **mirroring transference** (Kohut, 1984).

Through mirroring, we can support others to see themselves, to let go of the story and patterns that no longer serve them.

Crosbie Watler MD, FRCPC

Once we receive self-compassion through mirroring, we are attuned to its frequency. As a result we can keep tuning back in when we lose our way. It was psychiatrist and psychoanalyst Carl Jung who first popularized the term "unconditional positive regard." It means that despite our own discomfort, we accept others and respect their right to make decisions, trusting that even if we do not agree or understand their actions, they are doing their best with the resources (including their degree of congruence and sense of coherence) they have. To mirror this same acceptance inwardly (self-compassion), we can apply this same sentiment to ourselves by directing loving-kindness within, by using our voice to ask for what we need, by making decisions that align with our calling, and by setting boundaries that protect and empower our "roots."

Kristen Neff (2018), a pioneering researcher on self-compassion, has identified three main components of self-compassion:

1. Self-kindness: Talking to yourself the way you would to a good friend
2. Common humanity: Reminding yourself that everyone fails and suffers from time to time, and
3. Mindfulness: Observing any negative feelings you're experiencing rather than suppressing them.

Self-compassion teaches us that our passing thoughts and actions do not define us. It shows us that we do not need to be perfect to be enough, worthy of love, and accepted by others. For some fortunate people, self-compassion is gained during a childhood that enabled them to internalize unconditional positive regard from someone they looked up to. If not acquired in childhood, we must reprogram (referred to as reparenting in Chapter 8) as an adult by cultivating these relationships of unconditional positive regard with others.

The Duality of Self

By Crosbie Watler, MD, FRCPC, a Canadian thought leader and psychiatrist

A useful concept here is the *duality of self*. We are human *beings* first, but are conditioned to identify with our *doing* selves. The being self is our birthright—on the day of our birth, we are the silent witness. Awareness with no attachment, no judgement. No story about who we are—simply *I am*. Animals do not outgrow this awareness of essence, of being self. When we lack compassion for ourselves, it is simply because we have forgotten who we are. There can be no self-compassion without self-awareness. At the level of the doing, we have never and will never be perfect. Rather, we must anchor ourselves in being—the silent witness. We can strive to do better … but the outcome does not define us. We are already whole.

The Challenge: Orientation

By considering someone else's challenge, or working with another to consider ours, we cultivate nonattachment. We can often find comfort knowing we are not alone and that we can learn from and with each other. Working from this more objective space, we mitigate the stress response. We can then reorient from this position of strength, thus improving our ability to use all our biological, intellectual, and spiritual capacities. With this benevolent orientation, we can face adversities with confidence, knowing we have the resources and support necessary to navigate life's challenges.

The Challenge Orientation

Author, Elder, and Chief Phil Lane of the Ihanktonwan Dakota and Chickasaw Nations (Lane, 2019) reminds us that as humans, we are all indigenous to the earth. We are sacred, whole, and interconnected with each other and the natural world. To hurt or devalue, one hurts and devalues all. We are equal: equally sacred, equally important, and equally worthy of self-expression, love, and belonging. Many of us live and work in individualist paradigms that promote separation, but to realize our individual and collective potential, we need to experience the security of living as a community.

Operating as a cohesive community requires that we share a common belief in the sacredness of every living being, which cultivates an ability for the members to mirror unconditional positive regard to one another. This mirroring of unconditional positive regard promotes an inner knowing about the gift of life, enabling us to see the "signal" within the sacredness of our collective humanity. When the "signal" is strong, the details of our differences ("noise") are kept in perspective. No matter our colour, dialect, belief systems, or behaviours, the miracle of who we are in our **essence** overshadows the details of our vessel, the behaviours that flow from fear and shame, and the confusions in our conditioning. When we embody this sacred, unshakeable worthiness inwardly, we will naturally direct unconditional positive regard inwardly (self-compassion), filling ourselves up in abundance and enabling it to overflow onto the community around us. From this orientation, consider Sandy's challenge:

Sandy grew up believing that her worth was tied up in achievements, and this belief continues to be the primary driver of her *doing* today. She is in now her fifties and works as a lead faculty member at a postsecondary institution. Sandy is driven to attain success and notoriety, fueled by a deep longing for approval. She has a long, impressive history of awards, degrees, and appointments, highly motivated to prove herself. At work, she's known for her meticulousness, dependability; to those who fail to meet her high expectations, she's known as a critical taskmaster. She is proud of her ability to produce high-quality work and of her reputation as a "force" at work and at home. Sandy is typically the first one in and the last one out of the office each day. Other faculty members give her a wide birth, fearing her critical eye and socially dominant way of being. Sandy spends a good deal of her day perfecting her work, scanning for flaws, and going over and over her writing until things look just right. Unfortunately, these same relentlessly high standards are prescribed onto her co-workers and students. When mistakes occur, she feels angry. And while she manages her words carefully, her sense of disappointment comes through clearly in her tone. When she feels responsible for the mistake, she often ruminates on self-destructive thoughts for days. When others are to blame for mistakes or less-than-ideal outcomes, she reacts from the same sense of threat, causing her to direct this same shaming behaviour onto others. Because Sandy has such a dominant presence in the faculty and takes on a variety of leadership roles, her way of being has a significant impact on morale.

How do you feel when you read about Sandy's challenge? What is driving Sandy's way of being? Who is suffering as a result of her orientation to life?

Unconditional Positive Regard in Relationship

Unconditional positive regard is the chief characteristic of self-compassion. Without first attuning to felt sense of unconditional positive regard, self-compassion is simply not attainable. When we believe we are unconditionally and positively regarded, it is like tuning into a specific frequency on the radio. Until we find the right channel, we simply cannot receive what is being broadcast. Unconditional positive regard is the channel that we must tune into. Once we do, in times of insecurity—when we've gotten out of tune—we can often feel our way back to that same frequency. Better yet, when we cultivate relationships of unconditional positive regard, we can help tune each other back into that same frequency by mirroring unconditional positive regard. Receiving this form of unconditional acceptance from others reminds us that we are indeed good enough and that, despite our less desirable behaviours, we are worthy of love.

However, having someone in our life who shows us unconditional positive regard is not enough; we must come to believe it is true. We must come to trust it. And how can we believe that other people will care for us, no matter what, without testing that belief? Remember Robert Bly's piece "The Long Bag We Drag Behind Us" earlier in Chapter 4? Testing that regard means retrieving the innate qualities of our essence from the long bag, redeeming those parts of ourselves that feel forbidden. If we continue to play only the role we are prescribed, and do not behave in ways that may risk the disapproval of others, we simply cannot trust that we are indeed unconditionally accepted. Many people fear that being authentic, bringing those banished parts into the light, will lead to rejection. However, until we retrieve those repressed parts of ourselves from the shadows, testing our relationships as we do, we will not believe that we are unconditionally and positively regarded for our "real" self. As illustrated in Figure 5.1, as we come to experience a felt sense of our own worth, we begin to feel the same sense of others' worth.

Congruence is a natural outcome of a childhood characterized by embodied unconditional positive regard from a respected other. Once attuned to this felt sense, when suffering does occur, someone who embodies it is more likely to naturally direct the same frequency inwardly (self-compassion). The more fortunate ones received unconditional positive regard from a parent or guardian. However, in more competitive, individualistic cultures, through no fault of their own, most people are not exposed to the felt sense of this kind of unwavering regard and acceptance. You cannot attune to a frequency if it is not being broadcast. And even if it is being broadcast, sometimes the static ("noise") is too distracting to take in the message ("signal").

In my research (Dames, 2018a), I found that people can also find this safe and accepting place among friends, extended family, and faith communities. As long as it is believed to the point that it can be known in the body (embodied), we can also attune to this form of unwavering compassion from a pet or by believing in an unconditionally loving spiritual source. The source is not important; what matters

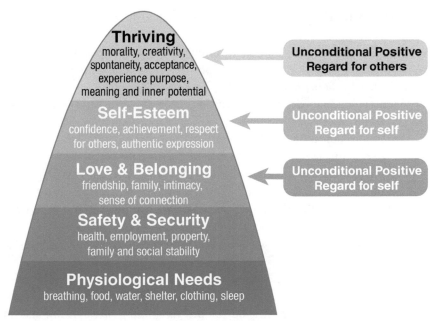

Fig. 5.1 Unconditional Positive Regard. Unconditional positive regard is the antidote to incongruent and hostile work cultures, and it is infectious. We learn it from others, which enables us to mirror it inwardly and then outwardly. The more unconditional positive regard we can embody, the less shame we will experience from the variety of circumstances where we feel a divide between the "real" self and "ideal" self.

is that it enables us to feel inherently worthy without condition. When we believe we are unconditionally positively regarded, we then have an ability to extend this belief system to others, reminding them of their inherent worth. Providing unconditional positive regard to others may be one of the most powerful things we can do to help promote thriving in others. When done without condition, both parties heartfully expand. However, our ability to serve others in this way hinges on our own capacity for self-compassion. In this way, the unconditional positive regard we experience in relationships reinforces that which we cultivate for ourselves.

Requirements, qualities, and facilitators of unconditional positive regard:

- Requirements of unconditional positive regard:
  - A perception that we are accepted as we are, quirks and wounds alike
  - An ability to see our own and others' inherent human worth, separate from behaviours and achievements, and
  - An ability to set boundaries out of kindness to ourselves and others, communicating our expectations and values, which prevents hostility and resentment.
- Qualities of unconditional positive regard:
  - A felt safety to "let our hair down" with room for mistakes without a looming threat of rejection

- Diversity is celebrated with the knowledge that the benefits far outweigh the discomforts
- A willingness to respectfully work through differences, agreeing to disagree and normalizing conflict as a healthy component of authentic relationships
- A focus on progress not perfection
- Vulnerability is a welcome and essential part of connecting and empowering ourselves and others, and
- Secure attachment (less anxious or avoidant attachment).
- Facilitators of unconditional positive regard:
  - A spiritual connection that provides us with unconditional positive regard
  - Doing our best and letting that be enough, with room to learn and grow from our mistakes and trusting that others are also doing their best with the tools/resources they have
  - Investigating our assumptions—just because it may have been true in a past situation, is it really true in this situation?
  - Speaking honestly and honouring our word, which cultivates greater self-trust/self-integrity, and
  - Cultivating nonattachment amid conflict, recognizing that our own and others' projections colour the current experience to the point where sometimes the emotional charge has little to do with the current event and a lot more to do with a past experience or belief system; therefore, it is not personal!

Healing Thy Caregiving Self: Self-Compassion as Medicine

Self-integrity is reflected in our ability to be true to our innate values and the things we stand for in life (congruence). If we claim to have a set of values, but do not manifest them in the world, then we lack self-integrity (incongruence). Integrity happens when our *do*ing flows from our *be*ing rather than the reverse. It stems from self-compassion. Conversely, perfectionism stems from fear.

We can think of self-compassion as looking at ourselves—our *doing* selves—with gentle acceptance. It enables us to connect to our inner world. It has two main requirements: objectivity and willingness. When we are both objective and willing, we can unconditionally accept whatever thoughts and emotions may arise, welcome them, and digest them. Digesting is a process of acknowledging the dissonance of difficult feelings as they come, validating the felt suffering, then stepping back to investigate the source. Oftentimes, the source of the dissonance relates to parts that we feel insecure about; the parts that were repressed in an effort to display a version of ourselves that felt more worthy of love and acceptance. When this happens, we are essentially trading our "real" selves for an artificial "ideal." When we do so, we live as imposters, haunted by fear and shame, never knowing when we might be exposed. Awareness and self-compassion enable us to reintegrate these previously rejected pieces of ourselves. Digesting and integrating all parts of ourselves, even those less culturally favourable parts, is the path toward congruence. With each step toward congruence, we are cleaning and clearing as we remember our wholeness.

Because congruence is the most loving action we can do for ourselves, when we are self-compassionate, we are highly likely to be more congruent. We are more grounded in who we are (deeply "rooted") and less likely to get blown about in bad "weather." When we are secure and congruent, we walk free of fear and shame. As a result of this more balanced physical and spiritual state of being, congruent and self-compassionate individuals have higher stress thresholds and fewer chronic mental health and physical issues.

Our level of congruence and ability to practise self-compassion impacts how we interpret stimuli in the workplace too. Caregivers who lack self-compassion are prone to incongruence, which happens when the "real" self is hidden to take on a more "idealized" display. When the display we put on in the world runs counter to who we "really" are, in that moment we are incongruent. Incongruence results in shame, and unmanaged shame leads to a felt insecurity that chronically activates the nervous system. As result of this hypervigilant, threat-seeking state, any passing stimuli, whether at work or at home, are far more likely to feel threatening (stressors). Conversely, those who are more self-compassionate, and thus have a greater sense of congruence, are more likely to view stimuli as manageable challenges rather than stressors. This objectivity promotes a greater capacity to resolve or at least manage feelings of dissonance, which improves the ability to engage in thriving (Dames, 2018a).

Caregivers suffering from burnout also tend to be deficient in self-compassion (Montero-Marin et al., 2016). Those that practice self-compassion are less prone to a variety of mental health conditions fueled by anxiety and depression; they can mitigate stressors; they are happier, more satisfied with life, and more self-confident; and they have better health outcomes (Bluth et al., 2017; Dames, 2018a; Gunnell et al., 2017; Homan & Sirois, 2017; Hwang et al., 2016; Kelly et al., 2014; Neff & Germer, 2018). Those with higher levels of self-compassion are more likely to manage workplace stressors with confidence as opposed to feeling overwhelmed by a perceived personal inadequacy in addition to the initial stressor.

In the thinking mind, self-compassion interrupts rumination on our feelings of inadequacy, saving us from the emotional exhaustion and self-destructive thoughts that might otherwise result. It enables us to accept all parts of ourselves, without condition, letting any judgements fall into the background. From this graceful state, we are more able to digest and even celebrate all parts of our personalities. This self-acceptance prevents us from carrying shame (for not being the socially prescribed "ideal" that we feel we should be).

Self-Compassion: An Antidote to Workplace Hostility

It almost goes without saying that when teams lack self-compassion, and thus collectively promote incongruence, shame and perfectionism run amuck, fueling hostile relations between co-workers (Dames, 2018a). Conversely, because self-compassionate and hence more congruent people carry less shame, they are less likely to project negative feelings onto others. In this way, self-compassion acts as an antidote for the hostility that stems from inadvertent shame spilling.

Those who habitually practice self-compassion can naturally extend the same compassion toward others. Self-compassionate employees are the fuel that enables and sustains flourishing communities. Father Greg Boyle, founder of a well-known gang intervention and rehabilitation program in the United States, asserts that "the answer to every question is compassion" (Sounds True, 2018). I would add that the answer to every question is *self*-compassion; from there, compassion for others is born. Establishing high levels of self-compassion in the workplace (or any community of individuals) has four core requirements:

- Establishing relationships where we feel unconditionally positively regarded for our "real" selves, which enables us to mirror the same inwardly
- Giving unconditional positive regard to ourselves, which occurs naturally in those who had it mirrored to them as children. The rest of us can develop it through community (as described previously) and through inwardly focused (and embodied) loving-kindness practices.
- Using stress management practices to open up space between ourselves and our experience of suffering; this cultivates nonattachment, which enables us to pause for a moment before we grasp onto, push away, or overidentify with a thought or action. This space is imperative to establish a sense of safety within ourselves, where we can accept ourselves without condition.
- Expanding awareness to notice the inner judgements that rule our inner space. When we investigate belief systems from a more objective space, we can decide whether they are congruent with our "real" selves as opposed to a belief system we took on from others. As we release belief systems that are no longer true for us, we also let go of the shame we carry as a result of them. Once our inner space is clear of shame, we develop a greater ability to drop in for self-soothing. As we develop the ability to soothe ourselves, painful emotions feel less threatening. From this place, our sense of meaning and personal power will overshadows our suffering, enabling us to resolve areas of dis-*ease*. Dropping in for self-soothing requires us to develop trust in the safety of the inner space (Chapter 9).

CULTIVATING THE CHOICE TO ACT CONGRUENTLY

If emotions are too stressful, it puts us at a higher likelihood of grasping for substances or activities to distract us, which provide only temporary reprieve from the pain. Instead of acting, we react. Doing this often leads to behaviours that are not congruent with our values. To interrupt this tendency, we must first address the felt threat, interrupting and/or resetting the activated nervous system. Once the inner space is free of threat (felt as shame or anxiety), we are more able to drop into our body. From this more empowered place, we develop a choice to act congruently.

Brain Chunking and Harmful Habits: Weaving in Self-Compassion

Brain chunking, which was introduced in Chapter 3, helps us understand how events are not the cause of stress; rather, it is how our brains interpret an event. A stressor develops when we consider an event as a threat to our primary human needs. It takes this form of rapid unconscious processing or patterning of information to function in life; however, sometimes the result of these processes (brain chunking) is snap judgements that can be inaccurate, overly simplistic, and potentially harmful. It was George Miller, a key figure in cognitive psychology, who coined the term "brain chunking" in the 1950s. The term describes our subconscious tendency to organize stimuli or information into patterns that represent a meaningful whole (Neath & Surprenant, 2003).

Brain chunking develops our intuition and forms our assumptions. As humans, we are constantly trying to identify patterns within what often feels like chaos, promoting a sense of control and order; this is a normal part of our humanity. There is a danger to this patterning and ordering, a danger of putting ourselves or others in overly simplified and controlled boxes that are inaccurate or that limit one's ability to move out of that box. For example, a medical diagnosis can emerge from identifying a specific pattern of behaviours or symptoms, which can be helpful if it educates and inspires us to receive a necessary treatment to resolve or manage our ailment. However, brain chunking can disempower us and others if we inaccurately label or box ourselves or others in, hampering the ability to evolve beyond the box we feel limited by.

Just like self-compassion serves as an antidote to hostility (shame spilling), it can also interrupt harmful habits. Self-compassion produces a higher level of consciousness at a slower pace than this default rapid unconscious thinking. We can cultivate this slower pace by intentionally transitioning from the reactionary thinking mode to the felt sense in the body—our sensing mode. In doing so, we tie our heart into the equation, enabling actions to stem from genuine kindness rather than a disconnected habit.

The difference between reacting, emerging from subconscious prejudgements and assumptions, and acting is mindfulness (conscious investigation). By engaging the heart through self-compassion, we develop an ability to choose actions that feel congruent.

Our subconscious prejudges (brain chunks) to make sense of our world, which promotes intelligence and intuitive capacities that are imperative to making everyday critical decisions. As with racism, when we make prejudgements, as in before our thoughts are mindfully investigated, facts may evolve into fixed and often harmful prejudices. For instance, consider your assumptions around gender and ethnicity. These assumptions form over time, patterned pieces of information we lump together to form beliefs about a certain group or type of person. These assumptions can help us to efficiently and intuitively make decisions and to help us navigate typical cultural preferences or to foresee events that are likely to occur amid a mix of certain types of people, events, and contexts. However, when this intuitive awareness lacks compassion, it can emerge as overly simplistic and often harmful prejudice.

As for caregiving, developing intuitive knowing through brain chunking is an imperative protective mechanism in the profession. It helps us to create a sense of order out of what could otherwise feel chaotic, making sense of our world (improving our sense of coherence). The capacity to make rapid decisions in critical situations is what separates the novice from the expert. Through experience, we hone these intuitive capacities. However, if we lack compassion, our prejudgements can go unchecked; lacking curiosity and conscious investigation, we can cause immeasurable harm to ourselves and others. To avoid misunderstandings and misinterpretations, it is helpful to step back, slow down, and remember to cultivate a sense of curiosity and compassion in a challenging situation. From here, we can hold our assumptions more lightly and remain open to surprise.

Mindfulness opens a door of awareness to who we are and character strengths are what is behind the door since character strengths are who we are at our core. Mindfulness opens the door to potential self-improvement and growth, while character strength use is the growth itself. (Niemiec, 2014, p. 344)

Emotions in the Workplace

An ability to manage emotions, defined here as an ability to feel and express them effectively in the world, is a form of human literacy and intelligence. It is largely subconscious and closely tied to the orientation to life and coping tendencies that we develop in childhood. How we perceive the outer world, and specifically whether it feels threatening versus manageable, impacts us personally and professionally.

Ninety percent of workplace success correlates with a person's ability to navigate their emotions and their awareness of the emotions of others (Taylor & Cranton, 2012). It requires us to mindfully hold our emotions, reflecting on what we are feeling and resolving areas of dissonance (Russ, 1998). As for work impacts, those with a greater ability to effectively feel and express their emotions will typically have lower rates of absenteeism, healthier coping choices and better psychological health and perform at higher levels (Sardo, 2004). Developing a greater ability to manage our emotions in an accepting, empathetic, and supportive environment may assist, even protect, those who are most vulnerable to the stressful nature of their work environment.

As a result of brain chunking (elaborated on earlier), we begin developing subconscious patterns that inform how we perceive and manage emotions. Changing our orientation to emotions as adults requires conscious action to forge new brain chunks. We can do this through the mindfulness practices suggested in this text (for example, "Escaping the Empathy Trap" in Chapter 3) or another source. We can mindfully manage our emotions at work by expanding our awareness of the boundary between our emotions and others', and with that a greater ability to recognize emotional transference and set healthy emotional boundaries.

Mindful Superpowers: Curiosity and Self-Compassion

We naturally become mindful when we cultivate a curiosity in the present moment. This curiosity then enables us to immerse in the felt sense, staving off boredom and the incessant dependence on rapidly changing external stimulation. Tolerating an embodied way of being (connected to felt sense) requires self-compassion. Without this unconditional positive regard for whatever emerges in the self, we are prone to getting frustrated, often spiralling into self-destructive thoughts. As a result, the mindfulness practice can feel more like self-punishment than self-care. Through curiosity, we gain the interest and resulting motivation to continue exploring the intricacies of our inner and outer worlds, even when uncomfortable sensations arise (i.e., emotional or physical pain). Through self-compassion, we attain the grace and patience to celebrate progress, despite our imperfections, and as a result we begin to trust the process. Later, we dive deeper into cultivating curiosity, accepting what is via unconditional positive regard for the self (self-compassion), allowing us to sustain a heartful practice and to develop our emotional management capacities in the process.

A Fresh Look at Self-Care/Self-Kindness

Self-care is a term that many of us have heard repetitively, perhaps to the point where it is now emotionally charged. When we lack desire to practise self-care, it becomes an obligation, just one more thing on our "to-do" list, and one more reason to feel like a failure when we do not do it. To pivot aware from obligational and therefore effortful *doing*, it helps to come to know what self-care means to us and how we can cultivate practices that stem from authentic desire.

Simply put, caring for the self is exactly that thing that will securely ground us, remind of us who we, reorient us, and expand us from an embodied (heartful) place.

If it erodes our sense of agency, we will contract and disconnect from our inner world, making us prone to once again prioritize *do*ing over *be*ing. Because self-care is tied to the needs of the moment, it is not helpful to hold on to any one practice too tightly. If we do, we will again fall into obligation. It requires a willingness to let the thinking mind ("noise") fall into the background while we prioritize the felt sense, desires, and promptings of the inner world ("signal"). To tune into "signal," we must feel our way through each practising moment, listening to our emotional messengers, correcting course when incongruence arises, and maintaining a willingness to flow with desire. To practise this fluid way of being, when you move through an experiential strengthening exercise in this book, remember to keep checking in with your felt senses. Each time we let something go that is no longer serving us, we free up space and energy. Furthermore, we cultivate congruence and develop a greater ability to act self-compassionately as we tune into our unique needs.

Attuning, Strengthening, and Clearing Practices
Attuning Practices

A. Relating to Self-Compassion
By reflecting on felt experiences, we expand our awareness of the belief systems informing our behaviours. Self-awareness is a form of mindfulness, and as such it requires the "figuring it out" mind to move into the background of what is actually happening in the moment. When the noise of the mind quiets, we are more apt to notice the sensations of the body and the subtle prompts from our essence. We can do this when our desire to engage in the process overshadows our fear of vulnerability.

- Think about the term self-compassion. What has it meant to you in the past?
- How has your perception of it changed?
- Consider the root of self-compassion—unconditional positive regard. How often do you apply it inwardly?
- Think about the last time you made a mistake or said something you regretted. How did you treat yourself?

A Note on Negative Self-Talk
We don't often recognize negative self-talk as the critical voice in our head. Instead, we feel a sensation in our body, typically characterized by shame, that represents a narrative that is self-destructive. Because the felt sense can be hard to name, it can be challenging to recognize it, and it can lead to our sitting in shame far longer than necessary. In time, as we develop our emotional and somatic (body sensations) literacy, we can catch these self-destructive spirals much quicker.

- Looking forward, considering your desires (what you actually want, not what you "should" want), what might you let go of?
- What needs to happen in order for you to make this change?

- What inner qualities or outer resources will support you to make the change?
- What actions are required to access those resources?

This is where we set an intention! Setting goals and intentions is how we choose a place to plant our seeds of change and is the way in which we prepare the soil to provide the most nurturing environment for successful growth. What do you need to do to develop the characteristic required to get what you want?

Make it count by staying embodied! This is not a "figure it out" exercise; rather, it requires your inner wisdom, which can only be accessed from an embodied space. To drop into this space, we move from thinking to sensing. If this is new for you, try it out; use the practices described next to "drop in" to the embodied inner world and hold an intention to be open to whatever unfolds. Learning to trust the process requires a willingness to live with questions. Trust that the answers will appear if and when you need them, at just the right time and in just the right way. The only thing required from you is your attention. As you prioritize shifting your attention to focus on the inner world, you are building self-trust, self-integrity, and ultimately congruence.

B. Self-Kindness Assessment
This self-kindness assessment was adapted from Saakvitne and Pearlman's (1996) self-care worksheet. It can be helpful to expand your awareness of various self-care activities. Please hold it lightly, being careful not to fall into obligation. The list is not exhaustive nor prescriptive, merely suggestive. Feel free to add areas of self-kindness/self-care that are relevant to you, and consider how often and how well you are taking care of yourself in a typical day. When you are finished, look for patterns in your responses. Are you more active in some areas of self-care but ignore others? How does this correlate with your desires in the area? Are there items on the list that make you think, "I would never do that"? Listen to your inner responses, your internal dialogue about self kindness and making yourself a priority. Take particular note of anything you would like to include more of in your life.

Rate the following areas according to how well you think you are doing by circling a number for each area listed:

3 = I do this well (e.g., frequently)
2 = I do this OK (e.g., occasionally)
1 = I barely or rarely do this
0 = I never do this
? = This never occurred to me

Physical Self-Kindness
_____ Eat regularly (e.g., breakfast, lunch, and dinner)
_____ Eat healthily
_____ Exercise

_____ Get medical care when needed
_____ Take time off when sick
_____ Get massages
_____ Dance, swim, walk, run, play sports, sing, or do some other fun physical activity
_____ Take time to be sexual—with myself, with a partner
_____ Get enough sleep
_____ Wear clothes I like
_____ Take vacations
_____ Other:

Psychological Self-Care
_____ Take day trips or mini-vacations
_____ Make time away from telephones, email, and the Internet
_____ Make time for self-reflection
_____ Notice my inner experience—listen to my thoughts, beliefs, attitudes, feelings
_____ Have my own personal psychotherapy
_____ Write in a journal
_____ Read literature that is unrelated to work
_____ Do something at which I am not an expert or in charge
_____ Attend to minimizing stress in my life
_____ Engage my intelligence in a new area (e.g., go to an art show, sports event, theatre)
_____ Be curious
_____ Say no to extra responsibilities sometimes
_____ Other:

Emotional Self-Care
_____ Spend time with others whose company I enjoy
_____ Stay in contact with important people in my life
_____ Give myself affirmations, praise myself
_____ Love myself
_____ Reread favourite books, rewatch favourite movies
_____ Identify comforting activities, objects, people, and places and seek them out
_____ Allow myself to cry
_____ Find things that make me laugh
_____ Express my outrage in social action, letters, donations, marches, protests
_____ Other:

Spiritual Self-Care
_____ Make time for reflection
_____ Spend time in nature
_____ Find a spiritual connection or community
_____ Be open to inspiration
_____ Cherish my optimism and hope
_____ Be aware of the nonmaterial aspects of life
_____ Try at times not to be in charge or the expert

_____ Be open to not knowing
_____ Identify what is meaningful to me and notice its place in my life
_____ Meditate
_____ Pray
_____ Sing
_____ Have experiences of awe
_____ Contribute to causes in which I believe
_____ Read inspirational literature or listen to inspirational talks, music
_____ Other:

Relationship Self-Kindness

_____ Schedule regular dates with my partner or spouse
_____ Schedule regular activities with my children
_____ Make time to see friends
_____ Call, check on, or see my relatives
_____ Spend time with my companion animals
_____ Stay in contact with faraway friends
_____ Make time to reply to personal emails and letters; send holiday cards
_____ Allow others to do things for me
_____ Enlarge my social circle
_____ Ask for help when I need it
_____ Share a fear, hope, or secret with someone I trust
_____ Other:

Workplace or Professional Self-Kindness

_____ Take a break during the workday (e.g., lunch)
_____ Take time to chat with co-workers
_____ Make quiet time to complete tasks
_____ Identify projects or tasks that are exciting and rewarding
_____ Set limits with clients and colleagues
_____ Balance my caseload so that no one day or part of a day is "too much"
_____ Arrange my workspace so it is comfortable and comforting
_____ Get regular supervision or consultation
_____ Negotiate for my needs (benefits, pay raise)
_____ Have a peer support group
_____ (If relevant) Develop a nontrauma area of professional interest

Overall Balance

_____ Strive for balance within my work–life and workday
_____ Strive for balance among work, family, relationships, play, and rest

List Other Areas of Self-Care That are Relevant to You:

_____

_____

_____

Strengthening Practices

A. Pause for Self-Compassion
Kristin Neff, a pioneering researcher on self-compassion, developed a short and affirming exercise called the self-compassion break (Neff, 2019), which I have adapted for your use here.

Before you begin, notice how anxious you are feeling. Anxiety is often the felt "signal" that arises when we forget who we are and lose sight of our inherent worth (unchanged by achievements and behaviours).

In this moment, on a scale of 1 to 10, how anxious are you? _____

Close your eyes and recall a recent person or event that brings up some stress (avoid starting with an intensely stressful situation). Focus on the situation, allowing yourself to feel the emotions that arise as you engage your heart and mind, bringing to life the inner experience of that moment. From this space, you will nurture yourself just like you would a dear friend.

Start by acknowledging that:

1. "This right now is a moment of stress" (or hurt, pain, suffering, whatever sounds most natural for you).
2. "You aren't alone, these feelings (pain, suffering) are a normal (natural) part of life." "Others struggle in this way too."
3. Think of a phrase that you most need to hear right now, something that expresses empathy and kindness. For this, you can speak in the "I," or continue to speak to yourself as you would a dear friend, whichever enables you to receive it best. For example, you might say:

"You deserve compassion in this moment."
"I fully love and accept you as you are right now."
"May you forgive yourself for not knowing then what you know now. Making mistakes and learning and growing as we go is a part of life."
"May you have the courage to be imperfect."
"Even though I feel [fill in the blank], I deeply and completely love and accept myself."

This exercise reminds us that difficult emotions are a part of life, that we are not alone, and that we are deserving of unconditional positive regard.

Take a moment to reflect on the activity. On a scale of 1 to 10, how anxious are you now?

_____
_____
_____

How might you incorporate or adapt this activity to make it feel more natural for you? How could you fit it into your daily routine? (For example, listening to a guided recording, going for a walk with yourself, setting a reminder, etc.)

_____

_____

_____

B. Body Scan

Sensations are different from the thoughts and emotions that activate them. When we focus on the sensations that move in the body, we train our brains to be present, to practise nonattachment and nonjudgement, and to connect to the inner world. You will likely label sensations you feel as good or bad, which often elicits an emotion. Notice the label and then let it go, stepping back from it and returning to the impartial observer role. As an additional option, if certain body parts seem tense or activate judgemental thoughts, try imagining that with each breath you are breathing spaciousness into those areas, softening with each exhalation. If focusing on a body part is pleasurable, stay there and enjoy it. By doing this form of gratitude practice, you are cultivating a sense of appreciation and connection with the body.

Practise loving-kindness by reminding yourself that this does not need to be perfect. Put your attention on intention and process rather than the end result. Focus on the principle, which is to be present with the sensations of the body, letting go of the details of how you get there. For the first few times, read the script below before you practise; each time you may notice something different and tweak your practice. No need to memorize anything. Trust that it will unfold just as it should.

The exercise begins with giving attention to the breath and moves into a full body scan. To move from your thinking mind to your sensing mind, if you want to stick to the below script, you will need to record yourself reading it or use another recorded version of your own. You can also work with your own version, allowing your intuition to guide you through the process.

If frustration arises, let it come, _be present_ with it, talk kindly to it. Remember that emotions do not define us; rather they are guests in our home, coming and going as they need to. If negative self-talk or sensations arise, practise _loving-kindness_ by reminding yourself that everyone struggles (_shared humanity_) in the beginning and that struggle is a part of being human. Every struggle that we consciously navigate is a worthy investment in our ability to sustain mindfulness.

Find a quiet place free of distraction and a comfortable position for your body to relax. Close your eyes. Release your shoulders, dropping them down and away from your ears. Bring your attention to your breath, observing the natural process of breathing, without needing to control it. As you relax, you may feel sleepy, or you may find that being this relaxed often sends you into a daydream. Each time it happens, simply bring your focus back to the exercise. This practice of pendulating your focus between your mind and your body is exactly the point. Just like we develop new muscles with physical exercise, so too is the case with mindful exercises. Just keeping coming back to the breath … in … out … in … observing how it feels as the breath moves in and out of the body, noticing as it transitions from the inhalation to the exhalation. Notice the space between each breath, then notice that you are an observer from this space.

Continue to bring your attention back to the breath, allowing each breath to come as it may, with no conscious effort to control it. Throughout the exercise, keep bringing yourself back to the observer role, noticing (not controlling) sensations that come and go. Perhaps you notice a lack of sensation; practise letting go of expectation. Cultivate a sense of curiosity about any sensations as they come and go, shifting their location, texture, and form.

Play with descriptive words that reflect how the sensations feel, look, and move. For example, are they dull or sharp? Light or heavy? Do they feel soft? Are they moving quickly or do they have a slow and flowing movement? Be open to whatever the experience brings. Your mind will often wander, especially in the beginning. When you notice that your mind has wandered, recognize it, practise loving-kindness, and return your attention to the body scan.

Now we transition to scanning the body, bringing awareness to the contact points between the body and the floor (or chair). With each breath, relax a little more. Imagine yourself melting into the surface below you. You can notice the sensations of your body in a variety of ways. Start by taking a deep breath, imagining the breath as it travels from your nostrils to your lungs and all the way down to your toes, gathering tension as the breath sweeps through your body and releasing the tension as you exhale.

Throughout the exercise, as tensions or discomforts arise, practise letting go of judgement, accepting the sensations as they are. If it feels too uncomfortable to continue, bring your breath to that area, softening it until the sensation can fade into the background. Now turn your attention to your toes, perhaps wiggling them, feeling the sensations against your socks, shoes, the floor, or the air as they move back and forth. Then move the attention across your toes and up your foot to your ankle, your lower calf, and up your thigh, moving up to your stomach, feeling the breath moving in and out, rising and falling.

Bring your attention to your heart space, perhaps even noticing how it slows as you continue to relax into the breath; turn your attention to your right hand, moving up the arm; bring your attention to your chest, scanning up your neck to your face. Feel the sensations in your jaw and your throat; notice the feeling of the back of your head making contact with the surface beneath it, moving up to the top of your head. Now, notice how your body parts are connected, taking notice of any sensations, welcoming them as guests and with curiosity. Watch how the sensations shift and change. Practise accepting all sensations as equally welcome guests in your inner home, neither good nor bad, just sensations rising and falling, shifting and changing. Turn your focus back to your breath, observing it for as long as you like. When you feel ready, gently open your eyes.

Take a few minutes to reflect on this practice. How did you feel during the body scan? What parts of the body held tension? Were some easier to sense and sit with than others? As you reflect, practise nonattachment, allowing and accepting every experience you had, observing judgements (labelling as good or bad) that flow in and allowing them just as easily to flow out.

You can use a shorter version of this practice by finding a few moments in the day to drop in and bring your attention to the body. You don't need to be lying down. You could do this practice while you're standing in line at the grocery store or while you are walking from one place to another. Practise moving your awareness from your toes on up, doing a scan for tension and breathing into those specific areas to soften them.

Experiential Strengthening Practice

A. Dealing With Tension in the Body—Softening Into Sanctuary

Moving through difficult emotions, which often manifest as stress in the body, is a common theme in this text. While this topic begins here, it will continue to come up in subsequent chapters, aiming to remind you of your inner and outer resources, all of which expand your capacity for healing. Making peace with the protective mechanisms of the nervous system (Chapter 3), cultivating nonattachment to be able to sit with discomfort (Chapter 4), and surrounding yourself with relationship(s) where you can tune into unconditional positive regard (Chapter 5) is the fuel that enables you to stay connected to your body in the process.

It's not about "figuring out" the story correlated with the past wound. Doing so only keeps us in our heads and often leads to disembodiment. Many times, the story doesn't matter at all. What matters is staying embodied. We must feel it to heal it.

As sensations, thoughts, and emotions change, coming and going like waves in the ocean, try to notice when they transition. Observe how sensations ebb and flow. As you notice the subtleties in the sensations in your body, you will learn to distinguish external energies from that arising from your essence (the "real" you). Connecting and grounding to your *being* cultivates resiliency and enables you to navigate passing events with more confidence and ease.

If we avoid emotions when they come up in the moment, we are prone to getting trapped in a superficial sense of discomfort. Adding to this, we miss the opportunity to resolve the dissonance of the moment and any related past wounds that the current moment has unearthed. If our deeper wounds remain buried, they will continue to manifest as a barrier to connection and will put us at greater risk for a host of mental and physical illnesses. This is simply a natural consequence of stuck emotional energy. Only when we allow ourselves to feel our wounds can we release them. As we release them, we gain a greater capacity to connect inwardly and outwardly.

Moving Through Discomfort by Accepting and Softening

Healing occurs in layers. The initial feeling is often the tip of the iceberg. Denying the existence of an uncomfortable emotion prevents us from healing the larger wound beneath it. Furthermore, even when we do lean into the discomfort, exploring and feeling the emotions that are bubbling to the surface, we will often find that there is more than one wound. Like layers of an onion, when we remove one layer, we uncover other unaddressed wounds. This can feel frustrating and even exhausting at times. This too is normal, particularly in cultures that encourage us to avoid emotions, leading to incongruent and disembodied states of being. Layers of unfelt and thereby unhealed wounds is a natural consequence of disembodiment (disconnected from the felt senses of the body).

Though hurts from the past can feel intense and too complex for the "figuring it out" mind, in time we can come to trust that in any given moment we will have what we need to navigate the challenge. When the sense of threat arising from the inner world pushes us beyond our window of tolerance, we cannot stay embodied and tend to the wound. Our internal protector, the nervous system, quite literally takes over. When this happens, it is time to tap our external resources. This is when our investment in relationships of unconditional positive regard is imperative! We cannot walk this journey alone. As described in Chapter 1, and captured in polyvagal theory (Porges, 2011), when we collectively resource, we expand and expedite our capacity to heal.

Trust your intuition. Notice and investigate the emotional messages that present. When nearing overwhelm, stop and take a break. It is time to focus on soothing the insecurity in the body. Doing so will expand our window of tolerance for the emotional stress and allow us to develop self-compassion in the process. Rushing the process can be a form of self-punishment, leading to emotional dissociation and further incongruence. Take it slow, stay connected, making peace with all parts of the work while you gain trust that your higher self, or a spiritual source you connect to, is holding you, providing you with the strength and resources you need to take the next step in your journey. Every self-compassionate and connected step moves you toward congruence with your "real" self. Trust the process, trust the pace. Accept that there are no shortcuts in this work.

Reorientation opportunity. Healing happens when we prioritize the means of getting there over the end result. By feeling our way through the experience, staying embodied in the moment, we will get there!

Self-care. Each layer we remove is a step forward on our healing journey. With each step, we are retrieving lost pieces of self that are tied up in the emotional energy trapped beneath our unhealed wounds. Every intentional and embodied moment is an investment in the healing journey. Like the onion, we remove one layer at a time. While this can feel slow, an equally important part of this process is the grace and compassion to enable the body to take all the time it needs. It is important, even essential, to take it slow, to listen to the body and tend to its needs. Not tending to the needs is what got us here in the first place. The healing process requires a new orientation centred on prioritizing the means of getting there over the end goal. To prioritize the means, we learn how to take care of our more insecure parts of self. Choosing to take the time to do something that feels good for the body is imperative to expanding our window of tolerance for difficult emotions and to build self-trust in the process. This is self-care!

Self-care is never a selfish act—it is simply good stewardship of the only gift I have, the gift I was put on earth to offer others. Anytime we can listen to true self and give the care it requires, we do it not only for ourselves, but for the many others whose lives we touch. (Palmer, 2000)

There will be days we avoid the discomfort brewing in the inner world. This is normal! Giving ourselves grace when we fall outside our window of tolerance for stress is our opportunity to cultivate self-compassion, trusting that we will be called back to it when we are ready. *Getting too deep too fast, ignoring inner cues to take a break, can further compound and reinforce trauma.* By leaning into the inner cues of the body, we are rebuilding self-trust. This requires a reorientation away from what we may have been taught. In this new orientation, we start recognizing the sacredness of the messages the body is sending. They are gifts, guiding us on our healing journey. While they may feel threatening if we attach or overly identify with them, their role is to show us, to alert us to areas of incongruence so that we can tend to them. Just as a splinter produces pain so that we can remove it, so do emotions provide cues so that we can work through new or old (trauma) dissonance. Cultivating self-compassion by stepping back (nonattachment) and talking to our pain, much like we would a child or a friend, enables us to take a break when that is in our highest interest.

Managing your biology is imperative in order to stay embodied in this process. In Chapter 6, there are a number of stress mitigation tools that can help you settle the nervous system.

Let's practise! You can read the material below and then make it your own guided journey by recording it so that your wiser, more nonattached, and secure self can coach the less secure self through the process. This is a great way to develop self-compassion and self-trust! Refriending/reparenting is elaborated on in Chapter 8.

Bring up a recent tension or difficult emotion you felt. When you notice it in your body, breath into it, softening the discomfort associated with the emotion or tightness.

Bring yourself back to the role of the observer, watching how the tension ebbs in and then flows out. Each time you notice yourself resisting it, breathe into the resistance. Soften it, welcome it, letting it rise and fall.

If the tension is intense, breathe space around the sensation in the body, clearly separating the sensation from the "you" who is experiencing the tension. Make the tension an "other."

If it feels too intense, stop by engaging your external senses. You can open your eyes, notice the smells in the room, listen to background noise, feel your feed on the ground, and so on. In doing so, you are stepping back from the sensation. Remind yourself that it is not you, nor does it define you. Your feelings are not threats; they are passing guests in your home. While they are perhaps confused, these guests have your best interests in mind.

To cultivate a greater sense of "otherness" with the sensation, speak to it like a dear friend. You might say something like, "I am with you, I love you, I'm so sorry for your suffering," and so on. Cultivate curiosity by observing how it moves, how it feels, what shape it is. Is it sharp or dull? Does it come in waves or is it nearly constant? Observing the sensation in this way helps us remain one step back from the discomfort, enabling space to exist between it and us, and settling the nervous system in the process. From here, we can touch on our judgements (defining thoughts and feelings as good or bad), and then let them go. This acceptance is part of unconditional positive regard for self, enabling what is to come and go, to be digested, and in time, to heal.

Attuning Practice

A Meeting with Your "Real" Self

Before I can tell my life what I want to do with it, I must listen to my life telling me who I am. (Palmer, 2007)

For many, dropping into the inner world will feel foreign and ambiguous, eliciting feelings of fear and anxiety. It is normal to feel threatened by the unknown. The only way to solve this is to refriend ourselves, enabling the unfamiliar to become familiar. If these unsure and insecure feelings arise, engage a breathing practice that settles your nervous system (elaborated on in Chapter 6), and remind yourself that it will pass. With repetition, as you develop comfort in this new space, the ambiguity and fear dissipate as you learn to connect to the peace and stillness within. These growing pains are a doorway to your inner home. But passing over that threshold can feel like a risk. I can tell you from personal experience that the risk is worth it and that you have all the capacities within and around you to navigate your way home.

Courage is not the lack of fear. Rather, courage is the ability to feel the fear and, when fueled with meaning, acting anyway, knowing it is the best thing for ourselves and others.

Think back to Robert Bly's "The Long Bag" in Chapter 4, where he describes how incongruence develops, often in childhood, and then persists into our adult years. Throughout our lives, we put every undesirable part of ourselves into a "long bag." To heal, we drop into our inner home, reach into the long bag, and retrieve those "real" parts of self that were left in the shadows.

To further illustrate how to access the "real" self, bring your attention to the 360-degree personality (Jung, 1954). Such a person is 100% congruent with their authentic self, unlike those who remain largely divided between the "real" self and a prescribed "ideal," and as a result are more incongruent (Rogers, 1959). We often fall prey to a mistaken identity, whereby we assimilate to the surrounding culture, and the prescribed expectations of those close to us. We mistakenly believe we are mere humans, having an occasional spiritual experience, as opposed to spiritual beings having a human experience. When we peel back the expectations that weigh on us, created by our habits, the habits of others, and the homogenizing culture we incubate in, we awaken to our "real" selves, our "real" purpose for being here. When we live into and out of our authentic selves, we can feel the richness of our inner and outer capacities. Our needs become evident, *because we are listening to the body*, and the resources necessary to fulfill those needs present, *because we are listening to the spirit (part of our essence)*.

For this practice, we will take a moment to remember what is "real." You can read the following passage and then feel your way through it on your own, or you can record it and play it back as a self-guided meditation:

1. Close your eyes to the outer world, allowing yourself to sink into the inner world. Focus on your inhalation as you get acquainted with yourself. Meet yourself. You are the observer of this "self." Observe yourself growing up, unencumbered by the pressure to conform to the standards and expectations of others. Instead, you are rooted in a deep sense that all your parts are worthy of love and celebration. What do you look like and act like when you are expressing yourself without any self-consciousness? Imagine that every piece of you, your strengths and shortcomings, your highs and lows—every part is loved and accepted as part of the package. There is no bar to reach, no role to fulfill, no condition to meet. You are free to be you. Being you is enough, more than enough. Tune into this feeling. Immerse in it for a moment longer.
2. Imagine that all parts of yourself are in the light. You are full of light, and nothing is banished to the shadows. What do you love to do with your free time? What activities do you get lost in? What makes time fly by when you are doing it? What makes you feel alive and connected to yourself and maybe others too?

3. Visualize your entry into adulthood, spreading your wings as you gain independence. What dreams do you have? Unencumbered by practicalities and expectations, what career entices you?

4. Visualize yourself as a more established adult. What activities are you drawn to? What desires do you have? What feels fun? Be cautious here: This is not about what others may pull you into, or what you think you should like, or what your culture might label as a fun, rewarding, or cool hobby. This is unique to you, that thing you may spend hours doing and yet it feels like time flies by. You finish feeling more energized than when you started.

5. Think about the social circle your true self would choose, where no conditions of worth are attached to popularity or to one's ability to attract a certain quantity or quality of friends and intimate partners. What does it feel like to be unencumbered by a felt need to ascribe to the ideal relationships and social life that many feel the need to attain to feel approved of? Where having one, none, or many friends or intimate partners is all valued with no condition or worth attached. If this were the case, what would your ideal relationships look like?

6. Connect to something you desire. This desire is yours alone. This desire is a connection point to your "real" self. It is not the desires of others. It is not the way you believe others have wanted you to walk, talk, and appear. Your desires pull at your heart, they ignite your passion, they energize you and make you feel alive. They are your unique doorway to thriving. Relearning about those desires requires us to drop into the inner space, heartfully connecting to the essence of who we are, free of the "ideals" we serve and the masks we hide behind.

Awakening to Our Highest Purpose

By Crosbie Watler, MD, FRCPC, a Canadian thought leader and seasoned psychiatrist

What is our highest purpose? Is it our work? Our family? Or it is some other role, relationship, or achievement in the waking dream of "my life"?

Muscling through our lives, our choices are often programmed and unconscious. We choose on the basis of fear, insecurity, greed. We reflect on "What do I want?" when what we want might not be what we *need*.

Let's begin our journey by reflecting on the following questions:
• Who am I?
• What do I need?
• What is my purpose?

These are the "soul questions." Whether we are aware of them or not, our answer to these questions will determine whether we stumble through life in a state of fear and reactivity or with clear purpose and calm intention.

Almost invariably, these questions provoke discomfort. We struggle with these questions, even when they are not in our awareness. They create angst and existential despair. We busy ourselves as a distraction, seeking just one more checkmark in doing mode to "make us happy."

This new job will make me happy. This move will make me happy—the geographic cure. This new partner will make me happy. Losing 10 pounds will make

Awakening to Our Highest Purpose—*cont'd*

me happy. How's that working out? We have boiled the ocean in doing mode. Yet here we are, with a pandemic of anxiety, depression, and existential despair.

We have been looking in the wrong place for our well-being. We have forgotten who we are—human *beings*, not human *doings*. If there is any satisfaction in doing mode, enjoy it. It won't last long. The endless quest for something out there to "make" us happy. Trying to fill our bucket, but it's never enough. There's a hole in the bucket …

The journey is not in seeking new landscapes, but in seeing with new eyes.

What exactly do we need to see with new eyes? Ourselves. Self-awareness. Everything that's righteous flows from there. This is the foundation of the whole enterprise, without which we will never awaken to our highest purpose. We are simply blowing in the wind, at the whim of ego, the conditioned mind.

We need to see ourselves—experience ourselves—as we did on the day of our birth. Awareness without boundaries. Free and clear space. The stillness of no mind. Simply "I am." No condition. Before we drank the Kool-Aid and started telling ourselves these stories about who we are:

- I am a failure.
- I am unlovable.
- I am—or will be—alone.
- I am lost.

Sound familiar?

The shift begins by looking beyond the veil of form. The external "reality" that we construct at the level of the conditioned mind and the illusion of our senses. At this level of consciousness—waking consciousness—we have the subject–object split. Here I am with finite boundaries and there you are. Fertile ground for me versus you, or us versus them.

This is the waking dream and it is a primary cause of suffering. The ancient sages called it *Maya*—the illusion of the senses. At this level of consciousness, we see just 4% of the visible universe. We see finite boundaries—disconnection—when in fact there is a continuous field of energy and matter where we merge with everything around us. In truth, we are never alone. *Aham Brahmasmi* … A Sanskrit mantra meaning "I am the Universe."

Ultimate truth—there are two of you—of me—in the game of life. The *doing* and the *being*. On the day of your birth, you were totally immersed in being. The silent witness. We say we "grow up." At the level of form we do grow. We develop a cortex. Intelligence perhaps, but not much wisdom.

We confuse achievement with worth—net worth. By the time we are out of diapers, we are already steeped in doing mode. We hear "hurry up" from a parent. "Put your thinking cap on" from a teacher. Well intentioned, but unconscious.

Who we really are is hidden by the veil of sensations, images, feelings, and thoughts. The turning of the conditioned mind. The monkey mind. Like clouds hiding the sun. We succumb to the collective delusion, "I think, therefore, I am." We were born into the sun. Clear blue sky is our birthright. It was all we knew. Before we lost our way.

We might not know who we are, but we know it when we see it. We see it—feel it—when we look into a baby's eyes. Or when a beloved pet walks into the room.

We love them because we see in them the essence of who we are.

Babies and small, furry animals don't say a thing, yet we feel their gravitational pull. Their healing field. Like medicine washing over us. Simply holding space.

We often worry about the right thing to say. In truth, our words carry little weight—less than 10% of human communication is the content of speech. It is where we show up from when we speak the words that matters. Or where we listen from. Are we listening deeply?

How do we hang out there more often? By holding space for others? For ourselves? Our parents might not have done it for us. That ship has sailed. They did the best with the tools they had—their own awareness—or lack thereof. Forgive them—they know not what they do—they were, or are, unconscious.

It is time to do it for yourself. This is too important to outsource ... looking for someone or something to "make" you happy. Make you whole. The time is now. Time to drop the stories.

In doing mode, you never were and never will be perfect. Get over it. At the level of being, you are already perfect. Anchor in that awareness, with an intention to do better. But the outcomes do not define you. Success and failure will come and go, like the weather. You are not the weather. You are the witness of the weather.

"It's time. You can feel it knocking. It's time to sit in front of the mirror where you can't lie to yourself anymore about who you are ..." (Community Elder and Circle of Indigenous Nations Elder, Duncan Grady).

Mirroring. I see you. No one else might have done it for you. Maybe they did and you lost it. What have you lost? The stillness of being. The silent witness. It is all that is truly yours—everything else is on loan to you. This role, that relationship, *my* body. Enjoy it, but don't identify with it. Whether you succeed or fail at any enterprise, *you* are not elevated ... or diminished.

This is the domain of "I don't mind what happens." Nonattachment. Whatever the challenge, anchor in nonjudgement, in spacious awareness. We can churn at the level of the mind and create a *problem* out of thin air, or we can drop in and access the wisdom of spirit ... the *being* self. The wisdom of the gut brain, the silent brain, where we feel into our bodies and make effortless, wise choices.

The challenges will come—life is not meant to be easy. Without challenges there is no evolution. It is not the challenges of a day that makes the day "good" or "bad." It is where we show up from. This will determine whether we are in flow or in a place of judgement and resistance.

In flow, we are connected with the silent witness and with everything around us. We are in that healing field of space and formlessness. A place where powerful unseen allies conspire to blow the wind in our sails. Not in the "muscling," but in the letting go. Where there is wisdom beyond our wildest dreams. In the stillness.

So, coming full circle:

- Who am I?
- What do I need?
- What is my purpose?

Ask any guru worth their salt and the answer will be the same:

Meditate on it.

The answer to each question is the same—thoughtless awareness. Alert thoughtlessness. It is the nonverbal *experience* of your authentic self when you shift attention from the thinking mind to breath and inner space. Your highest purpose is to anchor in that. And when you *lose it*, come back. When you feel the

> **Awakening to Our Highest Purpose**—*cont'd*
>
> stress response, the aching heart, the fear, the insecurity … the story, you've *lost it*. Come back.
>
> Whatever the challenge, whatever the question. It might seem "complex." The solution is not. Get out of your head and into your breath. Forget trying to resist the turnings of the mind. Simply change the channel. Step out of the ring and into the healing field of your authentic self. The stillness of being.
>
> This is the domain of spontaneous right choice, spontaneous right action. Where you will *feel* into the correct path forward.
>
> You are in yoga. Yoga—an ancient Sanskrit word meaning *union*. Union of body, mind, and spirit. What is our most important pose in yoga? Savasana. Corpse pose. In truth, no pose. Nowhere to go. Nothing to do. Just be. Attachment to nothing and yet full of everything. No one and nothing else is necessary. There are things I might *want*, but nothing I *need*. I am already whole. No condition.
>
> The sole purpose of a human life is to advance as far as possible along the path of consciousness.
>
> The more challenging life becomes, the more we need to walk the path and anchor in who we really are. Challenges then become rocket fuel for the evolution of our consciousness.
>
> Time to wake up. You are not here by chance. I see you. Your ancestors see you. They muse collectively, "We've got a live one." A rare one. A human being that is self-aware and conscious while in embodied form. They *will* blow wind in your sails, calling in all their benevolent allies.
>
> And all you need to do is get out of the way.

Strategies to Tune Into Your Highest Purpose

Tuning into the "real" self, one's essence, is particularly difficult in cultures that are cloaked in years of conditioning. If you are struggling to identify what is "real" against the prescribed "ideals" that you've been accustomed to taking on, try a few of these strategies:

1. Consider whom you admire. Often, the qualities in others we most admire are a projection of our own qualities that have not yet emerged from the shadows.
2. Find a picture of yourself as a young child (ideally before you started school). Reflect on what it was like at that age. Can you remember what drew you in, what captured your heart? Perhaps it is certain people, tasks, events, or activities that you remember getting lost in. If you can't recall any memories that young, can you think back to times as an older child where you were immersed in an activity/event/relationship? Consider what drew you, what called to you in those activities? What was unique about them? What made them special?
3. Contact someone who knew you before you assimilated to societal/cultural ideals (before school age if possible). Ask them what they recalled about you, what stood out to them? What did you like? What did you dislike/resist?

To add another perspective to the mix, best-selling author Cherie Carter-Scott (1998) provides some common human resonations that we are often quick to forget. Readings such as these help us reorient ourselves when we start to confuse the "signal" with the "noise." Or put another way, when the "real" is obscured by the socially prescribed ideals.

1. YOU WILL RECEIVE A BODY
   You may like it or hate it, but it will be yours for the entire period this time around.

2. YOU WILL LEARN LESSONS
   You are enrolled in a full-time informal school called life. Each day in this school you will have the opportunity to learn lessons. You may not like the lessons or think them irrelevant and stupid.

3. THERE ARE NO MISTAKES, ONLY LESSONS
   Growth is a process of trial and error: Experimentation. The "failed" experiments are as much a part of the process as the experiment that ultimately works.

4. A LESSON IS REPEATED UNTIL LEARNED
   A lesson will be presented to you in various forms until you have learned it. When you have learned it, you can go on to the next lesson.

5. LEARNING LESSONS DOES NOT END
   There is no part of life that does not contain its lessons. If you are alive, there are lessons to be learned.

6. "THERE" IS NO BETTER THAN "HERE"
   When your "there" has become a "here," you will simply obtain another "there" that will, again, look better than "here."

7. OTHERS ARE MERELY MIRRORS OF YOU
   You cannot love or hate something about another person unless it reflects to you something you love or hate about yourself.

8. WHAT YOU MAKE OF YOUR LIFE IS UP TO YOU
   You have all the tools and resources you need. What you do with them is up to you. The choice is yours.

9. YOUR ANSWERS LIE INSIDE OF YOU
   The answers to life's questions lie inside of you. All you need to do is look, listen, and trust.

10. YOU WILL FORGET ALL OF THIS.

Strengthening Practice

Remembering How to Play

Part of coming to know our essence is expanding our awareness of and feeling into desire. What sparks our desire? When infused with meaning, desire is stronger than fear. It is often how we lift the veil of cultural conditioning and tap into our unique essence. Often, it is not a specific activity or event that inspires us but rather a mix of qualities about that particular event. These qualities cause a resonant frequency within us, prompting our sense of meaning and desire. In a nutshell, this is how we engage in play. Besides the more obvious pleasure associated with play, engaging in play as adults is also a good stress management strategy.

Playfulness is the ability to transform our environment to make it more enjoyable. (Barnett, 2007)

People who are more playful are less likely to perceive stimuli as stressors and are more creative, adaptive, and less likely to devolve into isolating and escape-oriented reactions (Magnuson & Barnett, 2013). Adults who play are more likely to feel satisfied with life and are more inclined to seek enjoyable activities and be more active (Proyer, 2013). Finally, while the mental fitness benefits are obvious, those who self-identify as playful are also more likely to maintain their physical fitness (Proyer et al., 2018).

Reflect on what qualities spark your sense of desire. Think of one activity that excites you. Perhaps something that resonates with the frequency of the playful child within you. It can help to reach back to a time when you were more embodied, more in tune with desire.

- Do you remember getting lost in a specific activity as a child? Can you recall what qualities of that activity sparked your desire, the moments you caught yourself smiling, laughing, or immersed in a sense of timelessness?
- What quality of that moment captured your attention in this way?
- How might you expand this quality in your life?

Start small as you practise noticing and responding to what sparks your desire. Notice, without judgement, when you quench desire. Lean in to the moment—Can you hear or feel the belief system that is causing you to quench it? By exploring in this way, all actions and reactions are an opportunity to work more objectively and lovingly with what is.

If your desire is becoming clear (no need to rush!), try articulating the obstacles that keep you from engaging in play (letting yourself feel and respond to desire). What actions are necessary to navigate the obstacles that may be holding you back?

When will you take these actions?

The Challenge: Navigation

By considering someone else's challenge, or working with another to consider ours, we cultivate nonattachment. We can often find comfort knowing we are not alone and that we can learn from and with each other. Coming from a more objective space, we can step back, reorienting ourselves from a position of strength with access to all of our biological, intellectual, and spiritual capacities. With this benevolent orientation, we can face adversities with confidence, knowing we have the resources and support necessary to navigate life's challenges.

Let's circle back to Sandy's challenge and dig a little deeper into her story. Sandy did not believe she was unconditionally regarded as a child. As a result, she felt the need to earn approval by meeting any and all conditions necessary to be loved and accepted. Over time, her carefully crafted "ideal" self separated more and more from her "real" self. This separation was not a choice; it was a subconscious effort to survive, a necessary act of survival fuelled by a need to attain love and approval. The further apart the "real" and the "ideal," the more shame she felt. The haunting anxiety she felt caused her to overcompensate for this chronic sense of inadequacy. A natural byproduct of this common human pattern is perfectionism. Within this realm, there is no "good enough," only perfect or not perfect. Whenever her idealized standards were not met, she felt sick inside. This is her nervous system becoming activated, doing everything it can to get her attention, to alert her to the danger it is sensing. In this intense emotional state, Sandy tends to try to control everything and everyone in her world, holding tightly to a sense of order amid the felt chaos. In time, when the fear and anxiety have worn her thin, her nervous system will enter a state of freeze (see Chapter 3), protecting her from the ongoing fear and anxiety she feels lost inside of. In this frozen state, she quickly falls into her typical coping patterns, which only furthers her shame. And so it goes, again and again, like a loop she can't get out of.

Unfortunately, Sandy's story is a common one. When we get stuck in old patterns, we are often unable to attain the objectivity necessary to change course. We have become attached to the past wound, too close to it to see it for what it is. While Sandy may be unconditionally positively regarded by her loved ones, she doesn't believe it. She hasn't tested it by showing her "real" self, so she has not yet embodied it. While many will try to fix Sandy's behaviour through punishment, shaming her for shaming others, this is neglecting the root of the problem. Sandy does not need discipline—she needs direction. By getting to what lies beneath the wound she is living from, she can then meet the need at the root of her suffering, to recognize the need to feel loved for who she "really" is. Sandy will develop a new trajectory (Figure 1.3) by *coming to know* who she "really" is, *attuning* to her own unique frequency, *clearing* the barriers that separate her from inner and outer connection by *strengthening* her heartfulness and self-compassion and by *aligning* with the desires that enable her to live her calling.

Attuning/Reflecting Opportunity

We cultivate self-compassion by engaging in relationships and practices that help us see, feel, and talk to ourselves in ways that reflect the sacred and inherently worthy beings that we are. What relationships or practices help you tune into unconditional positive regard for yourself?

Attuning for the Journey Ahead: Attuning to "Signal": Clearing the "Noise" and Managing the Weather

We've come to know about congruence and self-compassion, attuning and applying the concepts to our inner world. Developing congruence and self-compassion cultivates a safe inner space, one in which we can find comfort and reprieve. As you develop more trust with your body, old wounds that were previously too threatening to feel will come up for healing. This is normal and something to celebrate! It is a sign of your progress. The wound that was too unsafe to feel is now feelable. Reorienting in this way will help you find the meaning within the suffering, to feel the release amid the tension.

Now that we've *come to know* about self-compassion, we will *attune* to the "signal" of who we are. From this more grounded place, we can better manage the "noise" created by the passing challenges we encounter.

CHAPTER 6

Attuning to "Signal": Clearing the "Noise" and Managing the Weather

Dropping into our roots connects us to our essence, the inner "signal" of the uncondi-tioned self. If we cannot ground ourselves when the weather feels threatening, we lose perspective, distracted by perceived threats that we cannot control. When we fixate on what we cannot control, we lose sight of what we can control.

Refriending the inner world is how we learn to distinguish what to attend to (signal) and what to let fall into the background (noise). Distinguishing signal from noise is a skill that has many benefits. For example, as caregivers, the ability to dis-tinguish emotional signals from noise means that we can we pick up on our own signals, but also distinguish between our energy and the energy transmitted from others. The ability to recognize the signal amid the noise is a natural outcome of mindfulness. Our emotions are signals that require interpretation. When we reflex-ively attach to, or identify with, emotions—assuming they are facts versus informa-tion to consider—they act as noise that hampers our ability to accurately interpret the message we are meant to receive (signal). Moving from thinking mode to sensing mode enables us to step back from the barrage of thoughts and emotions that occupy the mind. With this objectivity, feelings of threat move into the background, allow-ing us to discern what is worthy of our attention as opposed to a passing distraction.

Our "signal" to "noise" ratio represents the ratio of relevant to irrelevant informa-tion presenting in any given moment (Fig. 6.1; Table 6.1). When "noise" is cloud-ing the "signal in the body, it is time to regulate the nervous system. When external "noise" is distracting us, it is time to change our context. When the "signal" is hard to decipher, despite clearing the "noise," it is time to stop *doing* from an obligational place and to *be* in something we desire. The **significant thing/action**, referred to throughout the book, represents the action we are called to in any given moment that aligns with our "signal," despite the "noisy" distractions and social pressures.

The signal is the truth. The noise is what distracts us from the truth. (Silver, 2012, p. 17)

The Challenge: Orientation

Regulating the nervous system helps us develop congruence (the ability to distin-guish "signal" from "noise") and sense of coherence (the ability to move from victim to victor). When we lack space for introspection, it is hard enough to acknowledge

Signal to Noise Ratio

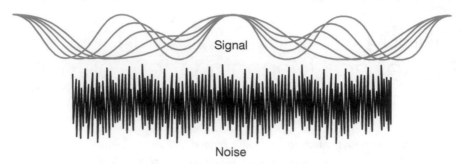

Fig. 6.1 The signal to noise ratio represents the ratio of relevant to irrelevant information presenting in any given moment.

TABLE 6.1 ■ Comparing the Signal and the Noise

	Noise	Signal
Defined as	An unwanted sound that feels too loud or too distracting	A stimulus that conveys meaningful information from one point to another
Perceived as	Not wanted	Wanted
Characterized as	An extraneous sound that obscures the original signal	The original stimulus
Quality/value	When signal to noise ratio is low (low signal, high noise): low quality	When signal to noise ratio is high (high signal, low noise): high quality

emotions (our "signal"), never mind tending to them when we feel triggered. This is exactly what many caregiving environments feel like—the parenting of young children included—we are surrounded by relentless stimuli ("noise"). Adding to this, many of us feel uncomfortable expressing emotions, even when we can find the space. Because we cannot tend to the emotion, owing to fear or lack of space, the energy ("noise") gets stuck in the body. As tension builds, the nervous system becomes activated. Enter the stress response.

As elaborated on in Chapter 3, when we are stressed, it hampers our ability to step back to navigate the perceived challenge in front of us. If the threat feels intense and we cannot respond to the associated emotion, we will likely react by fighting (anxiety and hostility), fleeing (depression and avoidance), freezing (disconnecting and dissociating), or fawning (pleasing others at the expense of our own needs, preferences, and desires).

Consider the analogy of the phone as the emotional messenger. Emotions are telephone calls bringing us information. If we answer the phone, we receive information about something happening in that moment. If we avoid answering the phone (or turn the ringer off) from freeze (Chapter 3), disconnecting from the feeling altogether, we block the message from coming through and lose the opportunity to resolve the body's felt need, which erodes self-trust. If we react to the ringing phone from a place of fight or flight, instead of answering it, we are likely to activate others by anxiously running around alerting everyone that the phone is ringing. We may even fuel shame by blaming ourselves for the ringing phone, or hit others over the head with the phone in anger. If we habitually block the message, ignoring (freeze) or reacting (fight–flight) to the phone of our feelings instead of answering it, we miss an important opportunity to connect to the emotion in order to tend to the wound that lies beneath it.

To make this challenge more practical, let's consider Mark's situation. Mark works as a first responder. These days, he feels a sense of dread before going back to work each day, and his anxiety is impacting his relationships with his co-workers. Lately, the workload feels relentless, and there seems to be more conflict and hostility between team members than usual. Mark has always enjoyed the lack of predictability in the workday—in his view, it adds adventure and challenge to the day. However, lately, the lack of predictability seems to fuel his anxiety.

There are two intertwining and equally important ways to address Mark's challenges.

First, Mark can adapt to the environment so that he can thrive. Much like trees need an adequate environment to forge deeper "roots," we too need environments that can support and nourish our ability to flourish. Second, Mark can adapt his orientation to the environment so that his triggers are less impactful ("weather").

There will always be components of our context that cannot be changed. When this is the case, we should accept it and reorient ourselves in a more empowered way. If we continue to feel victimized by external factors, we will fixate on the threat (that which is victimizing us), which then activates the nervous system. We then get "stuck" in this loop, one nervous system reaction after another. When we accept what cannot be changed, identify what can, and take action, we transition from victim to victor—this is how we become "unstuck."

Reflecting on Mark's challenge, what might be contributing to Mark's stress? What is it about Mark's situation that makes it difficult to "answer the phone of his feelings"? Consider these same questions for yourself.

Attuning Practice: How Do You Respond to Uncomfortable Emotions?

Consider your past tendencies. Which icon best resonates with how you tend to respond to uncomfortable emotions?

Avoidance/
distraction

Denial

Dissociation

Acceptance
and learning

The stress response can activate the nervous system to the point that we are so distracted (or altogether frozen) that we cannot feel, much less tend to, emotions. If we cannot tend to the emotional energy, it gets "stuck" in the body, causing us to become out of tune with our essence, the "signal" of who we are. In my experience, being present with an emotion can be like allowing the vinegar and baking powder to mix: the chemicals react, and the mixture bubbles up and out of us, leaving us in a more neutral, less volatile steady state. When the distracting "noise" clears, we can more easily tune back into the "signal," grounding once again in our most secure self.

When the inner world gets too "noisy," it feels too threatening to experience. The impact of the emotion is consciously *suppressed* or unconsciously *repressed*. Rather than reaching in to soothe, we are likely to reach out to substances or potentially harmful activities to distract us from our suffering. With mindful and self-compassionate practice, we rebuild trust with the body and the sensations within. As we gain trust with the body, we begin to recognize its messages as well-intentioned allies that fall prey to confusion. They are "others," separate from our essence, and as such, we can work with them compassionately without overidentifying with them (the source of "threat"). With the "noise" of fear cleared away, we welcome these emotional messengers as guests in our home, trusting that they hold important clues on this path of discovery of the "real" self.

Unhealed wounds from the past, presenting today as "trauma," are a particularly challenging source of incongruence. When a current-day event reminds us of a past event, our brain chunking superpowers can cause confusion between past and present threats. Memory is state dependent—even a small upset can recapitulate past memories of trauma, triggering a stress response far in excess of the objective present-day threat. It can feel even more threatening than when the core wound first happened. As discussed in previous chapters, this reactivity can be referred to as post-traumatic stress disorder (PTSD), where our sense of order in the moment becomes distorted based on a past event.

In this book, you will learn about "clearing" practices. These practices are about regulating the nervous system and cultivating nonattachment so that we can distinguish the "signal" from the "noise." Once we settle the body by clearing out the "noise," we can ground in and attune to the "signal" of who we are. From here, we can *be* with ourselves. From this state of *being* comes inspired doing, whereby we manifest our "real" selves in the world without effort. We simply flow in the currents of the energy around us; we are thriving.

Unfelt feelings, whether suppressed or repressed, remain trapped in the body as stuck energies. As we develop trust with the self and hold space for "what is," these stuck energies come up for healing. When we learn to experience these stuck emotions from a place of calm and grounding, we break the conditioned fear response. While having to "feel our feelings" may feel like a step backward, it is not. This is ultimately how we move forward.

Dropping into our inner world is sometimes easier said than done. If we get stuck in cyclical thought patterns characterized by self-judgement, criticism, and self-destructive thoughts, we buy into the idea that we aren't good enough. In our not-good-enoughness, we become a threat to ourselves. As a result, because a threat is sensed, the nervous system causes all sorts of uncomfortable "noise." As a result, the inner world will feel uncomfortably threatening and not a place where we will want to spend much time—and certainly not a place we will want to turn to for soothing.

Heightened cortisol levels support the fight–flight–freeze–fawn responses, reinforcing the feeling that our inner world is chaotic and unsafe. Substances and some impulsive behaviours provide external "solutions" to this internal problem. In an attempt to gain order by securing to an outside influence, we become disembodied, shifting out of *be*ing and into *do*ing. Because temporary distractions are generally not the result of conscious and compassionate choice, we are more prone to harm ourselves and others in our attempts to self-soothe in this disembodied state. The good news is, we have a reset button! By regulating the nervous system, we can step back from the perceived threat, creating a space between it and us. It becomes the "other." From this grounded state (tuned into "signal"), we can better manage the "noise" of the nervous system and the (often-misguided) narratives that are activating it.

Recognizing the Fight–Flight–Freeze–Fawn Responses

A fundamental reason why some people thrive, while others in similar circumstances suffer, is threat perception. Those who thrive are more likely to see new stimuli as manageable, whereas others might see danger. When we perceive stimuli in our lives as manageable, we are better able to navigate challenges without undue stress. As discussed in Chapter 3, most of us have heard about the fight-or-flight response, which stems from the sympathetic nervous system. Over the past decade, we have learned much more about the freeze (and fawn) response, which stems from the parasympathetic nervous system. Because their origins are different, we must manage them with a different set of tools.

Sympathetic activation sends us into a subjective spiral, even when it is more adaptive for us to stay objective, calm, and collected. We tend toward either fight or flight, subconsciously falling into one more often than the other. When neither option seems viable, we are prone to freezing or fawning.

Those who tend to take on a fighting posture often slip into critical and self-destructive thought programs ("I'm such a loser, I'm unlovable, I'll never get this right"). Here, the enemy we are choosing to fight is ourselves.

ANTIDOTE TO FIGHT: SELF-COMPASSION

Those who flee will typically avoid the discomfort by turning to outside distractions as a numbing agent or using substances, adrenalin, or busy activities to dissociate.

The antidote to fight is to recognize that we are not alone and to replace isolating behaviours with belonging and connectedness with others.

Those who freeze are prone to cyclical thought rumination ("I shouldn't have said that ... If I would have just ..."), causing us to fixate on what we could have and should have done. Mindfulness—presence—interrupts ruminative thinking by bringing our attention to the present moment through our senses. In the freeze state, the inner world sometimes feels too threatening to acknowledge. In this case, being mindful of how we are sensing external stimuli is often enough to deescalate our sense of overwhelm.

ANTIDOTE TO FREEZING AND FAWNING: MINDFULNESS AND SELF-COMPASSION

Besides recognizing our own defensive tendencies, it is helpful to recognize the tendencies of our loved ones and colleagues. When we can recognize defensive patterns, we are more likely to provide compassion because we see the nervous system as separate from the "signal" of who they are. Others are simply caught up in the "noise," driven more by fear than by choice. From this more compassionate place, we are less likely to get activated ourselves, and as a result, we can help to objectively deescalate the situation.

For instance, when two people are feeling activated, just by saying, "I'm feeling activated right now," we can interrupt an activating cascade in the other person. Or, when someone is clearly in a fighting posture, we could say, "I am not feeling safe right now. I feel like I want to protect myself by leaving this situation." Now that we've been "real," rather than trying to cloak our vulnerability, we immediately move into more of an empowered *being* state. By articulating the "noise," we are clearing a path to reconnect to our "signal" and helping others do the same in the process.

Interrupting Stress

A memory without the emotional charge is called wisdom. (Dispenza, 2012)

Knowing your defensive tendency can help you to recognize when it is happening, providing you with a cue to step back in order to interrupt the stress response. Doing so reduces perceptions of threat and allows the body to come back into homeostasis (free of dis-*ease* or threat). Essentially, when we regulate in this way, we return to feeling safe and secure in the "signal" of who we are.

Interrupting the Sympathetic Response: Fight and Flight

The balance between our sympathetic and parasympathetic nervous systems modulates our experience of stress. The sympathetic nervous system is designed to allow us to escape danger. Ideally, it cues us to take a *significant action*, which would then resolve the threat. Once the threat dissipates, the parasympathetic nervous system kicks in, helping us to relax and reverse the effects of the sympathetic nervous system. The problem is that in today's world, we are overstimulated by external stressors or by habitual rumination on imagined threats, and so we often end up chronically stuck in the sympathetic nervous system's biological loop. Without enough stimulation of the parasympathetic nervous system to rebalance us, we get no reprieve from daily tension and anxiety.

Reversing the chronic stimulation of the sympathetic nervous system has four basic steps: awareness, nonattachment, reorientation, and ritual. A breakdown of these steps follows.

1. Awareness

Awareness means recognizing when the sympathetic nervous system is activated. Step back (nonattachment) from the anxiety—detach from the emotion and instead position yourself as an impartial witness. To assist in the ability to step back, cultivate a sense of curiosity about the situation, whether it is something new about how you are perceiving the experience (impacting the inner world) or something new about the context (a difference in the outer world).

2. Nonattachment

Nonattachment means stepping back to objectively assess whether the situation actually poses a threat. Accept what is happening, *noticing and accepting* intense emotions (fear, anxiety) as a natural biological response to the sympathetic nervous system being activated. These intense emotional and now biological feelings are a normal chemical reaction within the human experience of stress (resulting from our interpretation of an uncomfortable emotion, which may or may not be based on accurate thoughts).

3. Reorientation

Reorientation means altering our perspective. This can mean changing the situation or changing our mind about the situation. Do something to *remove the stressor*. If you cannot remove it, *reframe the stress response* as a reminder to ground yourself in mindfulness. Every cue to practise mindfulness is an opportunity to assess the reality of the situation, deciphering whether it is an actual or imagined threat, and to resolve unhealed past experiences (i.e., trauma).

4. Ritual

Ritual means taking an action that activates the parasympathetic nervous system (relaxation response). There are a variety of techniques that activate the parasympathetic nervous system, cueing the body to relax. These techniques put us in sensing mode, enabling us to stay focused on the present moment. For example, we *feel* the floor or chair beneath us or the breath moving in and out of the body; we can *observe* our surroundings, letting any distracting stimuli rise and then fall into the background. When emotions feel intense, active relaxation and breathing exercises are most helpful, such as stretching or taking five long deep breaths or doing 4–7–8 breathing (described in the next section). Passive breathing, where the focus is to observe the breath rather than control it, is another great way to relax and practise nonattachment, but it is not always so helpful when cortisol levels are soaring.

Interrupting the Parasympathetic Response: Freeze–Fawn

According to Peter Levine's (2010) seminal Somatic Experiencing work, the body's freeze response is an involuntary survival mechanism that often results in emotional numbness and detachment, otherwise referred to as dissociation. In environments of unconditional positive regard, where we feel safe to express ourselves, we learn to regulate our emotions. If we did not have this environment in our developmental years, our nervous system may not have learned how to regulate when uncomfortable emotions presented. As a result, in high-stimulus environments where relationally safe connections are lacking, we are more prone to freezing (i.e., dissociating), as this was the mechanism that felt necessary to our survival in our developmental years. There are no quick fixes for these subconscious reactions; rather, it requires establishing an internal and external environment of safety, enabling the trapped emotional energy ("noise") to surface and discharge.

When faced with a real or perceived threat, the sympathetic nervous system is activated. But if in the split-second unconscious assessment of the threat we determine that fight or flight won't work—perhaps because it did not work in the past—then the parasympathetic freeze response kicks in, causing an inability to act at all. As a result, the energy becomes trapped. Once we unfreeze, the trapped energy that was created during the sympathetic activation will need to be released or else it will remain trapped, continuing to create inner "noise" until it can be released. We can facilitate this release by doing the *significant thing* to remove the threat or the perception of threat. Once the threat is managed, we can expand our window of tolerance for stress, enabling ourselves to refrain from freezing again. To further support the emotional/energetic discharge that can continue to activate the nervous system, we can use movement to shake off or stretch out the excess energy, much like animals shake after trauma.

Mindfulness is the key to noticing the process, making conscious what is unconscious, and working gently and compassionately with ourselves to rebalance the nervous system. Much of the work needs to occur *before* and *after* activation: establishing and becoming familiar with those practices so that we can use them right away; knowing and anticipating common sources of stress; demonstrating to ourselves that we have the resources we may not have had in times of earlier trauma; noticing the ways in which we unconsciously try to balance our nervous systems— some of which may not be healthy or effective, such as addictive behaviour; and replacing unhealthy behaviours with those that feel comforting. By navigating common pitfalls more intentionally and catching moments of activation, we are far more likely to find our way back to balance far quicker.

Feeling stuck? There is often a "significant thing" that we are putting off. This inspired action is how we reorient ourselves from feeling like a victim of life to a victor. We become empowered when we respond to this inner prompt.

CLEARING PRACTICE: INTERRUPTING THE FREEZE RESPONSE

When we feel overwhelmed by uncomfortable sensations in the body, in an attempt to minimize the stimuli, the body enters a dissociated or numb state. This response is the fight-or-flight response put on hold (Kozlowska et al., 2015). In this state, sensations are dulled, especially those related to bodily sensations such as emotional and physical connection. Because the freeze state is involuntarily linked to past trauma (stuck emotional energy), we can interrupt the response by reconnecting to the here and now. We do this by tracking physical sensations in the body, such as how the breath feels moving in and out of the body or how the air feels on our skin. The key is to keep the focus on physical sensations, taking our attention away from the activated emotions that relate more to past trauma than to current reality. Keeping the focus on physical sensations related to the here and now diffuses the sense of threat related to past trauma, bringing us back to what is happening in the actual moment.

When scanning our physical sensations, it is important to allow them to be as they are. While we might involuntarily label the sensations as good or bad, the most helpful thing is to recognize the label and then simply let it go. Again and again, we must come back to being the neutral observer. As stuck energy comes to the surface for release, it is not uncommon for people to experience tingling, shaking, and tremors as they release the energy (Levine, 2010).

If focusing on the body is too difficult because of the intensity of the emotions, tracking via the visual channel is another way to reground. When mammals feel immobilized because of the freeze response, their visual channel remains intact, enabling them to continue scanning their environment for potential threats

(Kozlowska et al., 2015). Using this visual channel to reconnect to the here and now is a gentle and effective way to gain perspective and reground.

 Attuning/Reflecting Opportunity

Recall a time recently when you felt acutely threatened. Which response was activated? Fight, flight, freeze, or fawn? Which response is the most common for you in stressful situations? What stress-busting activity seems to work for you now? What was it about that activity that seemed to work for you? What about it was pleasurable? What was effortful? What else might you try moving forward?

Tuning Back Into "Signal" With the Breath

By Crosbie Watler, MD, FRCPC, a Canadian thought leader and psychiatrist

Attention can only truly be in one place at a time. The default focus for our attention is the mind field. There is one addiction we all share—addiction to thought. We attend to thoughts and emotions even when they do not serve us or cause harm. We distract ourselves in desperate or harmful ways in order to change the channel, to get out of our heads.

One distraction that is omnipresent is the breath. Until you read this, were you aware of your breath? Simply switching attention *with intention* to breath or inner space immediately reduces sympathetic tone, allowing us to anchor and practise self-care.

Controlled breathing techniques improve mental function, help us focus, heighten our mood, and reduce cortisol levels (Ma et al., 2017; Perciavalle et al., 2017). In the next section, you will find examples of controlled breathing techniques that help to regulate the nervous system. Breathing in these ways requires concentration, enabling an ability to step back from self-destructive thoughts. As a result, these techniques deescalate our perception of threat. When the threat dissipates, a beneficial biological cascade results. Our muscles relax, our heart rate lowers, and our blood pressure goes down.

It is common to feel dizzy when doing these techniques, so remember to start slow and to titrate the practices if you are pregnancy or during certain activities that could pose a safety risk, such as driving. Inhalations are often done through the nose with the tongue on the upper palate (roof of the mouth). During most sitting meditations, both the inhale and exhale are done through the nose. However, during breathing exercises that promote cleansing/purification, regeneration, and the transmutation or release of difficult emotions, exhalation is often done through the mouth; this promotes a full exhalation and emotional release. However you choose to practise, there is no need to complicate breathing. Breathing deeply in and out of the belly is often enough to attain a mental, emotional, and biological shift. The following exercises promote a greater ability to interrupt the stress response (sympathetic nervous system) and activate the relaxation response (parasympathetic nervous system).

Intentional Attention

By Crosbie Watler, MD, FRCPC, a Canadian thought leader and seasoned psychiatrist

Attention is the fuel for the body–mind activation loop. When we anchor in spacious awareness, there is no fuel left to feed the fire of body–mind reactivity and somatic tension is metabolized.

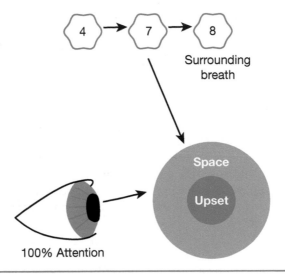

Regulating With Breath
The 4–7–8 Technique

As illustrated by Dr. Watler, you can use the 4–7–8 technique to create space around the upset (discomfort in the body), which interrupts the mind–body activation loop we often find ourselves stuck in. *This practice often causes dizziness (by design!). Do not attempt while driving or during other activities that require your full, unaltered attention.*

Begin by noticing how you feel. On a scale of 1 to 10, how anxious are you now?

Next, empty your lungs by fully exhaling through the mouth. With your tongue gently resting on your upper palate (roof of mouth), inhale for 4 seconds through the nose. Hold for 7 seconds. Exhale again through the mouth for 8 seconds, making a "whoosh" sound to exhale more thoroughly. Three rounds of this breathing are often enough to activate the parasympathetic nervous system (relaxation response). As a result, we are more able to drop into our bodies for self-soothing and to release stuck energy. If the initial threat is not managed, or we have not successfully reoriented ourselves to it, we will continue to get activated until we do.

It is normal, even a good sign, to feel slightly lightheaded. This light-headedness is what interrupts the stress response. If you aren't noticing an effect, try holding the counts for longer.

On a scale of 1 to 10, how anxious are you now?

The 4 × 4 Technique
Begin by exhaling through your mouth to empty your lungs. With your tongue gently resting on your upper palate (roof of mouth), breathe in through your nose for 4 seconds. Hold for 4 seconds. Exhale through your mouth for 4 seconds. Hold for 4 seconds. Start the next cycle by breathing in through your nose for 4 seconds. Start with four cycles of this 4 × 4 technique to begin and adapt according to your desire, timing, and ability.

Breath of Fire
To get the maximum benefit, I suggest you first practice this technique with a qualified teacher (online or in person). This is a yogic pranayama practice that invigorates the body and clears the mind. Begin in a seated position with a straight spine and closed eyes and mouth. Rapidly inhale and exhale through the nose with a focus on snapping the navel back to the spine as the breath is pushed out of the body. The breaths are quick, occurring at a pace of two to three cycles per second. To start, limit these sessions to 15 seconds.

Sighing
A long exhale followed by a 2-second pause before inhaling results in a release of physiological tension in those who are anxiety prone (Vlemincx et al., 2016).

Breath Counting
Breath counting facilitates the ability to focus on the breath, interrupting the thought rumination that often spurs the stress response. Breath counting also builds concentration by improving your ability to sustain mindfulness and meditation. Observe your breath as it enters and exits your body, counting to 5 for each exhale and then starting again at a count of 1. As your skills improve, increase your count up to 10.

Heart Breathing
Heart breathing describes the process of filtering every breath, thought, and emotion through the heart space. It is an excellent way to tune into your inner "signal." To practice heart breathing, first drop into the inner world, settling into quietness and letting external distractions fall into the background. Imagine the heart space, moving beyond the threshold of the thinking mind to focus on your physical and spiritual centre, deepening and slowing your breathing as you do. In this space, you connect to your essence, transcending the veil of the ego so you can see and feel your connection to self, to others,

to nature, and to a larger spiritual world. From this connected place, you can more easily distinguish signal from noise.

Using this technique prior to stressful events is a form of *priming* (see Chapter 8) that helps to lessen anxiety related to a current event or future challenge. You can do this by imagining yourself in the event while focusing on the breath as it moves in and out of the heart, reorienting yourself from a heartfelt lens (cultivating objectivity and relaxing your physiology), removing the emotional charge at the root of the initial stress response.

Focusing on your heart while you inhale and exhale helps to cultivate loving-kindness and supports the development of self-compassion. As we focus on a sense in the body, we strengthen our ability to stay in the current moment, connect to the inner world, notice inner sensations, and improve concentration and clarity of mind. As we learn (often through trial and error) strategies that help us feel connected, we can quickly drop in and self-soothe more easily when we need it most.

There are a variety of ways to promote heartfelt connection. Some prefer visualizing, or using the imagination, to reorient themselves, enabling them to view themselves and the world through a heart-centred lens. For example, imagine inhaling a cleansing, white light in through the crown of the head, and while exhaling, imagine extending love and compassion from the heart. Others find that mantras (quietly or out loud) quickly move them across the threshold. Take your time trying out different techniques, noting what you like so that you can add it to your tool belt. Based on previous life experiences, personalities, and sensory preferences, the key to the doorway of our inner worlds will vary. Having multiple tools at your disposal gives you choices that are based on your unique needs and the context you find yourself in.

Getting Unstuck: The Signal of the *Significant* Thing

We can counter the effects of stress hormones by taking a *significant action*, moving us from feeling like a helpless victim to an empowered victor. These significant actions are never the same; they change with every momentary challenge. Sometimes, it means saying "no" when we feel pressured to say "yes." Sometimes it means leaving a job that runs counter to our values. Sometimes it means saying "yes" to desire, despite our looming fears. Doing the significant thing is exactly how we get unstuck! By acting in a way that honours the body's felt need, you are sending a message to the nervous system. You are acknowledging the message and acting on it. This is all a part of building trust and ultimately refriending the body (including the nervous system).

How do you know what the significant thing is? As we become more accustomed to how the "signal" of desire and inner knowing resonates in the body, the significant thing becomes more obvious. At first, because we are getting reacquainted with the body, moving according to the felt senses, it will feel like trial and error. Adding to the challenge, often the significant thing is also the hardest thing, requiring the most vulnerability. As a result, we often subconsciously avoid the significant solution, turning to anything and everything else instead. When lesser solutions do not get us unstuck us, and our motivation to end the suffering overshadows our fear, we attain the courage to take our significant action.

Anxiety: Signalling Us to Remember Who We Are

Many of us are conditioned to avoid anxiety with a variety of creative distracting and sedating strategies. However, on this path toward greater congruence, anxiety can be an ally, signalling us if we stray from our values and calling. "Signal anxiety" is a barometer and requires enough bothersome intensity to get our attention. The term was initially defined as an instinctual tension that occurs when we fear losing love and acceptance (Freud, 1926, 1937). It happens the moment we stop feeling that we are unconditionally positively regarded by self or others. Soon enough, because we have forgotten our inherent worth, we lose sight of who we are and our inherent worth (**"signal"**). As a result, we turn our attention to feverishly decorate ourselves with external assets (**"noise"**), fixating on external approval to gain security. The noise is the conditioning (fixating on *doing* and *getting*), which can easily drown out the signal. The noise often presents as "should" statements that we prescribe to ourselves and others.

As a reframe of our typical fear of anxiety, viewing it as a signal that promotes congruence can prevent it from feeling like a stressful threat. From this more objective and heartfelt space, we have a greater ability to receive the message. The message may be difficult to hear, much like it is difficult to listen to an instrument that is out of tune, but its purpose is benevolent, illuminating an area of incongruence for us to tend to. Tending to the incongruence enables us to tune back in, to remember who we are. As we ground back into our values and calling, our fixation on *doing* dissolves and we can get back to *being*.

How do I make it go away? The signal is the frequency that flows from our inner world, providing the inner resources, wisdom, and courage to navigate the outer. We lose access to these inner resources when we aren't tuned in. If we get out of tune with our signal (forgetting who we are), we become ungrounded and, out of fear, we turn our focus to attaining external security. When this happens, anxiety is the messenger, signalling that we have forgotten who we are. Signal anxiety disappears when we remember who we are and when we respond by compassionately tending to the felt unmet need in that moment (the *significant* thing described earlier).

Strengthening Practices

A. Breathing Into the Noise
When we are surrounded by noise, we are unlikely to distinguish the signal. To gain the space necessary to step back so that we can tune into our signal (nonattachment), we must first recognize when we are consumed by it. Once we see our attachment, we can recognize it as separate from who we are, enabling us to disidentify and eventually let go. As we let go, a space develops between the felt conditions (imposed by self or others) prescribed by the world and the "noise" (pressure to earn our worth by doing). When we disidentify, we are more likely to see it as a stimulus we can manage rather than a threat. From this quieter, less threatening space, we tune back into our signal, navigating the outer world from this more meaningful, connected, empowered, and resourced inner space.

Breathing Into the Noise
- Bring up a situation in your current life where you are feeling insecure. Continue thinking about this situation until you notice an anxious feeling in your body. When the anxiety presents, get curious as you note where the anxiety is, what it feels like, and how it presents itself.
- Imagine that this felt sense has a double-walled balloon around it. With each deep inhale and exhale, fill the space between the two outer walls. As you are breathing with this visual, lean in to receive the message that is waiting to be heard. If you find yourself lost in noisy thoughts, go back to breathing into the space between the two outer walls, cultivating more space (nonattachment). From this more spacious place, revisit the message.
- Once the message is delivered, continue breathing into the space until it is so big that you can visualize the balloon slowly floating away. Now that you are aware of the noise, seeing it for what it is, you are more able to distinguish it from the signal.

B. Out of Tune? Attuning to your "Signal"
When we get out of tune from our inherent worth, our values, and our calling, we are likely to look for security in the outer world. When we can't love and accept ourselves (because we are lacking self-compassion), we look to others, settling for conditional acceptance and worth. Tuning back into our signal is about remembering the inherent worth of who we are, beneath our conditioned selves. How do you remember who you are? What resource reminds you that you are inherently worthy and loved?

Tuning Into Unconditional Positive Regard (Signal)
- Bring someone or something to mind, perhaps a person (present or past), your wiser self, a beloved animal, or a spiritual source. It is not important who or what it is; what is important is how they resonate with your inner signal. The more it ushers you into a felt sense of unconditional positive regard, the more likely it will allow you to sink back in tune with the signal.

- Taking it a step further, engage in a conversation, a prayer of sorts. Gain a felt sense of *being* with the source (feeling unconditional positive regard) and begin a conversation. Tell it what is in your heart, what is worrying you. Stay connected to the felt sense of love and compassion, allowing yourself to stay connected to your heart. When you have finished saying what needs to be said (releasing shame), take some time to listen and observe. Bask in the moment and celebrate yourself for walking through this exercise. With practice, you will come to know the voice that flows from signal. This wise, grounded voice will remind you of who you are. Practise just being with this source, engaging in prayer and really listening to the wisdom that emerges.

From this more grounded place, we can step back from the noise, navigating to the signal from a more nonattached and empowered place. Some days, comforting affirmations will come to mind. Some days, you will rest in the quietness. Other days, the conditioning (noise) will be too loud to distinguish the signal, making the experience more difficult. Every experience provides an opportunity to expand awareness, cultivate nonattachment when we need it most, and continue practising self-compassion (especially in the difficult moments) as we journey forward.

Desire as Signal, Obligations as Noise

Distinguishing the signal from the noise requires both scientific knowledge and self-knowledge: the serenity to accept the things we cannot predict, the courage to predict the things we can, and the wisdom to know the difference. (Silver, 2012)

When we step back from rumination and instead connect to our senses and the present moment, we obtain the space needed to keep thoughts and emotions in perspective. Within this space there is a doorway to desire, and through desire we can access our essence. Practically speaking, by not identifying with passing thoughts and emotions, we are better able distinguish between the barrage of noise we experience each day and the important signals to which we ought to pay more attention. These important signals include our primary needs that require tending to.

To deescalate the body's alarm system, we must believe that our primary needs are being satisfied. Until we do, we will continue to experience projections and impulses over which we have little conscious control. By identifying the noise, which often relates to past experiences rather than the present moment, we can turn the volume down. Once we can make distractions quieter, we are better able to navigate the current challenge.

Strengthening Practice: Finding Sanctuary and Responding to the Root of Desire

When we feel that a need is unmet, anxiety surfaces. In individualistic cultures such as our Western culture, these perceived unmet needs are more likely to concern love, belonging, and self-esteem. Those who have root systems that feel safe, enriching, and accepting without condition are more likely to engage in thriving, even when the going gets tough. Because of the stability of their root systems, they are less likely to perceive these events as threatening.

When we find sanctuary in the inner world, we are connecting to spirit, opening to feeling the longings and desires of our heart. If you trace these desires back to the source, you will find a basic need longing to be met. Ultimately, these longings are reminders of our fundamental needs—to feel safe, nourished, warm, and whole. We want to be truly seen and deemed inherently worthy, without the conditioning and protective displays that distorts our sense of self, fuelling incongruence. Some may fear desire, perhaps because they learned that desire is somehow selfish or dangerous. When we quench desire, we are likely to fall prey to many projections and compulsions, the natural result of the incongruence fuelled by the suppression of desire.

 Attuning/Reflecting Opportunity

To illustrate the power of desire, think about the last time you acted compulsively, satisfying what might have felt like a deep craving. Look past the surface, beneath the activity or substance that you craved, to the core desire that lay beneath. What need or longing did the substance or activity promise to satisfy? How could this core desire have been satisfied in other, perhaps more fulfilling ways?

Responding to desire requires us to act authentically, asserting ourselves in a way that is congruent with our values and desires. Those that can act, despite the vulnerability required, are doing so because they accept themselves to the point where they no longer value the opinions of others above their own wants and needs. The defining quality of this secure way of *being* is the belief that we are worthy of unconditional positive regard. Coming to accept ourselves happens naturally when we feel seen and accepted for who we are by others. After all, if others can love us for who we really are, maybe we really are inherently worthy, and maybe—just maybe—we can extend that same love inwardly. Within this self-compassionate space, we can step out from under the hats we wear and the shrouds we hide behind with a naked but gloriously emancipated sense of self.

Attuning/Reflecting Opportunity

Once grounded in your inner world, consider:
   Where do you *want* to be? This is not where you think you should be, or where you think others think you should be, but where you *long* to be.

It is unnecessary to effort to produce or to force results. In fact, gentleness is an important quality of self-compassion: we can trust that when we are ready, the answers to our questions will materialize from within. Self-compassion means releasing the need to control, trusting that our inner resources are being developed as we meet ourselves wherever we are, being present to what is, and practising unconditional positive regard inwardly and outwardly.

If you were unencumbered by feelings of guilt or fear and you lived the life you wanted to live, what would be different? How would that feel? How would it change your life? What would you be doing that you aren't doing now? What would you be allowing that you aren't allowing now?

- What qualities of self are required to attain this desire?
- What are the obstacles to attaining what you desire?
- What actions are necessary to navigate the obstacles?
- When will you take these actions?

Experiential Practice

This practice can be read by a partner or recorded. Whatever you choose to do, in order to promote embodiment, it's important that you listen to it rather than read it.

- Begin with your eyes open. Scan your environment for an object you feel neutral about, with no obvious positive or negative emotions associated to it.
- Close your eyes and envision this object in your mind's eye.
- Open your eyes and scan your environment for a neutral object, paying close attention to the details, such as texture and colour.
- Close your eyes and envision the object in your mind's eye.
- Open your eyes once again, scanning your environment, not focusing on any one object.
- Close your eyes and envision yourself in the here and now.

As you see yourself as you are in this moment, shower yourself with loving-kindness. You can do this in a variety of ways. What is most important is that it feels genuine. For instance, you may use your breath, blowing love and compassion on yourself with each exhale. For those who are more visual, you could shower yourself in a golden light, letting it warm and nurture you. Or you may resonate more with mantras, choosing words to nurture yourself in the here and now. As you immerse yourself in loving-kindness, try subtly smiling, providing a physical expression of this nurturing moment.

When you are ready to open your eyes, feel your feet on the floor.

Notice how your body is feeling now. If you feel ready to take this exercise a step farther, deepening your self-compassion while still in this safe space, build on the sense of connection by doing something that taps into desire, something you will enjoy. Choose an activity that is easy to attend to in the moment like making a cup of tea, having a hot shower, playing an instrument, or sitting in the warm sun.

Additional Stress Reduction Activities

Besides the stress mitigation tools described previously (comforting touch, subtle smiling, and reassuring self-talk), there are many activities we can use as rituals to reduce cortisol, enabling us to better manage stimuli before they become chronic stressors. The key is to find an activity that feels good, one that involves more reward than effort. Immersing in an activity that sparks embodied desire interrupts the thinking mind, which is often the source of stressful thoughts and emotions. There are common strategies that tend to work for many humans, usually a form of art that draws us into our heart space. Some do this by playing or listening to music, getting lost in the beat of a drum, poetry, sketching, sexual activity, dance, or journalling. Other moments may call for something more physical, such as intense cardio, yoga, or stretching. The list below offers a sampling of cortisol-lowering techniques that have shown promise in the literature.

Forest bathing, which comes from the Japanese word "shinrin-yoku" (森林浴), involves spending contemplative time immersed in nature, at a leisurely pace, paying special attention to the sensory experience. Also called "forest therapy," forest bathing is effective in reducing anxiety, depression, and anger while increasing vigour and boosting the immune system even after the immersion experience is over (Li, 2010; Park, et al., 2007).

Emotional freedom technique (EFT) involves tapping various energy points on the body while repeating a mantra that correlates with a desired emotional state. During the process, one addresses a current stressor or brings up a stressful memory from the past with compassionate awareness while tapping on acupressure points. EFT shows promise in the research, with over a 100 studies investigating its impact. Findings show that it reduces anxiety, can be used as a treatment for chronic PTSD (Church et al., 2013; Clond, 2016), and produces changes in molecular genomics such as microRNA expression (Yount et al., 2019).

Sustained stretching mobilizes soft tissue, improves flexibility and range of motion, and reduces cortisol levels, with effects lasting into the following day (Corey et al., 2014). Restorative Yoga, a practice centred around sustained stretches and meditation, reduces cortisol and improves immune function (Eda et al., 2018).

"Shaking it off" with self-induced tremors, intense bouts of exercise, or dancing can be useful to release acute and chronic stress and trauma. Much like animals will tremble after an acutely stressful event, we too can release stress and trauma in a similar way. There is a formal, self-induced form of "shaking it off" involving the stretching of major muscle groups in the legs followed by self-induced tremors. The stretching and tremors discharge negative energy and activate the parasympathetic nervous system, which some claim has significant impacts on one's perception of their health, wellness, and overall quality of life (Berceli et al., 2014). Informally, as elaborated on below, we can also gain some benefits by bringing awareness to the stress and tension and then vigorously shaking the body, imagining the tension falling away as we do so. Short bursts of exercise or dancing can have a similar "shake it off" effect.

Exercise is a more traditional "shaking off" of stress that is known to improve mental function, boost the immune system, and reduce the risk of developing numerous chronic diseases (Basso & Suzuki, 2017). In addition to stress mitigation, regular exercise reduces the risk for several health conditions, including cancers, diabetes, and heart disease (Kyu et al., 2016). In a large US study (Chekroud et al., 2018), physical exercise was strongly correlated with mental health burden. The greatest benefits seemed to be experienced by those who exercised three to five times a week for 45-minute intervals and for those who exercised with a sports team. While there are still debates about the benefits of different types, duration, and other impacting factors such as economic status and education, having an exercise practice that you enjoy can be an act of self-kindness that seems to promote a greater ability to thrive.

Acupuncture, which originated in China and has been practised for thousands of years, involves the insertion of fine needles into various parts of the body. The needles are then stimulated using the hands or electrical impulses. Though research exploring a number of possible mechanisms for acupuncture's pain-relieving effects is ongoing, there is some evidence that it can reduce cortisol (Eshkevari et al., 2013) as well as depression and anxiety (Carvalho et al., 2013).

Aromatherapy involves the smelling of extracts made from natural sources to calm the limbic system, promoting relaxation and reducing stress (Ahmad et al., 2019). Aromatherapy combined with massage has shown significant effects, decreasing stress and anxiety and improving immune function (Chen et al., 2017; Cooke et al., 2007). Research on the effects of aromatherapy alone is lacking and seems to show mixed and inconclusive results.

Reflexology is a noninvasive technique whereby practitioners apply pressure to points on the feet and hands that correlate to internal organs and other parts of the body (Embong et al., 2015). Research is limited and largely anecdotal regarding its impacts and ability to reduce stress, with some evidence indicating that it may improve quality of sleep (Li et al., 2011).

Reiki was developed over 100 years ago in Japan. The practice focuses on working with energy fields and can be an effective tool for promoting relaxation and reducing stress (Helali, 2016). Practitioners gently lay their hands some distance above or directly on the body and use various hand movements to work with the body's energy (McManus, 2017).

A reminder that it is not necessary or even advisable to adopt every one of these activities as part of your repertoire. However, if you do not already have some of these tools in your toolkit, try a few out and see what feels good.

Going Back to Move Forward—Using EMDR, CBT, DBT, and Other Exposure Therapies to Reduce Stress

When we fall into states of fight, flight, or freeze, we cannot objectively work through difficult thoughts and emotions, often leaving them unresolved and fuelling the same old cyclical event–response behaviour. However, the intention of exposure therapy is to reimagine the event at another time, when we felt safe and supported in our environment. In doing so, we get another chance to release emotional energy that may be stuck and to work through and update old belief systems (that we realize are no longer true). Because the aim of exposure therapy is to allow and sit with emotions that were previously too intense to hold, it is important that you have a trusted and skilled other to support you. These are the people that remind you of who you are when you forget. Please consult with a therapist before using any of the following techniques.

In addition to EFT (described earlier), three popular therapeutic tools that support re-exposure are EMDR, CBT, and DBT. **Eye movement desensitization and reprocessing (EMDR;** Shapiro, 2017) involves a variety of techniques that direct the eyes back and forth while you reimagine an activating event. Cognitive behavioural therapy (CBT) was developed in the 1960s and 1970s by Beck (1970) and Ellis (1962), bringing awareness to the relationship between our thoughts (conscious, automatic, core beliefs beneath) and behaviours. This technique works toward behaviour change through self-monitoring, scheduling, and exposure-response prevention. **Dialectical behavioural therapy (DBT)**, another evidence-informed reorientation tool (Linehan, 2014), is a modified version of CBT that combines emotional regulation, reality testing, mindfulness, acceptance, and stress tolerance.

In an extensive meta-analysis of research conducted in the last decade, researchers Khan et al. (2018) found that EMDR and CBT were equally effective at reducing depression, but EMDR was superior in its ability to reduce anxiety and PTSD symptoms. Ultimately, re-exposure practices, whether used as a part of formal therapy or not, are an excellent tool to work with past traumas that are being projected into the present day. These practices reduce the intensity of past traumatic experiences until they are no longer perceived as a threat by the nervous system.

Immersing in Felt Sense Through Expressive Writing

Expressive writing can be used as a standalone practice or as a supplement to psychotherapy. It involves writing freely and emotionally without worrying about technique (Reinhold et al., 2018). You name, feel, express, and release emotions; it is most effective when you feel a desire to do it and are free of distractions. Research shows that this practice can reduce symptoms related to anxiety and depression (Smyth et al., 2018) and improve cognitive abilities, prosocial behaviours, pain, fatigue, and overall well-being (Tonarelli et al., 2018). Those with more avoidant coping strategies can find it challenging to stay emotionally engaged, but to reap the benefits of the practice, remaining connected to the felt sense is imperative (Sabo Mordechay et al., 2019). For those on the more avoidant end of the spectrum, it may take some time and tweaking (distancing vs. immersion, as described in the next paragraph) to promote a sense of safety and to develop a greater tolerance for the uncomfortable emotions that may arise. Twenty-minute sessions are sufficient, with greater benefits accruing when sessions are longer and more frequent (Reinhold et al., 2018; Sloan & Marx, 2018).

There are different strategies that take into account our tolerance for uncomfortable emotions and whether we are prone to coping with this discomfort by avoiding our felt senses. Some will find that using a distancing strategy, whereby they reflect back on an event, can promote adaptive self-reflection and prevent avoidant tendencies (Sloan & Marx, 2018). Others will find that immersing in the topic or event, by imagining that they are going through it again, will promote a greater ability to feel, express, and release painful emotions (Sloan & Marx, 2018). There are no guidelines on the topic—what is important is the ability to feel the emotions related to the topic. For some situations, it may be helpful to write about the same topic or event multiple times, enabling deeper reflection and more opportunity to feel, express, and release related emotions.

Strengthening Practice
Reduce Stress and Promote Well-Being With Expressive Writing

The following activity is based on research by Tonarelli et al. (2018) on expressive writing. Find a quiet and private place. You will spend this time writing about the thoughts and feelings that arise when you think about a topic or event that continues to emerge in your present day (via projections), causing adverse impacts in your life. This might be a past or present event or topic that is causing you distress. Ideally, you will explore this topic or event prior to analyzing it with others, which enables you to drop in to connect with the felt sense of the event, rather than getting distracted by cognitive analysis, which often prevents us from feeling the associated emotions. Don't worry about grammar and spelling. Promote a sense of emotional safety by choosing an environment and process that ensures your writing will be confidential; to further instill this, you might even plan on disposing of (or burning) it when done.

When you are ready to begin, set a timer for 20 to 30 minutes. Write about the event or topic, then write about the emotions that emerge, and then write about what it means to you now. When the timer goes off, put your writing in a safe place or dispose of it.

For the next writing session, if the event or topic you wrote about previously continues to feel emotionally charged, repeat the same process. When it feels neutral, meaning that you are experiencing greater objectivity and have perspective, you are ready to move on.

SUBSTANCE USE: USING TO ESCAPE OR TO HEAL?

We all use substances in different forms and for different reasons. Both substances and activities can be medicine for us, helping us regulate the "noise" so that we can better tune into the "signal." Where we often run into problems is when we use substances to escape from stressful thoughts and emotions, ignoring our internal alert system and avoiding the pain of old wounds. Emotional pain, much like the pain produced from a sliver, cues us to deal with a potential threat. Whether or not it is an actual threat, if it *feels* like a threat, then it is worthy of our attention. Feeling our wounds is part of the healing process. Allowing ourselves to feel a wound (even if it involves suffering) is like saying, "I see you. I hear you. I feel your pain, and I am here for you." Like grieving, healing a wound is a process we must walk through, not around.

> *No tree, it is said, can grow to heaven unless its roots reach down to hell.*
>
> C.G. Jung

The question is not whether we use substances; it is *why* we are using them. Having a third party's objective perspective is helpful when we cannot attain it ourselves. For example, this can include using pharmaceuticals in partnership with a physician or taking advice from a counsellor, trusting that they have our best interests in mind.

Soaking in the Inner World: Moving Through the Layers

> *Your visions will become clear only when you can look into your own heart. Who looks outside, dreams; who looks inside, awakes.*
>
> C.G. Jung

For many, taking refuge in their inner world might feel vaguely familiar, as it recalls a time in childhood when they found refuge in a safe inner space. At some point, after pushing parts of our "real" self into the shadows (making us incongruent), we may have experienced shame or anxiety that we did not have the maturity to process, and so we stopped visiting the inner world. Overtime, as shadows grow, fueling the shame within, the outer world became a welcome distraction, luring us away from the mounting trauma within. As a result, the inner world evolved into a distant and nostalgic memory. We often hear the whisper, calling us back, but it can feel too dangerous to approach. We end up filling our lives with activities, media, and other noise to avoid the silent space within. When we avoid facing our inner pain, we are actually missing out on a great gift, a sacred retreat that is available to us at all times, no matter the passing weather. While not quick and certainly not easy, dropping into the inner world and moving through our emotional layers is necessary to thrive.

So far, I've mentioned quite a few times the idea of "dropping" into the inner world. Let me explain a little bit more about what I mean by that. For me, and for many others, the inner world is what I experience when I calm my body and let external stimuli fall into the background, turning my attention to internal stimuli. I call it an inner "world" because of the complexity of sensation and experience I perceive when I focus internally. I use verbs like "dropping," "soaking," and "sinking" to describe the experience of this quiet inner centring because it feels like settling deeper into myself. Some people do the same by following a formal practice or rituals, taking regular time to go inward through meditation, contemplation, or even prayer. The term is not so important as the experience and the effect of supporting our congruence, that is, closing the distance between our "real" and "ideal" selves.

Based on my experience, the inner experience presents itself in layers, intertwining with our states of consciousness as we drop deeper into the inner world. The first, or most palpable layer, is the physical. The physical layer is often represented by sensations related to tension, pain, and restlessness.

Once our thoughts and physical sensations fall into the background, we can quietly draw our attention into our inner world, creating space for unresolved emotions to bubble up for healing. Many people stop at the emotional layer, unable to witness their emotions objectively. When our emotions bubble up and we can't step back, we are prone to interpreting our feelings as facts rather than information. In turn, when we experience our emotions as facts, we are likely to feel threatened and insecure, making us less equipped to resolve whatever challenge is at hand.

To move through the emotional layers of our inner world, we need to engage:

- Mindfulness to keep us in the present moment
- Curiosity to cultivate nonattachment between the sensation and us, the observer of the sensation, and
- Self-compassion to soothe the wound that has come up for healing.

With objectivity and self-compassion, we can now allow unresolved emotions from the past to come up, stay as long as they need to heal, and dissipate when ready. As we practise softening through the physical layer, sinking deeper into the emotional realm, releasing stuck energy as we go, we clear space within. The more space, the less "noise." Within this spaciously safe inner world, the more vulnerable parts of ourselves—those parts that faced rejection at some point in our life—can emerge from the shadows.

Finally, once we've moved through the stuck energy, we connect to the stillness of our essence. It is here that we taste, even if for fleeting moments, reprieve, peace, and a sense of euphoria that erupts from an endless sea of love within.

THE DISCONNECTED SELF

When we lose our connection with the inner world, we lose contact with the compass that guides us and aligns us. The disconnected self feels threatened by emotional messages; these messages feel ambiguous, confusing, and haunting when we cannot view and interpret them through the lens of the higher, connected, and empowered self.

The disconnected self yearns for the love that can only come through connection; as a result, it feverishly seeks belonging and approval from the external world. When events or people in the external world threaten our sense of belonging and approval, the disconnected self's very being feels threatened, ushering in acute feelings of stress. Love and acceptance are primary human needs, and because of this, we often do whatever it takes to attain them, including rejecting and hiding the parts of ourselves that we believe are unlovable. The disconnected self, believing it must conform to an "ideal" to be worthy of love, becomes more and more incongruent, and within this incongruence shame festers. The emotional messages that make it across the disconnected threshold cry out, sending warning after warning. Each warning feels like an ultimatum that, if articulated, may sound something like this:

> *Something is wrong, the authentic parts of you, the magic you hold, the power you wield, it longs to walk with you in the light; to hold you in suffering, to help you in uncertainty … it waits to be called out from the shadow. The thoughts and actions you are serving do not align with your essence. You are not living because the "real" you remains in the shadows. The fictional character (the "ideal") that you are projecting into the world is powerless, lonely, and terrified of being exposed for the illusion it is.*

Yes, bringing your "real" self into the light comes with risks. Change can be difficult for many, and as a result, some will disapprove of your actions. For a time, they may grieve the loss of what was; this is normal, and it will pass. They may feel irritated; this too shall pass. You are part of a much larger puzzle; as you move your puzzle pieces into place, you push against the edges of the pieces around you, unearthing all sorts of projections; this is normal, and it will pass. The risk of remaining disconnected, not manifesting who you are in the world, unable to really live, is a far greater risk than the temporary "noise" that emerges on the surface.

> *We live in the light, where the beauty of the real self can be seen and celebrated. Step into the light.*

REFRIENDING THE BODY: LEANING INTO THE INNER WORLD LIKE A DEAR FRIEND

With practice, we gain confidence as we come to see the benefit of being present with our emotions, even and especially the uncomfortable ones. As we step back to witness our emotions as messages, as letters to open, we gain insight into wounds that are ready to heal. This compassionate reorientation infuses our effort with meaning, which is exactly what we need to be willing to do to invest in the vulnerability of the process. As we remove a layer of stuck energy, there is often another layer underneath—one that, until now, we were not ready for. With each release, we feel lighter, more whole. Piece by piece, we retrieve another part of ourselves from the shadows.

Remember, we spent many years pushing components of our "real" self into the shadows; it can take just as many years to retrieve them. Patience is difficult, but slow and steady is definitely the quickest route there. When we move too fast, the body contracts in fear. Healing occurs when the body feels ready, titrated to enable us to digest past traumas in layers. Recognizing that this is how healing works, we can endure suffering with a sense of meaning and hope, trusting that we will be held and resources ourselves in whatever way we need.

You are not your emotions. They are "others," benevolent messengers. While they may be misdirected, they always have your best interests in mind.

 Attuning/Reflecting Opportunity: Resourcing From the Inner World

Consider your own tendencies. When you consider your orientation to life, how confident are you in your ability to manage the weather of the outer world? How often do you look inward for guidance as opposed to relying solely on the advice of others?

Recall a recent event where you felt threatened by a person or event. How did your mindset or perception of a potential threat to a primary need impact your experience of the stimulus or stressor? How did it affect your decisions and relationships? Now that you have space between the event and this moment (nonattachment), would you say that the stimulus was an actual threat to a basic need?

Clearing Practice: Reframing Thoughts and Uncomfortable Emotions

We delight in the beauty of the butterfly, but rarely admit the changes it has gone through to achieve that beauty.

Maya Angelou

With the rise of trauma-informed care initiatives, we as care providers are increasingly aware of the impact that trauma has on our clients. However, we rarely acknowledge how our own traumatic personal and professional experiences impact us. As we develop our roots, gaining a sense of safety in our inner space, past adversities that we didn't feel equipped to integrate will often come up for healing. Recognizing and reframing this as a normal part of healing enables us to embrace it as a good sign; it means we are now ready to digest experiences we didn't feel comfortable or ready to address before. As we practise allowing these experiences to bubble up, we gain a sense of confidence in our ability to welcome them, digest them, and when we are ready, let them go.

We cannot control when or which thoughts will spring up. However, we *can* control how we manage them. If we assume thoughts are true, we are likely to react. Conversely, if we interpret thoughts as information to consider that may or may not be true, we are more likely to manage the thoughts objectively, which will lead us to taking mindful action that mitigates the stress response.

The work of Katie and Mitchell (2003) provides a simple technique to objectively investigate the veracity and impact of our thoughts. There are six steps:

1. Acknowledge the thought by saying it out loud or writing it down.
2. Cultivate curiosity by asking yourself if it is true.
3. Go deeper by asking if it is *really* true.
4. Ask yourself how the thought, if it is true, is impacting your emotions and the resulting reactions to those emotions.
5. Explore what you would feel/be like without the thought.
6. Consider alternative statements to challenge the initial thought.

Katie and Mitchell's (2003) simple approach is an excellent way to interrupt old thought patterns, creating an opportunity to reorient via a renaming or reframing process. When the chaff of untrue self-deprecating thoughts is cleared, our sense of the "real" self and "ideal" self converge, improving our sense of coherence. With a strengthened sense of coherence, we are better positioned to confidently navigate perceived challenges so we can get back to thriving.

Managing Our Emotional Weather

If we do not tend to our inner weather, ignoring inner warning signals, the stuck energy often manifests as chronic anxiety. Furthermore, when we are more prone to subtle deceptive distortions (noise), failing to attune to the priority signal at the moment, we will tend toward lower-quality social interactions (Hess et al., 2016). When we deny our emotional messages, subconscious projections emerge, resulting in reactions and impulsive behaviours. Resisting inner messages and reacting out of fear leads to incongruence and fuels shame. The more shame we feel inside, the more likely we will avoid the inner world, fearing the discomfort that we find there. This cycle of denial, shame, and fear persists until we interrupt it. We can interrupt the cycle by checking our "emotional inbox."

In this day and age, we spend a lot of time "checking in," taking stock of our inboxes and social media accounts to stay current on external happenings. However, managing emotional weather means keeping up to date with our internal happenings. Emotions may feel good or bad, but they are neither. Rather, emotions are biological responses to life events, based on previous life experiences and our resulting interpretations of whether the event will threaten our basic needs.

When viewed in this way, we can maintain objectivity, receiving the information that emotions provide us, without feeling attached, identified with, or threatened by them (this is practising nonattachment). It is helpful to view our emotional messages as alerts, enabling us to recognize that dissonance is speaking. When we check our emotional messages, we are less likely to store them as trauma. Engaging with our emotions in this way improves our emotional intelligence too. For instance, with practice, we will start to recognize a primary emotional signal (such as fear), distinguishing it from the noise produced from secondary emotions (the anger that flows from fear). When we recognize the primary emotion, we can direct the appropriate self-compassionate response to tend to the felt insecurity.

Using Humour to Cope With the Weather

Humour can promote connection and congruence, but it can also do the opposite. At its best, humour promotes objectivity and our related ability to keep things in perspective and optimistically reorient ourselves in situations that play out in unfavourable ways. Optimistic reorientation is a characteristic of sense of coherence and when successful, it can prevent stimulus from feeling threatening (i.e., stressful). Without this objective reorientation, we are prone to attach to thoughts and emotions that can produce unnecessary suffering. Similar to the stress mitigation strategies described earlier, humour can interrupt the stress response (activating the parasympathetic system), shaking us free from our attachment to uncomfortable emotions that result when we ruminate on threatening thoughts. All of these benefits—objectivity, perspective keeping, and optimistic reorientation—promote a greater ability to manage our emotions.

When used productively, humour actually promotes deeper learning by helping us to relax and focus, resulting in greater motivation to actively take part in the learning process (Savage et al., 2017). Another benefit of humour is that it can promote social connection by underscoring common ground such as shared understanding, shared stories, and the common primal desires to laugh and experience pleasure (Savage et al., 2017). Humour connects us to others by engaging our hearts with laughter and by promoting authenticity through expression of the "real" self. Like a spoonful of sugar mixed into medicine, humour can make communication easier to deliver and more palatable to others. Because of its healing power, humour can be seen as sweet medicine itself.

Despite all these potential benefits, we can also use humour in ways that do more harm than good. For instance, if we use humour in a self-depreciating manner, which reinforces incongruence, we are at greater risk of feeling depressed (Rnic et al., 2016). In the same way that using self-destructive humour promotes disconnection within ourselves, humour that mocks is a form of "othering" that disconnects us from our fellow humans. Humour that dehumanizes us is never helpful. Even relatively benign humour can be unhelpful when we overuse it for escapism. Plus, if we use humour to distract ourselves from inner discord (unresolved trauma or an area of incongruence in our life), we may miss opportunities to address the wound that is coming up for healing.

◎ *Experiential Practice Opportunity*

When you experience uncomfortable feelings, which is common during sustained mindfulness, try a few of these techniques. See what works best for you. While you are focused on your inner world, if an emotion is too difficult to observe, then you can:

- Focus on your exhalation, which helps to discharge emotions
- Imagine breathing white light in through your belly and out through your heart, transmuting anxiety through and out of your heart, or
- Imagine breathing in white light through the top of your head, then moving it deep down into your belly (or the place in your body where the emotion is felt). Then, on your exhale, imagine discharging the emotion out of your inner space via powerful rays of light.

These breathing and visualization practices help us to get unstuck from the experience of overwhelming emotion.

Clearing Practice: "Shake It Off"

Have you ever noticed that after an animal has an altercation with another animal, or after an animal has an unpleasant experience, they perform a whole-body shake? This is the way that animals reset after the stress response has been activated. We, too, are animals, and we can get relief by doing a few minutes of any vigorous activity that enables us to let our energy loose. Examples are jumping, running, dancing, doing a full-body shake down ("wiggling it out"), and so forth. Shaking off tension can be done alone where we don't feel inhibited and can just let loose. To shake off tension, do what feels right in the moment—the key is to follow your instincts, be authentic, and release. As a bonus, the exercise of moving freely and spontaneously is an excellent way to practise authenticity.

As children, we engaged in these authentic activities spontaneously. As adults, we often have to consciously go through the motions, relearning what it feels like to follow our bodies' cues, and to do so authentically and freely.

◎ *Experiential Practice Opportunity*

Clearing Practice: "Stretch It Out"

At times, tension will feel stuck, especially in the major muscle groups of the lower body; for example, hips are a common place where tension gets caught and stored. Holding stretches or yoga positions that release those areas is an excellent way to release pent-up energy. The key is to hold the stretch for an extended period and to soften the tension with your inhalation, releasing it bit by bit with your exhalation. Stretch until it is uncomfortable, holding it there and breathing into the discomfort. The discomfort we feel when stretching is an excellent way to practise nonattachment, accepting, and softening our resistance or tension. Wait for the release as your body opens and you feel the energy shift. Go deeper into the stretch, hold, breath into it, and let it go. Take time to reflect afterward:

- How did it feel during the activity?
- How did it feel when you finished stretching?
- Did any shifts occur?

When we hold a stretch, letting the physical discomfort linger, we practise nonattachment (taking a mental step back), enabling our experience to be as it is. Use the breath to soften the tension. Practising in this way builds our emotional management skills and sense of coherence, teaching us how to work with discomfort without identifying and attaching to it.

Navigating Hostility and Horizontal Violence Among Co-workers

Violence is what happens when we don't know what else to do with our suffering. (Palmer, 2004)

Self-oriented perfectionism can lead to other or socially prescribed perfectionism. The perceived unmet need from which perfectionism arises is a felt lack of acceptance and belonging for our real self—a lack of congruence. Perfectionism is on a spectrum, and many of us take on perfectionistic tendencies at various points in our day and in our lives. Mild bouts of perfectionism can bring positives, such as high-quality work, dependability, and a strong work ethic. Extreme perfectionism, on the other hand, becomes toxic.

The tendency toward perfectionism is born in childhood from the belief that our "real" self is not good enough, not worthy "as is" of love and acceptance. As an act of survival, we push down the "real" self and replaces it with an "ideal" that will be more palatable to those from whom we feel we need approval. Our felt need to be an unrealistic "ideal" compensates for the shame we experience when we believe our "real" self is not good enough.

In maladaptive perfectionism, we set perfectionistic standards unsustainably high. To fall short of the ideal feels like a personal failing and perpetuates incongruence, leading to shame, anxiety, and depression (Flett et al., 2002). As a result of the shame born from individual incongruence, co-workers project their shame onto each other through competitive and socially dominant ways. Social dominance and the horizontal violence that often results is a natural outcome of the snowball effect of shame. Social dominance breeds a hierarchical orientation to the world. Those coming from a socially dominant orientation are motivated to wield power over others. When motivated by a hierarchical, or "power over," orientation, we are more likely to pursue self-interest over group interests. As a result, if work environments are full of social dominance, there is often a lack of empathy for co-workers, more exclusion and scrutiny of those with less status, a lack of desire to help co-workers unless it results in personal gain, and a high degree of hostility toward anyone who might challenge the hierarchy.

When we understand that the horizontal violence is fuelled by incongruence, the way out becomes clearer. Those who are perpetuating socially dominant ways of being are victims of shame. Those who have the most shame are at the greatest risk of perpetuating the **victim–perpetrator cycle**. Shaming them even more by witch-hunting workplace "bullies" (becoming determined to find a perpetrator) only works to heap more shame on a person and fails to address the suffering at its roots. Those who project hurt were also victims at one time, and when we fixate on labelling a person in black and white terms, we fail to connect to the human and the suffering beneath the label; as a result, we perpetuate the victim–perpetrator cycle. Relational dynamics are complex and often involve unresolved traumatic events from the past. (Remember, trauma is the stored-up energy from painful experiences that were not fully processed and healed/released.) When we project unresolved trauma from the past onto our current experience, our ability to keep events in perspective is limited; this is known as *emotional transference*. Practically speaking, emotional transference happens often. It is evident in those moments when someone or something *activates an emotion that is out of proportion to the event.* While the underlying trauma may not be immediately evident, the intense emotional response makes it difficult, even impossible, to react only to the situation before us. This form of emotional transference is a significant component of our experience of shame and our subjective interpretation of events (Dzurec et al., 2017). Cultivating awareness in these moments is necessary in order to step back (nonattachment). We must work with our fear, not resist it, and then objectively investigate the deeper source of our emotional angst.

As for how to address social dominance, even though our efforts to confront "bullies" head on may have good intentions, "shaming the shamer" only perpetuates the victim–perpetrator cycle and promotes incongruence for the shamer and in the workplace. So, what does actually work? Recognizing the suffering behind the shaming behaviour and responding with compassion; this is unconditional positive regard and is the antidote to shame (Sanderson, 2015). Because shame is at the roots of incongruence and horizontal violence, unconditional positive regard solves the ongoing problems associated with workplaces ruled by these competitive and socially dominant ways of being. While it may sound trite, perhaps even impossible, when we understand that co-worker hostility results from personal shame and suffering, offering compassion as a solution is not so far-fetched. Environments characterized by *conditional regard*, where employees must assimilate to a prescribed way of being (i.e., meet "ideal" conditions) to gain acceptance, promote incongruent cultures, which in turn promote incongruent employees and vice versa.

To illustrate this how acting incongruently can play out in the workplace, consider Tom's experience.

Tom's Story

Tom works as a caregiver. He's had some compounding emotional challenges lately. He's been grappling with back pain that distracts him most days, and his father recently passed away. He's having a hard time sleeping, feeling overwhelmed by work and funeral arrangements, and trying to manage the emotional strain in his grieving family.

Tom feels anxious all the time. He knows that he is edgier than normal but does his best to put on a cheery display during work hours. He arrives at work feeling exhausted, is distracted by his back pain, and because of stress has only had a few hours of sleep. The angst he is feeling hovers just below the surface of his cheery display.

Today, Tom comes to work and learns that, for the third day in a row, the team will be working short. Partway through what feels like another chaotic day with no breaks, Gary, a colleague who moves slower than average and often appears disorganized and frazzled, asks Tom to help him with his work so that he can keep up with demands. In the past, when asked to take on extra tasks, Tom hasn't felt like he could say no (playing to the cultural "ideal"); as a result, he complies with others' requests. Albeit, even when he says "yes," Tom makes a point of communicating his disapproval with shaming gestures (looks of disapproval, sighing, exclusion from conversations). Today, Tom's fragile emotional state gets the best of him, and when Gary asked him to take on extra tasks, Tom erupts. Without even thinking, he gives Gary a piece of his mind. Fed up with the frequent shaming gestures and now Tom's harsh words, Gary storms off to the manager's office to file a formal complaint. While Tom would typically mind his language, today, he has lost control. Besides his back pain, losing his father, and his exhaustion, he now also feels ashamed of his reactive behaviour and fears he will be labelled a bully by his colleagues.

Tom's story is a composite of several stories I have seen on the frontline and heard about through my research. After we've spent enough time in the field, most of us can relate to both sides of Tom's experience. For example, we may have felt edgy or volatile because of personal or work pressures. We may also have felt the need to keep a lid on our angst out of fear we will be shamed (and rejected) by others if we appear weak. These pressures cause us to push down our "real" emotions, taking on an "ideal" but incongruent display. Our true emotions fester in the shadows and eventually spill out of us, causing us to involuntarily transmit our suffering onto others. Shaming Tom's reactive behaviour only perpetuates more shame. Workplace policies that prevent verbal aggression are essential, but they are not effective at managing cultural shaming. As in Tom's case, when we feel hostile toward another, we will find subtle ways to let them know (think of the judging glances, sighs, and exclusion). Passive aggression can have the same impact as direct expression of disapproval, and can sometimes be worse because it makes it more difficult for the other person to respond.

When hostility between co-workers plays out, we can break the cycle of shame by bringing unconditional positive regard. For instance, even though Gary is slower to complete his tasks, Tom can accept that he struggles in this area, but also appreciate the extra time Gary takes to care for his patients, frequently bringing a positive attitude to the workspace. Tom can accept this downside of Gary's, knowing he is doing his best and that he has plenty of upsides too. This acceptance of Gary prevents him from feeling resentful of his shortcomings. Furthermore, because Tom is largely congruent at work (feels safe expressing himself), he can say "no" to extra requests when he is falling behind in his own work. Flipping the lens, if Gary can tap into unconditional positive regard, he would have a greater ability to step back from Tom's projection (nonattachment), recognizing that Tom is not himself lately and that his overreaction isn't personal. We all need to take responsibility for our actions, or more accurately, our *reactions*, making amends when necessary. Unconditional positive regard does not excuse abusive and shaming behaviour. However, when we recognize the suffering beneath the projection, we are more able to tap into the compassion required to offer grace and forgiveness when we and our colleagues need it most.

When another person makes you suffer, it is because he suffers deeply within himself, and his suffering is spilling over. He does not need punishment; he needs help.
Thich Nhat Hanh

Self-compassion is unconditional positive regard for self, which is a precursor to providing compassion and unconditional positive regard for others. How we view ourselves informs how we treat ourselves, which in turn determines how we treat others. Self-compassion enables us to have compassion for others, which is the antidote to work cultures entrenched in socially dominant, competitive, and hostile ways of being and relating. When we understand that the projections of others often activate our own projections, we are more likely to recognize the opportunity to heal our unresolved dissonance rather than fixate on the other person's problems. This willingness to use projections as a mirror, reflecting our own unresolved wounds, is a core principle within the healing framework of many 12-step programs. If you aren't familiar with the 12-step framework, their three underlying tenants are as follows:

1. Personal responsibility
2. A focus on progress over perfection, and
3. Communities of unconditional positive regard.

The steps that people use to steer clear of substances and co-dependance can also help us steer clear of our shaming practices. When the community in which we belong provides unconditional positive regard, social dominance becomes unnecessary and unappealing. When someone tries to bring social dominance behaviour into a strong community, they are met with compassion. This compassion shows that we are unconditionally regarded—the threat that usually activates our need to dominate in order to avoid rejection is simply not there (see Chapter 5, Figure 5.1).

Attuning to Self

If you don't heal from what hurt you, you'll bleed on people who didn't cut you.

Author unknown

 Attuning/Reflecting Opportunity

Reorienting: Learning to Welcome and Digest Unresolved Emotions One Layer at a Time.

Imagine a recent experience where you felt hurt or threatened by a co-worker's words or behaviour. Recall that shaming behaviours, the root of horizontal violence and hostility, are often a subconscious projection of one's own suffering. From this lens, how might your response toward someone else's projections change? How might you react differently, knowing that their behaviour is essentially the spilling over of their own shame and suffering?

Self-destructive thoughts are a natural byproduct of incongruence and low self-compassion. How we treat ourselves is how we view and treat others.

Taking it one step further, intense feelings of threat are usually the result of unresolved pain and trauma resurfacing. At every opportunity, the body will attempt to heal. If the body is reminded of an unhealed wound, it will present the wound for us to heal it.

When we feel victimized by someone else's behaviour, we are taking their behaviour personally, interpreting it as a threat. When we bring awareness to the perceived threat, we have an opportunity to reorient ourselves in the moment and heal unresolved issues from the past. The moments when we are activated or threatened act like a beacon, illuminating our old wounds. This illumination enables us to mindfully and compassionately validate where we feel hurt, digest the feelings, and let them go.

How might viewing moments of threat as a beacon, or a call to heal, change your feelings about people and events that seem threatening? What reminders or practices might help you take on this perspective when conflict arises in the workplace?

Instead of asking, "Why did this happen to me?," ask yourself, "What is this experience trying to teach me?"

Clearing Practices: Coping With Bad Weather

By reflecting on personal experiences, there is an opportunity to develop awareness and acceptance of unique belief systems, values, resources and/or barriers that impact the ability to practise self-compassion and engage in thriving. Self-reflection breeds self-awareness, which is a component of mindfulness.

 Attuning/Reflecting Opportunity

Recall your typical day and think about your typical routine. When do you feel anxious during your work and personal life? Are there common stimuli that seem to activate feelings of anxiety? Can you name the need that is going unmet and producing a feeling of threat?

Whether real or imagined, a perceived threat produces as stress response.

 Experiential Practice Opportunity

Try connecting to a feeling of threat that you often encounter at work, perhaps a person or an event that activates a stress response. Once connected, try a new cortisol-lowering tool (one of those described earlier or one of your own). Sit for a minute or two after engaging in the activity. Consider how you feel and notice whether you feel any shifts. Pick a word or phrase that describes how you feel. Reflecting on how each activity resonates (or fails to resonate) with you is an essential part of attuning to the tools that work best for you. A technique you try today may not stir you, but you may feel drawn to it in the future; consider it a new tool in your tool belt.

There is not one path for all. It takes courage to trust and prioritize the whisperings of the inner voice as the wisest counsellor. The inner voice aligns with your calling, directing your path according to your unique needs and desires.

Strengthening Practices

A. Generating Unconditional Positive Regard

Breathing in, I smile. Breathing out, I release. Breathing in, I dwell in the present moment. Breathing out, I feel it is a wonderful moment.

Thich Nhat Hanh

Generating unconditional positive regard for self (self-compassion) requires us to refriend the inner world. To do this, we must spend time there. In the mental health world, this activity would be considered a form of priming, whereby we attune to the desired *being* state, enabling us to come back to this frequency in situations when we feel less secure. Keep it simple and make it your own. I'll provide some ideas, but ultimately you know you best. Play with creating a scenario that your body enjoys.

For example, drop into the inner world by closing your eyes and taking natural breaths in and out of your nose. You can move your focus from your head to your heart by imagining the breaths flowing in and out of your heart. Perhaps you can even quietly repeat words that resonate with you, like *grace* or *mercy* (sending loving-kindness to yourself) on the inhale and *compassion* (pouring out loving-kindness to others) on the exhale; or, if you are a visual person, you might imagine white light coming in and out of your heart, purifying as it comes in and blessing others as it flows out.

Imagine somebody from whom you have felt a sense of unconditional positive regard. This can be a person, pet, or spiritual figure—whoever resonates for you as unconditionally loving. You know that no matter what you have done, what you are doing, or what you will do, they emanate a sense of unconditional positive regard for you. While your eyes are closed and you continue to breathe through your heart, imagine this person or being in front of you, emanating love and compassion. Breathe in their atmosphere; embody their love and compassion.

B. Using Music to Stir and Deepen Desire
Music is a powerful tool to stir our desires. We all require and therefore desire to be loved for our "real" self. It is a powerful way to cultivate feelings of connection for the self, promoting self-compassion.

Next time a song stirs you, turn your focus to your inner self, kindling a sense of appreciation for your essence, offering loving-kindness to all components of yourself. Think about the journey, the suffering, the triumphs, and the humorous side of life too. Send love and compassion to yourself: the self of the past, the present, and the future. Have your more secure self soothe your less secure self, much like you would comfort a dear friend. Reach out to another, reminding yourself that you are not alone—we (humankind) are all in the same boat, longing to be congruent and experiencing shame in times of incongruence.

C. Reconnection to the Body

Your body is your first home: 'Breathing in, I arrive in my body. Breathing out, I am home.'
Thich Nhat Hanh

While dropped in, imagine three or four ways in which you are grateful for your body. How has it served you? Move through the events of your life, acknowledging the journey you have travelled with your body. Recognize the resilience, forgiveness, and persistence of your body. Now, affirm yourself by saying to yourself, "I am grateful for this body." Feeling a sense of gratefulness is key. If you lose touch with the feeling, go back, imagining and immersing yourself in the events for which you are grateful. Then go back into focusing on the phrase, remembering how you experience the beauty of this world through the senses of the body.

Other examples of affirmations that promote connection are:

"I am free to love and accept this body." (Promotes acceptance.)
"I have everything I need within; I already know all of the answers." (Promotes trust.)
"I am a beautiful, self-expressed being." (Promotes self-expression/congruence.)

Quietly repeat each phrase to yourself. You can choose one for an entire sitting or transition to another phrase that feels right to you. If it feels more natural to create your own phrase, then please do so! The more you can connect to the feeling underneath the words, the more effective this exercise will be.

Clearing Practice Tip: Using "I" Statements

Be mindful of using first-person statements when self-soothing. It often feels more natural, but it isn't helpful when intense emotions present. "I" statements can cause us to overidentify with thoughts and emotions, limiting our ability to objectively manage them. For instance, when anxiety wells up, if I say, "I have anxiety" or "my anxiety," I am more likely to feel held hostage by the emotion, producing a felt threat that makes it difficult to impartially investigate its origin. However, if I say (or think), "There is anxiety. Tell me about yourself. What thoughts or past experiences are you emerging from?" I am more likely to cultivate a sense of curiosity and nonattachment, which will mitigate feelings of threat. When we aren't caught up in a nervous system response, we are far more able to provide acceptance and compassion toward the emotion and to identify the thoughts or area of incongruence at its roots. There are no hard and fast rules here, only suggestions for you to try, enabling you to identify what works best for you.

The Challenge: Navigation

Let's circle back to the example of Mark, a first responder who is struggling with a heavy workload, co-worker tensions, and a lack of control in life. Some of Mark's contextual challenges may not be immediately changeable, but he can adjust how he receives and tends to his internal world. What could help him feel, hear, and adequately tend to the information that his emotions are trying to relay? How can Mark respond to and navigate the challenges that are causing a stress response at work?

Because stress results from a primary need that feels threatened (or reminds us of a past event where a need was indeed threatened), it is helpful to understand where it is coming from. Stepping back enables us to come to know the source of the activation so we can take action to defuse it.

The RAIN (Brach, 2013) framework provides a process that can help Mark receive and respond to emotions. When Mark feels empowered to tend to his emotions, he will feel a sense of agency that will buffer him from chronic stress and hostility, both of which emerge as a result of feeling out of control.

The components of the RAIN framework are as follows:

- **Recognize:** He can recognize and cultivate an awareness of when he feels anxiety and resentment.
- **Allow:** He can allow whatever emotions emerge to fully surface (refraining from labelling them as good or bad), staying with his body as they come and go instead of resisting, distracting himself, or dissociating from them.
- **Investigate:** He can cultivate nonattachment by exploring the felt sense, following its ebb and flow, noticing how it presents in the body, and getting a sense of the core fear beneath it.
- **Nonattach:** Investigating enables Mark to see the emotion as an "other." It is not him nor does it define him—it is simply a messenger for him to consider. Nonattachment diffuses the sense of threat, as we are no longer identified and stuck to the feeling.
- **Nourish:** Once in a position where he can step back, Mark can come to the emotion from a place of agency. With agency, he can provide unconditional positive regard inwardly (self-compassion), the core ingredient necessary to enable the emotion to pass and the wound beneath it to heal.

Once Mark tends to the emotion on the personal level, he is more likely to feel empowered to tend to the changes necessary on the systemic level. A focus on the systems and contexts surrounding us is just as important as the inner work. Working on the outer from an empowered and whole inner place promotes agency and ensures that the contexts in which we live and work promote, or at the very least do not prevent, human flourishing.

 Attuning/Reflecting Opportunity

As we continue to reconnect, moving from the disconnected thinking mind to a deeper heartful way of knowing, we improve our ability to distinguish the signal from the noise, enabling us to align with what resonates and to let go of unnecessary distractions. What in your life feels like an obligation (noise)? How can this obligation be altered to better align with signal (desire, meaning)?

Attuning for the Journey Ahead: Strengthening Sense of Coherence

We are coming to know how to mitigate stress, the noise that distracts us from the "signal" of who we are and the wealth of resources we have within. By tuning in this way, we are more able to navigate the weather systems that swirl around us, seeing them for the "noise" that they are. We do this by attuning to the inner world. In this embodied state, with nonattachment and compassion, we can tend to and release stuck energy. Ultimately, we improve our ability to reorient ourselves to the weather, preventing it from becoming a distracting stressor.

Now, we dig deeper, *strengthening* our sense of coherence through mindful reorientation.

CHAPTER 7

Strengthening Sense of Coherence: Mindful Reorientation

In any given moment, we are either in a mindless state or a mindful state. When antici-
pating what might come, anxiety creeps in. When replaying what has passed, discontent-
ment creeps in. When attending to the present moment, we accept and rest in what is.

Strong roots develop from personal authenticity and in connection with who we are and how we connect to and navigate life. From this deeply grounded place, without self-consciousness, we can *be* in the moment, enabling us to live with joy and purpose. In Chapter 6, we focused on distinguishing the "signal" from the "noise." Mindfulness is exactly how we develop our skills to do just that. When grounded in the present moment, with no thoughts of the past or future, we can reorient ourselves from thinking to sensing, from *do*ing to *be*ing. By reorienting in this way, we connect to our life force, allowing us to be rooted in a more optimistic and confident way of being in the world. From this place, how we manifest in the world is congruent with how we feel in the world. We can self-compassionately resource in times of need and abundantly give in times of plenty. Ultimately, we know that we will be okay, that we have what it takes to navigate passing challenges, and that life is meaningful and manageable. This is what our most congruent and coherent selves look like. Stepping into the stream of mindfulness is the current that moves us along in the process.

We are coming to recognize when we get caught up in thoughts as we learn to listen to the body's cues. We are attuning to what it feels like to be in the flow of *be*ing and to quickly clear out the "noise" that disembodies us. Now we strengthen our sense of coherence through *mindful living*, helping us shift from the scarcity that flows from obligational *do*ing so that we can step into the stream of abundant *be*ing.

While the term *mindfulness* suggests that it is a form of thinking, it is in fact the opposite. *Awareness* is a more accurate term for this state of consciousness than *mindfulness*, as it is not limited to the thinking mind. We can observe the thinking mind, just as we can our emotions, sense perceptions, and intuition, energetically sensing and noticing things both internally and externally. Mindfulness is a container for the various perspectives from which we experience life. What we attend to literally *constructs* our reality, and what we attend to grows. We can *choose* to cultivate a watchfulness or awareness of swirling thoughts versus cultivating more thoughts about our thoughts. By being aware, we transcend the thought cycle, empowering us to use thoughts as a tool rather than letting ourselves feel oppressed by them.

Meditation could then be defined as sustained mindfulness, or mindfully tending to our *being* state for sustained periods of time. Conversely, mindful awareness brings the quality of meditation into any activity.

The Challenge: Orientation

By considering someone else's challenge, or working with another to consider ours, we cultivate nonattachment. We can often find comfort in knowing that we are not alone and that we can learn from and with each other. Working from this more objective space, we mitigate the stress response. We can then reorient from this position of strength, thus improving our ability to use all our biological, intellectual, and spiritual capacities. With this benevolent orientation, we can face adversities with confidence, knowing we have the resources and support necessary to navigate life's challenges.

Let's practise by considering Robert's challenge. Robert is in his early thirties and is wearing a variety of hats, including his newly minted family physician hat, his father hat, and last but certainly not least, his hat as a life partner and his caregiving hat for this life partner, who has become progressively more disabled with a terminal health condition. Every day seems to bleed into the next as Robert tends to daily urgencies, leaving little to no space to tend to his own needs. Most of his days are filled with anxiety about the unknowns ahead, with growing uncertainty and insecurity about what might unfold. Overtime, Robert has become more and more disconnected from friends, whom he rarely feels he has the time or energy for. He spends as much time as possible with his family, but he finds that the time is increasingly haunted by a sense of guilt and a growing feeling of helplessness to navigate what lies ahead. He sees how this deepening sense of despondence and disconnection from self and others is starting to impact his children. When Robert does have time to rest, he finds himself filling the time with additional tasks or picking up extra work, which feels like a necessary distraction from the uncomfortable feelings that await him when he pauses all the *do*ing. With the rising incidence of mental health challenges that he is learning about and tending to in his patients, Robert feels ashamed that he too is struggling. However, he fears that if he is honest about his feelings, his reputation and livelihood will be at stake. Tokenized terms such as "self-care" and "mindfulness" feel like luxuries that Robert cannot afford right now, and they only fuel his growing feelings of inadequacy. The career that once felt so promising now feels like one more daily box to check amid a sea of unending boxes. Each day runs into the next as he robotically goes through the motions of life. Robert feels deeply stuck.

What feelings arise when you read about Robert's challenge? Sense of coherence consists of one's sense of meaning, predictability, and comprehension of life.

Viewed through this lens, how is Robert's sense of coherence? What is driving Robert's way of being? In what ways can you relate to Robert's challenge?

Sense of Coherence and Mindfulness

When I first studied the concept of sense of coherence, I was struck by its profound parallels with the concept of mindfulness from Buddhism. Sense of coherence, like mindfulness, emphasizes a sharpened awareness of present phenomena, free of insecure attachments. The focus is a constant practice of moving from the subjective thinking mind to the objective sensing mind. From the sensing mind, we can objectively and compassionately work with passing thoughts as nonthreatening "others," emotions, and external stimuli with acceptance and nonattachment. We can objectively orient ourselves to the outside world, distinguishing the "signal" from the "noise," and we are empowered by a deep sense of meaning and purpose in life (Grevenstein et al., 2018). Sense of coherence and mindfulness underpin our ability to manage external stimuli in both our personal and professional domains. When our sense of coherence is high, we are less likely to feel threatened or stressed by the events and feelings that inevitably come our way. When low, we tend to feel victimized by life, too caught up in potential threats to see the opportunity in the path forward.

The concept of sense of coherence (Antonovsky, 1987) is made of up of three components:

1. The ability to understand and predict life events
2. A person's belief that they have the resources to meet the demands of life events, and
3. A person's ability to derive meaning from day-to-day activities.

Those with higher sense of coherence scores are more likely to have positive long-term outcomes for their mental and physical health, while those with lower sense of coherence scores are more likely to feel stressed, use substances to cope, and be affected by a variety of chronic mental and physical health conditions.

When guided by intention and grounded through mindfulness, we develop an awareness and trust in the abundance of our resources (Super et al., 2016). We come to believe that in any moment we have what it takes to succeed. Even in the moments that look less favourable, whether owing to circumstances or our reaction to circumstances, we can appreciate the learning opportunity. This relentless sense of optimism and gratitude causes the vast majority of life to feel rewarding. We can accept what *is*, stepping back from the "noise" as something that is separate from us, a construct of the thinking mind. From this more objective space, we keep things in perspective, maximizing our ability to creatively manage challenges.

Examples of assets (internal and external) that promote a sense of coherence and ultimately a greater ability to thrive are material resources, social supports, a positive childhood upbringing, and roles that bolster self-efficacy (Dames, 2018b). When available, these resilience resources buffer us from stressors and can improve sense of coherence in two ways:

1. By empowering us to acquire the resources needed to manage stimuli by modifying the context and/or by teaching us how to apply our resources to resolve the stimuli. Examples include establishing supportive relationships, adapting our work context to better meet our needs, and gaining financial stability.
2. By enabling us to feel confident that we have the resources to navigate stressors, as opposed to feeling overwhelmed by them; recounting past experiences of success; and mindfully using gratitude and optimism. For example, developing self-compassion and self-efficacy through mindfulness and goal achievement prevents difficult emotions and events from feeling threatening, bolstering our confidence to manage difficult emotions and to resolve or navigate stimuli before they become stressors.

To cultivate a higher sense of coherence, we can expand our awareness and ability to access our inner and outer resources. It requires us to live in the embodied moment, connected to our innate and intuitive intelligence.

This book uses mindfulness practices as the primary tools to expand our awareness, enabling us to recognize what is happening around and within us. From this expanded awareness, we cultivate curiosity and, as a result, nonattachment. When less attached to passing "noise," we can stay embodied, connected to our spirit and all our creative capacities. From this optimistic orientation, we have the confidence to navigate life. Practising mindfulness not only improves our focus by training our attention, but it also cultivates an open and accepting attitude toward life events, impacting our life orientation (Slutsky et al., 2016). Our life orientation (sense of coherence) determines whether we interpret stimuli as threatening or stressful, and so it impacts our ability to accept and manage the resulting emotions. This occurs because if we are in a state of threat, we are prone to mindless reactions (fight–flight–freeze–fawn), which only fuel further insecurity and harmful projections.

We become mindful when we make the conscious choice to shift from thinking mode to sensing mode. If we do not make the choice, our untrained mind will habitually slip into thinking mode, fixating on thoughts of the past or the future. This mindless thought rumination is a breeding ground for anxiety and depression. When we assume that our thoughts are facts as opposed to subjective judgements, we limit our ability to be present and see things as they "really" are. In every moment, we are either in a *mindful* state (sensing) or in a *mindless* state (thinking). The average person spends 50% of their waking hours in thinking mode, ruminating on thoughts of the past or the future (Killingsworth & Gilbert, 2010). Thinking enables us to plan, remember important events, and set goals. Sensing enables us to live and remain open to what is "actually" happening at the moment. By staying in sensing mode (being mindful of the present moment), we are strengthening our intuitive knowing. When combined with loving-kindness, we can compassionately and optimistically reorient ourselves, enabling us to integrate new understandings in our day-to-day lives.

Where the magic really happens is when our thinking emerges from our sensing or when our doing manifests from our being. This is mindful living in a nutshell.

Moving deeper into how we engage with sensing, let's look at how our emotions act as powerful cues telling us what mode we are in. For instance, when we are caught up in threatening thoughts of the future, anxiety results. Using the anxiety as a mindfulness cue transforms uncomfortable emotion into an opportunity. We may not be mindful when anxiety creeps in, but we may be signalled by the tension in our shoulders or back or by an upset stomach—these powerful cues can help us interrupt the stress response. When we experience the world through our senses, we remain tethered to our "signal," which cultivates nonattachment and enables us to stay open to what is happening at the moment. It helps us let go of the need to cling to security in the thinking mind. This skillfulness prevents us, or quickly helps us pivot away, from attaching to thoughts of the past or the future. As a result, we are more objective, creative, flexible, adaptive, and confident in our ability to manage our thoughts and navigate challenges.

Shinzen Young (2016a), a noted mindfulness researcher and the developer of Unified Mindfulness, defines "self" as the sum of our mental image (inner seeing), our mental talk (inner voice), and our body (feelings). By intentionally observing these sense components, we create space. From this space, we have a choice to act in ways that are compassionate and beneficial to all. Nonattachment is a key component of mindfulness, where we act as an impartial observer of the coming and going of different moods, thoughts, and mental states with acceptance and without judgement. Nonattached mindfulness promotes choice, shifting our orientation from subjective to objective, deescalating the reactions of the nervous system, and improving our ability to navigate obstacles without feeling threatened by them.

Space between the "signal" and the "noise" is the secret sauce of mindfulness.

When we attach or identify with an emotion, thought, or action, we are prone to feeling threatened by external stimuli, which turns them into stressors, compounds our suffering, and hampers our ability to thrive. When we run into what Shinzen Young (2016b) refers to as the "Icky-Sticky Creepy-Crawly It-Doesn't-Really-Hurt-But-I-Can't-Stand-It Feeling," we often assume we are doing something wrong. If misunderstood, these feelings will make us avoid embodied mindfulness at all costs, which many of us do by distracting ourselves throughout the day with *doing* rather than *being* (living incongruently). However, having these feelings emerge is actually a sign that we are doing something right! We are creating a safe space, an inner sanctuary, where we are ready to heal past wounds that would otherwise continue to haunt us from the shadows. The more we resist emotional pain, the greater our suffering will be. Young (2016a) came up with this succinct equation:

$$\text{Suffering} = \text{Pain} \times \text{Resistance}$$

We can dissolve resistance by (1) accepting that suffering is a part of being human, (2) accepting that emotions are the doorway to healing, (3) knowing that emotions will dissipate in time, and (4) cultivating a sense of gratitude for the healing opportunity within the challenges.

Another pathway to resolve resistance is to cultivate nonattachment between our "signal" and the "noise" of others' hostile behaviours. This is *rational detachment*, and it is an important skill. This form of nonattachment is characterized by an ability to not take the behaviours of others personally. It enables us to recognize that the hostile behaviours of others are less about us and more about unresolved hurts from the past being projected into the current situation. From this vantage point, we can keep things in perspective, without getting stuck in our own assumptions and fears. Because whatever is happening *out there* isn't personal, it also isn't threatening to the nervous system. When grounded in this rationally detached position, we can shift our focus from what is wrong to what can be done about it. On a related note, rational detachment can also be applied to past hurts that we are projecting onto our present day (see Chapter 10). If we confuse one with the other, we are apt to spiral into stress states simply because the thinking mind is conflating a past event with present-day stimuli.

The Science of Mindfulness

Mindfulness is not just a way to gain objectivity and ground in "signal." It also has immediate effects on the parts of the brain that buffer us against anxiety, depression, cognitive decline associated with aging, and the experience of pain (Laneri et al., 2016; Yang et al., 2016). By strengthening neural connections, research shows that our ability to control emotions improves, our tendency to react out of fear diminishes, and because it improves the volume of the brain's grey matter, we become more self-aware and introspective (Schwartz & Gladding, 2011; Vestergaard-Poulsen et al., 2009).

Cultivating mindfulness through loving-kindness practices regulates the neural circuitry of emotion. Those who develop meditation and loving-kindness skills activate the amygdala and the temporal lobe, which promotes emotional regulation and empathy (Lutz et al., 2008). In a nutshell, sustaining loving-kindness practices improves the brain's grey matter, impacting the area responsible for empathetic engagement, buffering us from anxiety, and improving our mood regulation (Leung et al., 2013). Changes in the brain can occur after just one mindfulness session, and with ongoing practice, it creates lasting changes in grey matter in the hippocampus and a decrease in brain cell volume in the amygdala (Hölzel et al., 2011; Kral et al., 2018). These changes translate into lower stress and cortisol levels, improved memory, and an improved ability to focus.

Mindful breathing also has powerful physiological effects. For instance, working with the breath increases performance, reduces stress, improves emotional management, and has a host of other short- and long-term health benefits (Rozman et al., 1996; Sarabia-Cobo, 2015). By focusing the attention on the chest, imagining the breath moving in and out of the heart, and then slowing down the rate and increasing the depth of the breath, we shift into a more coherent state. As a result, mindful breathing positively impacts vagal activity and heart rhythm (McCraty et al., 2009).

Studies continue to underscore the impact that our minds have on our physical health. Sense of coherence demonstrates how our confidence to manage life's challenges directly influences our risk of developing a number of physical diseases. For example, a dissertation study of 50 healers and physicians from 11 countries and 20 cancer survivors who went into spontaneous remission (without medical treatment) found that there was a strong mind–body connection that facilitated the survivors' remission (Turner, 2010). Those who went into spontaneous remission focused on improving their diet, taking herbal and vitamin supplements, and following four mindful focuses: (1) spiritual connection, (2) body/intuition connection, (3) cultivating an awareness of repressed emotions and then working to release them, and (4) cultivating joy (Turner, 2010). Though this study was published in 2010, more studies have built upon it, underscoring a similar message. A more recent study found that using mindful practices to reduce stress improved the early stages of wound healing (Meesters et al., 2017). Dozens of studies demonstrate the power of mindfulness, confirming that it can help us manage stress, optimistically reorient our thoughts and emotions, and as a result, prevent disease and promote healing.

Experience is not always tethered to the here and now; instead, it ebbs and flows between mental contents from both intrinsic and extrinsic sources. (Smallwood & Schooler, 2015).

Mind Wandering

While moving from thinking mode to sensing mode seems relatively simple, the reality is that, based on our unique subconscious assumptions (brain chunking is described in Chapter 5) and the highly stimulating environments many of us live and work in, there are numerous challenges to face. This section outlines a few of these challenges and some ways in which we can reorient ourselves when it feels tricky.

The flipside of mindfulness is mindlessness, or mind wandering. The typical person spends nearly half of their waking hours thinking about anything but the present moment (Killingsworth & Gilbert, 2010). Mind wandering is not all bad— in fact, it is an important part of how we process and digest information, often the breeding ground for creative insights and future planning efforts. When done with intention, we can minimize the downsides of mind wandering (fruitless rumination on past events or future worries) and maximize the benefits. While we can always use some fine tuning, gaining more moments of mindfulness, we need not berate ourselves for letting our minds wander. With practice and time, we can sustain mindfulness for longer periods. When our minds wander, it is an excellent opportunity to give ourselves grace and self-compassion, redirecting our focus back to the moment.

WANDERING INTO JUDGEMENT

Speaking of wandering, when doing so, we frequently wander right into judgement. As you observe your thoughts, notice how they gravitate to judgements. Our prejudices, which are subjective, limit our ability to give people the benefit of the doubt and stay open to seeing things as they are. Judging is a *normal* part of being human and a necessary component of making critical decisions. It is not helpful, however, to judge ourselves for being judgemental, as it only results in unnecessary shame. By engaging in mindfulness to switch into sensing mode, we take a step back from our initial judgements. From this place of nonattachment, we cultivate a sense of curiosity about our prejudgemental and prejudicial thoughts, taking stock of the uniqueness of the situation. Reorienting in this way puts thoughts and emotions in perspective—they become information for us to consider rather than facts. From this grounded place, we can freely respond rather than be held captive by our reactions.

WANDERING TO ACTIVITIES AND SUBSTANCES TO COPE

When we are caught up in threatening thoughts, the nervous system becomes activated and takes over. As a result, we commonly react by wandering right on over to our most trusted distractions, attaching feverishly to activities and substances to cope. Awareness and management of emotional projections enables us to challenge the self-destructive programming that deters us from reaching inside for self-soothing. To illustrate how deterrence works, let's say you have a friend who criticizes you when you are at your most vulnerable. They chastise you whenever you make a mistake and dismiss your opinions and emotions. Would you feel any desire to go to them the next time you are suffering? Or would you do everything possible to avoid crossing paths with them when you feel vulnerable? As long as the critical cast of characters continues to dominate our inner world, we will avoid it at all costs. As a result, because it feels unsafe and therefore not possible to securely attach inwardly, we will keep trying to find our security in external attachments, often perpetuating coping tendencies that do not serve us in the long run.

Training the Brain to Be Mindful

Rituals are simply the habits that bring us back to our bodies, where we engage in an intentional form of *doing* as a bridge to get us back to the business of *being*. There are two general meditation styles, which differ according to how we direct our attention. One involves orienting ourselves as the impartial third-party observer to thoughts and sensations as they arise and dissipate. The other focuses the attention on specific objects such as the breath or mantras (short, repeated words or phrases). Try a variety of practices and go with whatever resonates for you. What you desire and what is workable in the moment will change depending on your environment, your state of mind, and your time allowances. Here are some options to try:

- Focusing on the breath (see Chapter 6), which can vary from belly breathing, heart breathing, or observing the breath as it moves in and out of the body
- Focusing on short, repeated phrases or mantras that are either spoken aloud or silently, with or without movement
- Focusing on the internal world, observing the passing thoughts and feelings
- Focusing on the external world, experiencing the world through one (or more) of the senses
- Attending to a gratitude practice, forgiveness practice, or loving-kindness practice, and
- Following a guided meditation.

Rather than using mindfulness to stop the mind, which would be a futile and frustrating effort, we instead use it as a tool to calm the mind. Concentrated effort can be difficult at first, but with regular practice, the brain develops the ability to easily transition to the sensing mode and will sustain focus for longer periods. Each time you practise mindfulness, you are investing in your brain's development. When the mind wanders, remind yourself that it is a normal part of the training process; take comfort in knowing that each time you redirect your focus, you are on the right track! Practising mindfulness develops not only concentration but also patience and self-compassion.

On a practical note, as much as we may prefer to lump our meditation time into a long sitting or two a week, the frequency of our practice is more important than the duration. (Cebolla et al., 2017; Soler et al., 2014)

One of the simplest ways to calm the mind is to focus on the breath. Rather than controlling the breath—as we learned about with the regulating breath work described in Chapter 6—breathing in this way involves simply being the observer of the involuntary process of breathing. Mindful breathing means cultivating curiosity about the relationship between the breath and our physiology and emotions, noticing the details of each breath—the speed, the depth, and the rhythm of the inspiration ending and the expiration beginning. Joseph Emet (2012) described it as follows:

> When we are daydreaming, the breath follows the rhythm of our thoughts. That rhythm can be irregular, because we are going from thought to thought, from one thing to another. As we continue to follow the breath instead of our thoughts, the breath gets into a steady, regular rhythm.
>
> Usually we follow our thoughts without any attention to the breath. Here, we reverse that—we follow our breath. At the beginning, we treat our thoughts a little bit like the way we treat the radio in the background. As we do other things, we are aware that the radio is playing, but we do not follow it actively. For example, when the announcer says, "Go and buy that car right now, because it is so amazing," we do not drop everything and rush out to buy it. We have learned to take an attitude of sophisticated detachment with regard to the radio. Now we cultivate the same detached attitude toward our thoughts.

Attuning Practice
Observing the Breath

Observing our breath is a simple form of meditation (sustained mindfulness) that is accessible anywhere, for any length of time. How we breathe impacts the activation of our sympathetic and parasympathetic nervous systems (mitigating stress and promoting relaxation). There is no "right way" to observe your breath—do what feels most natural to you. To begin, most people gravitate toward nose breathing, as it facilitates relaxation, and mouth breathing dries out the mucous membranes. Here are a few more tips:

* Notice the sensation and temperature of the air passing in and out of the nostrils
* Feel it move down into the chest
* Feel the belly rise to make room for the fresh air
* Feel the shifting of your clothing as the belly rises and falls, and
* Feel the breath transition: notice the moment the inhalation ends and the exhalation begins.

You may notice how the breath follows a regular rhythm. Emet (2012) describes the rhythm of the breath as that of waves on a beach:

> Like the waves, the breath comes from somewhere we don't know. Then it goes inside, and gets lost, like the waves that get absorbed into the sand. Some of the water gets

returned back to the ocean, but it is not exactly the same. Now it has cleaned the beach and is carrying back some debris and also the warmth of the sand with it. The breath has also just cleaned the body, and the out breath is warm and full of carbon dioxide. You can let yourself be guided by this mental imagery. Involve all your senses and now bask in the sunshine on that beach for a few minutes and enjoy the whish of the waves ... What is happening in the mind at this point is also a little bit like the difference between city driving and long-distance driving. In city driving, there is much stopping and starting and emotions like impatience or irritation. When you settle into long-distance driving, all those calm down. The rhythm changes.

Making and Breaking Habits

Motivation is what gets you started. Habit is what keeps you going.

Jim Ryun

Mindfulness is a way of being, an ongoing practice of waking up to what is actually happening in any given moment. As outlined earlier, we become mindful by transitioning from thinking mode to sensing mode. For instance, ruminating on thoughts of the past (where discontentment is born) or future (where anxiety is born) is done in thinking mode. Focusing on what is happening in the moment through our senses (sounds we hear, sights we see, feelings we feel, etc.) is done in sensing mode. One mode is fixated on thoughts and the other is fixated on what is happening inside and around us. Neither is all good or all bad; in fact, both are necessary for us to process and digest information.

For mindfulness to be effective, we must develop habits that act as cues to activate the transition from thinking to sensing. For instance, noticing anxiety in the body cues us to notice what is happening in the mind. Or setting a physical reminder cues us to notice what is happening in the moment or helps us do from a *be*ing state, rather than the other way around. Mindfulness efforts are cumulative. Every mindful moment is an opportunity to invest in habits that promote sense of coherence (how we orient ourselves to the external world) and congruence (manifesting our "real" selves and inspirations in the world).

We can all relate to the frustration that accompanies fruitless attempts to form and break habits. Habits are those repetitive behaviours that stem from subconscious thought processes that are cued by internal and/or external stimuli. Once a behaviour moves from being a conscious effort to an automatic response to a stimulus, it frees up our mental resources for other tasks. Unfortunately, many habits persist even after our conscious motivation has dissipated, which is why even though we may know that a habit is no longer serving our best interests, they are often difficult to change. It can be particularly challenging when social and self-**stigma** enter the picture. When perceived social stigmas exist, it often evolves into self-stigma, which then turns into shame. When we feel the shame associated with stigma, it often prevents us from asking others for support (Hammarlund et al., 2018).

Ironically, despite the impulse to self-isolate that accompanies feelings of shame, *the antidote to shame is authentic connection*. That means reaching out to those whom we trust we will give us unconditional positive regard. When we genuinely believe that we are receiving unconditional positive regard from others, despite our shortcomings, shame dissipates.

Habits intertwine with tendencies to use substances and activities to cope with or avoid suffering. We reach out for external objects when we do not feel safe reaching inwardly. Suffering occurs when we fixate on thoughts about a real or imagined threat to our basic human needs. While many of us avoid labels such as "addiction" and "substance use," which are complex and cloaked in shame, we all have habits and can relate to the power they can wield. Focusing on strategies to break habits we aren't proud of often ends in failure and fuels shame, further perpetuating self-destructive thoughts/sensations and incongruence. By focusing on forming habits that develop deeper roots, which moves us toward congruence, we improve our ability to make objective choices that serve our highest interests. Congruence improves our ability to act in ways that nourish our roots as opposed to feeding habits that leave us feeling trapped in a subconscious impulse loop. Old ways of being that no longer align with our values lose their grip and fall away.

Coping mechanisms that don't serve us in the long term are a symptom of getting caught up in the "noise," leaving us unable to tune into the "signal" of our life force and the wealth of resources at our disposal. They are a reflection of incongruence (behaviours not aligned with our values and inspirations) and low sense of coherence (lack of confidence in our ability to navigate challenges). Focusing on the symptom will not deal with the "root" problem.

While the amount of time and effort it takes to form habits depends on many factors, on average it takes 66 days to make a behaviour automatic (Lally et al., 2010). In other words, habit formation involves repeating the behaviour, in the same context each day, for over 66 days for it to become effortless and automatic (Gardner et al., 2012).

Applying basic principles of skill development (Fitts & Posner, 1967) to mindfulness habits requires effort in the beginning. We need to repeat the practice of operating from sensing mode over and over until it becomes familiar. We notice our mind wandering and make corrections as needed. With a newfound awareness of tensions, we can soften them and often let them go. Taking on the impartial observer role, we notice the difference between letting things be and trying to control them. With time and intention, it becomes easier as the rewards begin to overshadow the effort. With more repetition, it becomes automatic, and soon we find ourselves minding the moment without cueing. Because it feels good to move in this liberating way of *be*ing, we lean into it without any conscious effort. This is what it means to awaken to the moment. To be free of what was or will be. To be content in the here and now.

Attuning Practices

A. Creating a Habit/Ritual

The law of harvest is to reap more than you sow. Sow an act, and you reap a habit. Sow a habit and you reap a character. Sow a character and you reap a destiny.

James Allen

Most people will overestimate their ability to accomplish tasks in the short term (6 months to 2 years) and underestimate what they can accomplish in the longer term (3 to 5 years). When setting an intention for the long term, it's okay to dream big! However, when creating a habit, think small and simple. Each small step will move you closer to your long-term goal:

1. GOAL: Decide what you *want* to accomplish. Example: I want to be more present.

   _____

2. PLAN: Choose a simple daily action that moves you closer to your goal. Example: I will ground myself by checking in with my inner self several times a day.

   _____

3. SPECIFICS: When and where will you do this chosen action each day? Example: Every time I enter my home or office, I will drop in by observing three cycles of breathing before I begin a task.

   _____

If helpful, keep a record to motivate and remind yourself to do the action until the behaviour becomes automatic. Remember to keep the focus on progress, not perfection.

If you make a mistake, no need to ruminate on it. The practice here is to notice when you are stuck (ruminating) in critical thinking. Stop. Celebrate that you caught yourself in the muck, enabling yourself to see it, then step back from it. Remind yourself that the practice is in getting back on track. This is all a part of the process, and you are exactly where you're supposed to be. Practising self-compassion is exactly what will get you unstuck so you can keep moving toward your goal.

If you forget and slip back into your old ways, don't use it as another opportunity to berate yourself. Instead, reassess your goal. Is it one that you truly desire or did you set the goal because you felt you "should"? If the goal does not align with your desires, your are far less likely to invest in yourself in the process of achieving it. Is your plan simple enough? In order to consistently apply effort to completing an action each day, it has to be simple.

Start small! Moving toward your goal often happens in small, incremental steps. With each successful step, confidence/self-efficacy (a core component of sense of coherence) grows and you move closer to your goal. The repetitions will get easier over time, and you will be far less likely to forget. When you make a mistake, it will become more natural and believable when you continue to remind yourself that challenges are normal and that your process is good enough (and that *you* are more than good enough!).

B. Breaking Habits With Mindfulness

Making a habit requires enough repetition to transition from conscious effort to conscious ease to subconscious automaticity. Breaking a habit is the reverse of the process of forming one. Rather than working toward automaticity, we are working toward consciousness *by bringing mindfulness back to the action*. From this expanded awareness, there is an opportunity to interrupt the habit. Noticing something new about a situation or activity cultivates curiosity, deepening mindfulness. As a result, new neural pathways form.

Think of an activity you do on autopilot. Challenge yourself to bring a renewed sense of mindfulness to it. Look for something new, cultivating curiosity and bringing your focus back to the activity each time your mind wanders. For example, eating habits are a great way to practise a mindful habit, bringing more consciousness back to an action that is often automatic and mindless. It is common for our attention to wander while we eat. We focus on a screen or get lost in thoughts of the past or the future.

Experiential Strengthening Practice

A. Mindful Mealtimes

In a review of five weight-loss studies in the United States, focusing on mindful eating improved participants' felt awareness and connection to their body and hunger and satiety cues, improved self-compassion, decreased cravings, and decreased their tendency to use food as a coping mechanism (Dunn et al., 2018). Another study involving 59 000 participants with type II diabetes found that those who slowed their rate of eating were 42% less obese than those who continued to eat quickly (Hurst & Fukuda, 2018).

We often eat in autopilot mode, mindlessly consuming food without paying much attention to the sensation of eating and the body's cues. As we bring mindfulness to the experience, we gain trust in the body's cues and listen to our desires. Mindfulness enables us to notice what is new and to pick up on subtle cues. For instance, we might notice a desire to push our plate away or that what we are eating no longer has much flavour. Remember, mindfulness is a practice that takes time to develop. Your ability to develop the habit will take time, persistence, and self-compassion. When you slip up, mindlessly eating until you are uncomfortably full or forgetting to pay attention to the what and how of eating, flex your self-compassion muscles and use the experience as a learning opportunity. Each step forward (or backward) is an investment in our lifelong journey of learning.

Now, try eating a meal with a degree of ceremony:

1. Choose a comfortable spot, ideally one that is clean and free of clutter and distraction.
2. Look for food that appeals to your palate. Choose it not because it is a rational choice or because you "should" eat (i.e., because it is healthy, budget friendly, easy to prepare, etc.) but because it is truly something you desire.
3. Plate your food so that it looks appetizing to you. Is it colourful? Interesting?
4. Plan mealtimes in such a way that you can relax while eating rather than waiting until you are overly hungry or have just a few minutes to eat.
5. Infuse the act of eating with loving-kindness (Chozen Bays, 2009), perhaps not every time, but as a regular practice. For instance, using breathing to settle yourself and silently repeat the following phrases: "May my body be at ease" (as you immerse in feelings of ease), "May my body be happy" (smiling slightly as you repeat the phrase), and "May I be free of anxiety about eating." Play with phrases that resonate with you, and if time allows, expand these loving-kindness phrases to considering others ("May others with anxiety about eating be at ease," etc.).
6. Slow your eating down. To slow down, you might try setting your fork or spoon down between bites or intentionally taking a few breaths between each bite and chewing the food slowly and thoroughly before you swallow.
7. With a sense of curiosity, engage all your senses. Notice the aromas, the flavours, and the textures of your food.
8. Cultivate gratitude by immersing in the pleasure you are experiencing, including your emotional state and your degree of hunger and satiety. Reflect on how each bite of food is nourishing your body.
9. Connect to your desire partway through the meal: Do you want more or has the flavour waned? Are you still enjoying the experience or are you losing interest?

B. The Raisin Exercise

This exercise, adapted from by the University of California, Berkeley's (2010) "Greater Good in Action," requires 5 minutes, a raisin (or something similar), and an open mind. The original author suggest practicing it once a day for a week to develop a more mindful way of being with food.

- Holding—Take a raisin and hold it between your finger and your thumb.
- Seeing—Take the time to really focus on the raisin, giving it your full attention. Examine the unique texture and colour; look at where the light shines; notice the darker hollows, the folds, and the ridges.

- Touching—Close your eyes, focusing on the wrinkled texture of the raisin and how it feels in your hand.
- Smelling—Hold the raisin up to your nose and smell the raisin; notice any effect that this has on your mouth and stomach.
- Placing—Gently place the raisin in your mouth and leave it there without chewing. Focus on the sensation of what the raisin feels like in your mouth.
- Tasting—Very slowly and consciously, chew the raisin once or twice. Fully experience the waves of taste emanating from the raisin, how these change over time and change the raisin itself in shape.
- Swallowing—See if you can detect when you first have the intention to swallow, and then consciously swallow the raisin.
- Following—Sense how your body is feeling as a whole after eating the raisin.

Handwashing: Cleaning the Hands, Cleaning the Heart
Handwashing is a well-ingrained habit that is often done multiple times a day. What a great opportunity to use these frequent moments mindfully! As you step up to the sink, find your breath. As you begin the process of cleaning your hands, imagine this cleansing is also happening in your heart and mind. As you lather the soap, a practice meant to stir up the bacteria on the skin's surface, imagine you are stirring up the negative thoughts and moral injuries of the day. As they all come to the surface from a good lather, you can now rinse them off with ease. Try putting your own words to the practice, making sure you engage your heart when the energetic release and letting go occur.

A few final words on making and breaking habits. The process requires patience as well as an ability to stay open while maintaining a self-compassionate and non-judgemental approach. Making or breaking a habit takes time, and slip-ups are expected. There is often a gap between when we gain spiritual awareness and when we embody the newfound insights. Rituals provide a bridge between where we are and where we are going. Rituals act as a physical reminder to take a moment, enabling us to consciously transition from thinking to sensing. It is important to hold rituals and habits lightly, to consider and reconsider how they are helping us and when it is time to let them go.

Let Go Early if It Is Not Resonating

None of us wants to ritualize tasks that feel more effortful than rewarding. We want options, but too many options can feel overwhelming. Given that we are all unique and will have varying preferences, pay attention to what your body is telling you when you try them on. When you engage in the ritual, how does your body respond? For instance, when we remember who we are and the vastness of our spiritual resources, we tend to feel more connected, grounded, and confident. If we are performing a ritual from a place of fear and obligation, we are more likely to encounter resistance, which causes more effort. Because the nervous system gets activated when it feels oppressed (threatened or overpowered), it is more difficult, if not impossible, to remain open hearted. Without an open heart, we perpetuate our felt sense of disconnection from self, spirit, and others, which is what drove us to the ritual in the first place.

Expect It to Be Messy!

Making and breaking habits is a messy process characterized by fits and starts. If we fixate on perfection, we will find ourselves attached to black and white thinking, which fuels incongruence, shame, and a low sense of coherence; getting stuck in this rabbit hole dampens our confidence and momentum. Accepting slip-ups enables us to use them as opportunities to practice self-compassion and optimistic reorientation. The key to success is keeping at it and focusing on progress.

Ritual is to the soul what food is to the physical body. (Some, 2009)

The Why and How of Meditation Practice

Feelings come and go like clouds in a windy sky. Conscious breathing is my anchor.
Thich Nhat Hanh

Sustaining mindfulness throughout the day tethers us to *being* and helps us catch ourselves when we fall into disembodied *doing*. From this space, we receive important messages from the body in the form of physical sensations, emotions, and spiritual inspirations. It is through meditation (sustained mindfulness) that we come to know the unconscious parts of ourselves, those parts that have not yet emerged from the shadow (Jung, 1970). Eventually, repressed emotions get activated, causing us to project our suffering onto others. *Nearly every enduring irritation we feel about others is a projection of the shame we feel about our incongruence,* which can be traced back to an unaccepted and therefore unintegrated part (including repressed emotions) of our "real" selves. The more of our "real" self that remains repressed, the more we project our shame (a natural byproduct of incongruence) onto others (Jung, 1970).

The "shadow" (negative and positive) is a metaphor for the place in which the disowned parts of the self are hidden from the light of day. In other words, we do not let these parts of ourselves manifest in the world because they have been deemed unworthy of expression. Who deems them unworthy? We do—but this is not a conscious choice. In childhood, we do what we have to do to meet our survival needs. These needs include the need to be loved and accepted by others and to feel a sense of belonging in the world. If these primal needs are threatened, we adjust course, pushing the parts of ourselves that may risk our survival into the shadow. While we try to hide these parts of self, they do not stay hidden. They tend show themselves when our nervous system is activated, causing them to pop out in all sorts of unpredictable fashions. As we mindfully feel our way through the layers of our conditioned incongruence, these parts come up for healing, and if we feel safe enough (embodying unconditional positive regard), we reintegrate them. This mindful process is how we come to realize our wholeness.

We know *why* mindfulness is important, so let's dig deeper into the *how* of it. Depending on your intention, there are three overarching categories of meditation:

1. **Focused attention**—Focusing attention cultivates concentration on a singular event. You can focus on your breath or a sensory experience such as objects you see or sounds you hear. This practice works to minimize the impact of distractions, reducing mind wandering by bringing the attention to a singular event (Dahl et al., 2015). This form of meditation trains your attention, improving focus, concentration, and memory.

2. **Open monitoring**—During open monitoring, you expand your attention, staying open to whatever experience arises (internally or externally), refraining from labelling, overidentifying, and judging (Dahl et al., 2015).

3. **Compassion meditation**—Often incorporates open monitoring and focused attention, with a focus on extending loving-kindness to others. As a result, these practices impact your relationships and ability to resolve conflict, which are socially beneficial behaviours (Goetz et al., 2010).

These examples cover the overarching meditation categories. The following list will help you refine your intention even further. Be sure to try a variety of approaches before you decide that meditation is not for you. If one causes great effort, try another; experiment until you find one that resonates with you. The following list illustrates the overarching categories, which vary according to what one's needs and goals are. Each of these is included in this book in different forms:

- Relaxation meditation (body scan, passive observation of the breath, yoga)
  - Progressive relaxation (body scan)
  - Releasing tension by focusing on the breath and letting emotions and tensions fall into the background
  - Active muscle relaxation (and release of tension) via stretching and yoga
- Visualization to improve performance (imagery meditation)
  - Improving performance for a future task (athletics, public speaking, etc.)
  - Creative visualization
- Connection to self and others (loving-kindness practices, yoga, body scan)
  - Working through areas of resentment and conflict
  - Improving the ability to be compassionate to self and others
  - Connecting mind, spirit and body, including gratitude for what is
- Transcendental Meditation (intuitive meditation, entering altered mind states)
  - Using mantras and breathing exercises to access the intuitive self and deeper brain waves, resulting in alchemical healing

- Reprogramming and shadow work
  - Working through unresolved trauma, noticing and reparenting/reprogramming old and incongruent thought patterns
- Forgiveness practices reorient us, releasing us from the role of the victim and empowering us as survivors
- Using open monitoring with nonattachment, witness projections from past trauma and unresolved events, and work to accept every emotion that springs up. Welcome them knowing that this is part of the healing process. Practise acceptance, refraining from identifying, labelling, or judging them as good or bad. Successful reprogramming/reparenting requires self-compassion and nonattachment (enabling unconditional positive regard for self), soothing ourselves like we would a small child or close friend.

Dr. John Yates, a former professor of neuroscience with over 40 years of Buddhist meditation experience, describes 10 stages and four milestones in the development of one's mindfulness abilities in his book, *The Mind Illuminated: A Complete Meditation Guide Integrating Buddhist Wisdom and Science for Greater Mindfulness* (Yates, 2015, p. 6):

The Novice Meditator
  Stage One: Establishing a Practice
  Stage Two: Interrupted Attention and Overcoming Mind-Wandering
  Stage Three: Extended Attention and Overcoming Forgetting
  Milestone One: Continuous Attention to the Meditation Object
The Skilled Meditator
  Stage Four: Continuous Attention and Overcoming Gross Distraction and Strong Dullness
  Stage Five: Overcoming Subtle Dullness and Increasing Mindfulness
  Stage Six: Subduing Subtle Distraction
  Milestone Two: Sustained Exclusive Focus of Attention
The Transition
  Stage Seven: Exclusive Attention and Unifying the Mind
  Milestone Three: Effortless Stability of Attention
The Adept Meditator
  Stage Eight: Mental Pliancy and Pacifying the Senses
  Stage Nine: Mental and Physical Pliancy and Calming the Intensity of Meditative Joy
  Stage Ten: Tranquility and Equanimity

Technology: Supporting Mindfulness

While technology can distract us from connecting to our inner selves, it can also remind us to be mindful. A variety of meditation apps have been designed that provide guided meditations and check-in reminders throughout the day. You can even set reminders on your phone. For example, in a scheduled notification on your mobile device, you might ask yourself, "In this moment, are you mindful or mindless?" Mindfulness generally happens through conscious intention, so having environmental cues are helpful to form mindful habits.

Mindfulness Tools: Neurofeedback and Binaural Beats

Binaural beats are an auditory tool that uses two different beat/tone frequencies in each ear. As a result, it can alter brainwaves, enabling people to enter specific brain wave states. For instance, depending on the different beat combinations, binaural beats can be used to improve cognitive flexibility and focus (Fischer et al., 2016), reduce anxiety (Chaieb et al., 2017), or promote the ability to enter relaxed/meditative states (Jirakittayakorn & Wongsawat, 2017). In addition, long-term altering of the brain network has effects that are similar to those of meditation (Seifi Ala et al., 2018).

Neurofeedback tools, such as electroencephalogram (EEG) headbands, provide instant feedback on the electrical activity of the brain. The theory behind using neurofeedback, similar to biofeedback, is that by connecting our brain states to specific activities and feeling states, we are more likely to enter our desired states quickly and confidently. Research shows that neurofeedback has significant positive effects on cognitive performance by promoting the ability to focus and concentrate, allowing us to enter mindful states at will (Gruzelier, 2014). Using neurofeedback tools has significant potential to augment mindfulness-related capacities (Navarro-Gil et al., 2018).

Attuning Practice
Awareness Through Mindfulness

When we are mindfully reflecting, as opposed to mindlessly ruminating, we develop awareness and acceptance of our unique belief systems, values, resources, and/or barriers that impact the ability to practise self-compassion and engage in thriving. Therefore, self-awareness is an outcome of mindfulness. Conversely, focusing on the future and the past prevents us from minding the moment and often provokes feelings of anxiety and discontentment. To cultivate curiosity (and thereby non-attachment), we can step back as an impartial observer, letting our thoughts and emotions fall into the background.

If you are on the move, you can also apply mindfulness to your activities. Find a rhythm with each step, or in the case of passive activity, sit mindfully. Repeat the practice and notice any changes that occur with your sense of mindfulness and the feelings that result.

If you are having a hard time staying in the moment, drop into the inner world, to the place where you see, hear, and feel internally (letting external stimuli fall into the background). Using your natural breath, silently breath the words "right here, right now" in and out.

Or, close your eyes and focus on how the mechanics of your breathing impacts the felt sense of the inner world. Focus on our inhalation for a few cycles. Take notice of how you feel inside. Now, focus on your exhalation for a few cycles. Take notice of how you feel inside. Do you notice a difference between how you feel during inhalation versus exhalation?

Remember to take a moment for reflection after each session. Note what came with ease and what felt good. Note what was more effortful. Through reflection, you attune to the unique practices that suit you. In time, you will form your own practices, which often are a mosaic of many. Keep what you like and let go of what you don't.

When we expand our awareness through mindful practices, we can investigate how varying environments are impacting the felt sense. For instance, when you are in loud and busy environments, do you notice any physical and/or emotional changes? How about in nature? Can you practise focusing on the sensation/stimuli, observing with a sense of curiosity, reminding yourself that emotions, sensations, and thoughts are only messengers to consider, not facts or threats? Doing this enables you to step back from the initial judgements and tendencies to label things as good or bad. Let them come and go, being careful not to attach or ruminate. Doing this as you go about your daily activities promotes an ability to cultivate non-attachment, which buffers you from stress and improves your ability to creatively navigate challenges.

Focusing on the inhalation tends to promote an ability to sink into self for deep inner listening. Focusing on the exhalation tends to promote connection to others, relaxation, and emotional discharge.

Attuning and Strengthening Practices
Strengthening Practices

A. Mindfulness in a Pinch
When we are on the move, it is difficult to find a time and place to drop in for any extended periods. There will be times when we find ourselves overwhelmed with our thoughts, perhaps caught in a cycle of thought/emotional rumination that is difficult to break out of. While bringing our focus to the breath is often effective, when emotions are strong we may need a few other strategies to shift us, enabling the strong emotions to fall into the background (notice that we are not resisting them). Try on a few of these short mindfulness activities, picking one or two (or combine a few into one practice) to support you in your day-to-day life:

- Pause, feel your feet on the ground and be aware of the earth below. Look to the sky. Breathe in the spaciousness of the sky with a deep cleansing breath, in through your nose and slowly out through your mouth.
- Bring your focus into your body by placing the flat palm of one hand on the top of your head. Focus on the feeling of gentle pressure, bringing yourself fully into your body, into the present moment.
- Bring your focus to the bottoms of your feet. Move your toes around in your shoes to feel the earth beneath you. You can go one step further and imagine your feet growing roots into the earth, deeply grounding you.
- If intense emotions emerge, place a hand(s) on your heart or your belly, whichever feels comforting. As you do, straighten your back and subtly smile, empowering yourself and connecting to the joy of your heart. From this empowered place, imagine bringing the felt discomfort into your heart. Nurture the discomfort by speaking to it from your heart space or just surround it with light until it softens.

B. Using RAIN

As described in Chapter 4 and summarized again below, the RAIN framework provides a structure to expand your awareness (see Figure 4.1). Adding the cue to practise self-compassion to our sensing (mindfulness) practices is self-soothing and promotes congruence. When you complete the practice, take a few moments to be still, reflecting on the helpfulness of the practice and paying attention to any subtle shifts. Taking notice deepens and integrates the changes that occur.

The acronym RAIN is helpful to anchor you as uncomfortable emotions or sensations come up (Brach, 2013). The framework provides a process to help us receive and respond to emotions, preventing chronic stress and hostility (and related subconscious projections), both of which emerge when we feel out of control. Once we tend to the emotion on the personal level, we are far more likely to confidently enact the changes necessary to reorient ourselves to the "weather," either changing our environment or reorienting ourselves to stressors so that we successfully resolve them. Resolution does not always mean the stressors go away, but they will no longer feel threatening. Once we tend to the emotion on the personal level, we are far more likely to feel empowered to enact the changes necessary on the contextual, cultural, and systemic levels.

After taking a moment to observe yourself, choose a word or phrase that describes how you feel. Taking notice after each practice will help you decipher which tools and practices resonate with you. Those that resonate will promote connection and the ability to rest in the inner world. Hold the tool lightly, as in time another tool may call you. When you need it most, the right practice will call. Your job is to take notice when it calls, answer the call, and trust the process as you intuitively feel your way through the practice. Building awareness and focusing on the benefits of these mindfulness and meditation practices will remind and motivate you to pull the most fitting practice out of your tool belt when you need it most!

C. Improving Concentration With Breath Counting

In addition to realizing wholeness, meditation improves our awareness of the connection between thought rumination and emotional states (enabling us to interrupt self-destructive thoughts) and improves concentration and thought clarity (Jung, 1970). Breath counting is an excellent way to flex and track the growth of our concentration muscles and to practice self-compassion.

- Begin by finding a comfortable position that allows you to focus on your breath, in a place free of distractions.
- Observe your breath, letting go of the urge to control it.
- Count each exhalation until you have completed 10 breaths.
- Once you have counted to 10, start the cycle over again at one.

This exercise requires concentration. Whenever you catch your mind wandering, start over again at one. Even if your mind wanders for a brief moment, start back at one again. You can think of it like a game, challenging yourself to stay focused. Remember, it takes practice to build concentration. Mind wandering is a normal part of the practice. Each time it happens, bring your attention back to your breath. As you gain concentration, frequently making it to 10, switch it up and start counting backwards from 10.

Practise self-compassion by reminding yourself that the journey forward is about progress, not perfection.

D. Improving Restraint by Working With Discomfort

When we drop into the inner world, creating space for inner prompts, we experience a variety of thoughts and sensations that tug at our attention. These range from physical discomforts, itches, restlessness, and boredom, to tasks and insights that compete for attention.

When sensations and thoughts arise, knocking on the door of your consciousness, try taking a step back from them by breathing into the felt sensation. Creating a space by stepping back from the stimulus enables you to objectively investigate the distraction and prevents you from reacting. Practising restraint as a mindfulness practice improves our ability to exercise the same principles in our daily activities. Noting stimuli that tug at our attention and that activates uncomfortable emotions before we react to them gives us the space we need to critically think and to keep events in perspective, preventing a stimulus from becoming a stressor.

Attuning Practices

A. Pause for Grounding and Connection

Taking pause has become a widely adopted strategy to practise mindfulness as a group or individually across many academic and health care facilities. It is an excellent example of a mindfulness/presence practice that is meeting a need as it gains traction within our health care culture. The practice provided here is adapted from Demers and Roper (2018) for use in team huddles, before administrative meetings, and among individual providers as they transition between tasks and breaks. If completed in full, this practice takes about 5 minutes. As noted earlier in the discussion about creating effortless habits, the more the practice is repeated, the more quickly we are able to "drop in."

Posture
Keep your posture relaxed and spine upright, with feet on the ground and eyes closed, if helpful, to focus inwardly.

There are three parts or movements to the pause:

1. Settling or grounding
2. Expanding awareness, and
3. Generating love and compassion.

Part 1: Settling
Become aware of your breathing. Follow your breath as though you were watching waves on the ocean rolling in and out. Follow your breath as closely as possible so that your mind aligns with your body. Notice and allow a greater sense of inner quiet and stillness. Breathe more deeply to relax further; this settles the heart and nervous system. Now imagine drawing your breath down to your feet. Feel your feet on the ground and the stability of that. You might imagine yourself as a tree growing roots into the earth.

Part 2: Expanding Awareness
Listen deeply for what else you are aware of internally in this moment. Notice sensations in your body … Notice how you're feeling emotionally … Notice the thoughts come and go. Now notice what you're aware of externally, such as sounds inside and outside the room, the light, the temperature. As you scan your field of awareness, touch each thing that comes to you lightly, then let it go and continue to scan. Notice how vast your field of awareness is.

Part 3: Generating Love and Compassion
Now draw your attention back inward, to your heart—your physical, emotional, and spiritual centre. Notice the feeling of warmth and energy there (you may want to place your hand on your heart). Breathe into your heart, and as you exhale fill your body with love and compassion. As you breathe in again and exhale, extend love and compassion outward, toward each other, to fill the room. Breathe in again, and exhale to extend love and compassion throughout the hospital (or wherever you are) … and beyond.

Completing
Gently bring your awareness back into the room, to your body and the feeling of your feet on the ground. When you're ready, gently open your eyes.

Benefits of Pausing
- Nurtures and protects our health by settling the nervous system and relieving stress
- Allows space for us to process our experiences (vs. letting unprocessed or repressed experiences build up)
- Refreshes us
- Cultivates resilience
- Serves as an antidote to the common tendency to be dissociated or fragmented in our heads, whereby we feel disconnected, hold our breath, and so on, as a way of coping with chronic stress, exposure to trauma/suffering, feeling unsafe or unsupported
- Cultivates mindfulness and connection by bringing more of who we are to our work and relationships, drawing on our broader capacities such emotional intelligence and intuition, and
- Allows us to tune into what is happening in an expanded field of awareness, enabling us to act from a grounded, heart-centred place.

B. Imagination/Orientation Defines Experience

Imagination, the power to form an image of something, impacts our emotional states and enables us to reprogram old thought patterns that are no longer serving us. To illustrate the emotional impact of the imagination, notice what happens as you imagine different colours:

- Drop into the self by breathing through your heart or your belly, whichever you prefer.
- Now imagine yourself filled with the colour red. How does that feel?
- Now imagine yourself filled with the colour blue. How does that feel?
- Now imagine yourself filled with the colour green. How does that feel?
- Now imagine yourself filled with the colour yellow. How does that feel?

This activity shows the power of our thoughts. The images we focus on, our imagination, impacts our emotions. It reminds us to be mindful when an emotion bubbles up, noting the thoughts and images at their roots. Stepping back, cultivating curiosity (nonattachment), enables us to investigate subconscious thought patterns. From here, we can interrupt negative thought patterns.

C. Sweeping the Mind Clean of Debris

Most of us spend a good deal of time lost in our thoughts. From this space, we are more prone to react rather than objectively act to resolve or reorient ourselves to a perceived threat. When we bring awareness to the thoughts that are bubbling to the surface of our minds, we recognize them as "others," which enables us to take a step back. This stepping back offers us another perspective. From here, we can talk compassionately to the thoughts, much like we would talk to a dear friend whose suffering is due to loss of perspective. There are a variety of ways to step back from the thoughts that are keeping our brains in a hypervigilant state. One of these strategies is to visually sweep or vacuum the mind clean.

To begin, find a place and space that allows you to settle down with minimal external distractions. As you breathe in, imagine your breath is sweeping or vacuuming your mind clean, gathering up old and no longer useful thought patterns. When an area is clean, take a deep breath in for 4 seconds, hold the breath in for a count of 7, and with a long exhale (typically 8 seconds, but no need to count) imagine that you are releasing the old thoughts from your inner space into a dustpan or vacuum bag. Take a moment to reflect on the old belief patterns that are in the dustpan or vacuum bag.

Next you can move to other parts of your body where you may sense stress/trauma, which often feels like uncomfortable emotions or physical tension. Sweep each area with your breath, gathering and exhaling the debris out of your safe inner space. After each area is clean, focus on your natural breath and take a few minutes to notice how you feel.

D. Practice: The Power of a Smile
Breathing in, I calm body and mind. Breathing out, I smile. Dwelling in the present moment, I know this is the only moment.

Thich Nhat Hanh

Our disposition has similar effects to imagery. For instance, studies show that a subtle smile improves mood. When developed into a habit, smiling subtly has long-term social, mental, and physical benefits (Johnston et al., 2010; Lin et al., 2015; Tuck et al., 2017).

Observe how your biology and resulting emotions respond when you smile during meditation. Taking the exercise a step further, try smiling as often as you can (keeping it subtle) throughout the day, observing the impact it has on you and how others respond to you. Use mindfulness to turn this practice into a habit and reap the long-term benefits.

Attuning to Self: Goals That Align With the "Real" You

Imagine a world where we all got to incubate in a culture that prioritized well-being over materialism, the pressure to assimilate, and the fear that comes with social dominance and competition. Without going too far into the ripple effects, keep it close to home and ask yourself, "What if I held my own well-being as sacred?" Imagine it. What would you do differently? With whom would you spend your time? What would you let go of?

Dropping into the inner world enables us to decipher between that which comes from genuine desire versus that which feels like a socially prescribed obligation. Goals and actions that align with the "real" self stir us; this may feel like a *gentle pull*, a *want*, a *longing*. Accessing desire is imperative to aligning our goals with our essence. When we own our goals, ensuring alignment with our desires, we are far more likely to reach them. When obstacles arise, we are more likely to stay motivated, knowing that our efforts are a worthy investment and that we are propelled forward by a power greater than ourselves; this is living a calling.

WHAT SOIL ARE YOU GROWING IN? FROM ENCULTURATION TO EMANCIPATION

Through no choice of our own, we have had informal rules, social stratification, and prescribed etiquette imposed on us as conditions of acceptance in the world. We are handed these conditions from those that raise us and the larger culture we take direction from. These conditions are imbedded in us, and as such, they subconsciously inform the typical mindset. Our mindset is the orientation from which we interpret stimuli and make meaning. Our way of being springs in large part from this conditioning, impacting our typical mindset. For example, when raised in an environment where the dominant belief is that there is abundant opportunity for all, we are more likely to cheer others on in their success, bolstering our colleagues' efforts whenever possible. When raised in an environment where a scarcity mindset reigns, we are more likely to see colleagues as threatening competitors. When we can understand that we did not choose our typical mindset, it provides the self-compassion necessary to keep things in perspective, keeping shame at bay and the nervous system in check.

> ### Attuning/Reflecting Opportunity
>
> Circling back to "real" goals (i.e., goals led by desire), consider what it would be like to be unencumbered by feelings of guilt or fear. Imagine that you lived the life you wanted to live—What would be different? How would that feel? How would it change your life? What would you be doing that you aren't doing now? What would you be allowing that you aren't allowing now? What obstacles are in the way of attaining what you desire? What actions are necessary to navigate the obstacles? What qualities of self do you need to acknowledge or cultivate in order to take these actions? When will you take these actions?

The difference between our dreams and goals is that goals are dreams with actionable timelines and a felt sense of accountability to reach them.

Common Challenges With Mindfulness

Mindful presence, internal focus, and meditation can all be difficult, especially in the beginning, but working through the challenges is a worthy investment. I guarantee there will be times when you feel you are not "doing it right." Don't worry, this is a normal part of the process as you gain familiarity with what works and what doesn't work for you. The following are the most common challenges you'll encounter.

INCONSISTENCY

We have plenty of distractions throughout the day that encourage mindlessness, and relatively few cues that remind us to be mindful. As a result, unless we set up our own reminders to be still and present through the day, mindlessness will sabotage our efforts. Many of us are adept at multitasking and live highly sched-uled, overstimulated lives. As a result, we are more familiar with using busyness to distract us from our discomforts, and less familiar with responding to discomforts by dropping into our inner worlds to resolve them. These distractions work against our efforts to stay connected to our senses, desires, and emotions.

Ensuring variety—for instance, by sampling the practices listed earlier—is nec-essary to find practices that are enjoyable and self-soothing, but too much jump-ing around prevents us from progressing from effort to ease. Just the buildup to a nurturing ritual settles our biology and ushers us into a state conducive to self-soothing. For instance, when anxiety wells up, if we have an established routine response, the emotion will activate a self-soothing response. When self-soothing in the face of suffering becomes a habit, effort subsides and we begin to engage in the ritual automatically. Without practice, however, switching from thinking mode to sensing mode takes great effort; as a result, in a moment of stress we often reach for relief in whatever form we are most comfortable with, which for many makes external distractions an enticing option.

Here's a solution to consider. Just as we carve out time for appointments, meet-ings, events, brushing our teeth, meals, and so on, we can schedule time to medi-tate. Just like brushing our teeth is a habit that now feels easy, so will mindfulness and meditation. They might start with a great deal of effort, but with consistency over time, these practices will become easier, even automatic. Begin small, start-ing with as little as 3 minutes. Create a ritual; consistency is more important than duration. The best time to meditate is unique to each person; play with a few time slots and reflect on the impact. For example, many people find that the morning is a good time to set mindfulness intentions for the day. Another great time is after work, as it enables us to switch gears from work mode into relaxation mode before dinner and evening activities.

EMOTIONAL DISCOMFORT

If we experience a rush of negative emotions every time we sit down to meditate, it would be natural to feel resistant to it. It is important to remember that meditation is an opportunity for emotional healing. In other words, those emotions that we did not or could not feel in the past—the ones that got stuck in our bodies—will fill our inner space. They need to be felt before they can be discharged. When we meditate, we become more connected to our emotions, our desires, and our longings. Unresolved emotions from past events or traumas will often spring up during meditation, providing an opportunity for healing. Knowing that the experience of uncomfortable emotions is often a pathway to healing them can help us to avoid avoiding them. However, knowing that our focus is on healing does not always take away our suffering. Suffering is a normal part of being human. While not all suffering is necessary, at times we must walk through suffering, doing the necessary grieving work, to resolve our past traumas.

When feeling emotional discomfort, try to remember that meditation is about letting things be as they are. Your practice provides an opportunity to cultivate nonattachment, openness, patience, and loving-kindness. Rather than focusing on resisting or changing what is happening, try letting things be. When emotions are too intense or "sticky" to observe with objectivity, turn your attention to an object of focus (breath, mantra, visual sense, auditory sense, olfactory sense, etc.). Let the emotion fall into the background. Build the strengthening practices described earlier into your habit.

PHYSICAL DISTRACTIONS AND DISCOMFORTS

When we drop in, we slow down, get quiet, and tune into the inner world. However, when busyness subsides, every itch and ache seems exponentially more pressing. This too is normal.

With practice, we become adept at noticing distracting sensations and our thoughts about the sensations. We can validate them and then let them fall into the background. As we do this, we continually bring our attention back to our object of focus. Another approach is to bring our focus to the discomfort, whether an emotion or a sensation, cultivating a sense of curiosity as the emotion or sensation rises, falls, and evolves. Both strategies, whether moving our discomfort to the background of our consciousness or making it the object of our focus, enable us to view thoughts, emotions, and sensations as an impartial observer, accepting what is without feeling threatened. Creating a space between us and the discomfort is imperative (nonattachment). When we attach and identify with thoughts, emotions, and sensations, we often feel threatened and oppressed by them, which typically leads to disembodiment. However, when we recognize them without identifying with them, they do not threaten who we are. They are simply passing stimuli that we can manage. In times of frustration, it can help to reorient yourself by remembering that each difficult meditation session is training our brains and is also an opportunity to practise self-compassion. The next time an uncomfortable emotion emerges at work, we are more likely to step back from it, recognizing it as a stimulus to manage rather than a threatening stressor.

UNREALISTIC EXPECTATIONS

Meditation is a fluid, sometimes cyclical, process. There is no finish line. Some days will feel easy, while other days will feel like hard work. Sessions that are difficult, full of seemingly unproductive mind wandering and boredom, can feel like frustrating setbacks. These sessions are not failures. Quite the opposite—after a long period of mindlessness (immersed in thoughts of the past and future), taking time to meditate is an excellent way to switch gears, reset, and reorient by moving into sensing mode, attending to what is happening in the moment. Meditation enables our overstimulated brains to relax.

By cultivating an optimistic perspective (and thus improving our sense of coherence), we are more able to view all meditation experiences as worthy investments, trusting that it is all a necessary part of our development process. With consistent practice, the habits of mindfulness and meditation will become more automatic, but it is not a linear journey.

SELF-DOUBT AND SELF-DEPRECATING THOUGHTS

"Is this even working?" "Am I doing this right?" "I'm getting worse at this, not better!" "There must be something wrong with me." "This doesn't work for me." These are all common thoughts that crop up when we start something new. Feelings of incompetence are normal as we take on new habits! Practising breeds familiarity, resulting in feelings of competence and confidence; this means your practice is moving from effort to ease. Some people's brains and habits give them a greater ability to relax into meditation, resulting in greater feelings of ease in the process. Others will have to work at it more, especially in the beginning. There is no "right" way. Just as there is no magic bullet prescription that works for all people and all conditions, there is no single effective approach to meditation. What is most important is holding intentions for mindfulness/meditation that motivate us to practise consistently.

Rather than judging the self-doubt and self-deprecation that spring up, practise nonattachment. That means recognizing that any of these thoughts are just that—passing thoughts. They are not facts. When negative thoughts arise, consider it an opportunity to practise self-compassion and cultivate openness and patience. Speak kindly to the negative thoughts that spring up, acknowledging them and investigating them with curiosity. When we step back from the thoughts, we transform judgement into curiosity, creating a safe space for emotions to come and go without causing an immediate reaction. With reorientation, even the emotions that result from self-deprecating thoughts can be seen as a gift, as they can prompt us to step back, interrupt rumination, and practise self-compassion.

The Challenge: Navigation

Let's circle back to Robert's challenge. As a resident in training, a father, and a family caregiver, Robert is under immense pressure to perform in multiple roles. If Robert does not have the time and space to tend to the emotional messages he is receiving, they will eventually start to feel more like threats than neutral messengers. The more he feels that he needs to ignore his own needs and desires, the more incongruent he will tend to feel. As a result of the shame that comes with living incongruently, he is likely to avoid dropping into his inner world for soothing. He will quite likely turn the emotional volume down or off all together. Unfortunately, while temporarily spared from emotional suffering, he has also turned down the volume on his desires, sense of meaning, and passion for life. This robotic way of living enables Robert to focus on tasks without the distraction of emotions, but his ability to make meaning, creatively resource, and find joy in his day is hampered as a result.

Finding ways to mindfully *come to know* and *attune* to what provides a sense of reward in life is essential to ensure an effort–reward balance. Too much effort with too little reward leads to emotional exhaustion, disconnection, and depression. Clearly, Robert's context and commitments are promoting an imbalance that requires attention. Because Robert is subjectively stuck in the "noise," he may need outside help to address his stressors in order find his way back to the "signal" of what matters most, someone who can support him to creatively resource to navigate his daily challenges.

> ### Attuning/Reflecting Opportunity
> We are strengthening our sense of coherence by building mindful habits and aligning our goals with the desires that we are connecting to as we drop into the inner world. What activities are helping you stay heartfully connected, infusing a sense of meaning and desire in your daily tasks?

Mindfulness opens a door of awareness to who we are, and character strengths are what is behind the door since character strengths are who we are at core. (Niemiec, 2014)

Attuning for the Journey Ahead: Strengthening by Tilling the Soil of Our Childhoods

We are coming to know how mindfulness bolsters sense of coherence. From an empowered and resourced orientation, we can manage passing stimuli before they evolve into chronic stressors.

Now, as we *attune* to the felt senses in the inner world, we continue *clearing* areas of incongruence. Without getting stuck in narratives that disempower us, we can gently feel our way back to our upbringings, tilling the soil of our childhoods.

CHAPTER 8

Strengthening Our Roots as We Till the Soil of Our Childhoods

When we retrieve the lost parts of ourselves from the shadows of our youth, connection to the inner world strengthens, empowering us as we continue our journey toward wholeness.

To evolve into our most authentic selves, we need to step out of our comfort zones and into vulnerability. Vulnerability is a requirement for the authentic expression of who we really are. Relational containers that engender a sense of safety do so because they allow us to feel unconditional positive regard. Unconditional positive regard is a core primary need in childhood and beyond. It is a requirement of thriving. When we experience unconditional positive regard, we then naturally mirror the same felt sense inwardly. Once we sink into the felt sense of it, we can then take on the vulnerability necessary to express who we are more authentically. If we did not believe we were unconditionally positively regarded as children, when ready and resourced we can go back as the healer, the protector, and the parent (interchangeable with guardian) we needed in the past. In this way, we can rewrite the story, **reparenting** ourselves by tending to old wounds that continue to show up in the present moment. From this conscious and intentional place, we can now give ourselves the unconditional positive regard necessary to allow the pain, kindly tend to it, and when ready, let it go.

In this book, reparenting describes the process of directing unconditional positive regard inwardly, from a well-resourced and relatively nonattached place, to work *with* the wounded self rather than *as* the wounded self. We get to go back as the adult who now has the capacity to tend to our inner child. As we do so, we can feel the wound again, allowing the pain to arise so we can tend to what it needs. We replay the adversity, but this time we are the empowered and resourced adult, providing the love and protection needed in that moment, transforming and transmuting the pain with loving-kindness. We tend and we tend until the wound is fully healed. Once healed, projections into the current day cease, and we are able to move on from a place of wholeness.

The Challenge: Orientation

By considering someone else's challenge, or working with another to consider ours, we cultivate nonattachment. We can often find comfort knowing we are not alone and that we can learn from and with each other. Working from this more objective space, we mitigate

213

the stress response. We can then reorient from this position of strength, thus improving our ability to use all our biological, intellectual, and spiritual capacities. With this benevolent orientation, we can face adversities with confidence, knowing we have the resources and support necessary to navigate life's challenges.

In Chapters 3 and 6, I discussed typical nervous system responses (fight–flight–freeze–fawn). To learn how we can better orient ourselves, let's consider Wendy's challenge. Outside of her role as a law enforcement professional, Wendy is a 40-something single parent of two children. She had what she describes as a turbulent childhood that lacked a felt sense of unconditional positive regard from her parents, coupled with several adverse events that seem to surface in a variety of projections in her work and family life. When she feels threatened at work, she gets activated, which feels like an overwhelming rush of anxiety. This intense emotion typically leads her to feel dissociated as a result of the **freeze** response. Wendy recognizes this challenge and is becoming more aware of the anxiety when it presents, but her nervous system is too overwhelmed to allow her to sit with it.

Like Wendy, how we perceive current events is often informed by events from the past. Unhealed wounds do not go away; they remain as they are, continually reminding us of their existence via current-day emotional projections. When we recognize what is happening, we can circle back to the original wound and employ our current-day resources to heal it. We all have these projections and opportunities for healing. This is a normal part of being human!

Emotional projections show us our core (unhealed) wounds, illuminating healing opportunities. These projections include those stemming from core physiological needs (finances to support core needs, food, warmth), to safety (physical and emotional security), to esteem (feeling good enough as we are, having a sense of agency). The core wounds we carry are often the product of more than one event. There is often a pattern of events that leads to an impression or belief that we carry forward. For this reason, it is helpful to look beyond the details of any particular event, focusing instead on the core need that went unmet. It is the same unmet need through which we tend to interpret future events as threats.

What is an example of a projection that continues to show up in your life? How does this impact you at work? What people or events tend to remind you of that core wound?

Before I launch into what the research has to say about our childhoods, it is important to understand that many of us did not have a **child-centred upbringing** and that many of us struggle to provide this to our children. We are in good company! No parent is perfect, and expecting perfection from ourselves or others only fuels shame and incongruence within ourselves and others. Embracing this "progress not perfection" approach shows others and our children that we too make mistakes, have difficult days, and say and do things we regret; that this is part of being human. In this environment, it is less about avoiding mistakes and more about learning from them and doing our best to make amends when necessary.

From this vantage point, we are more apt to extend grace to ourselves and others, recognizing that holding each other emotionally hostage only perpetuates suffering for all.

The good news is that, as adults, we get another chance to retrieve those forbidden and neglected parts of ourselves, those parts we felt we needed to leave behind as children. When we reconnect to the inner world, we have the ability resolve past trauma, reparent our less secure self, and spur on the growth of the underdeveloped/childlike parts of ourselves in the process. In this environment of unconditional positive regard aimed inwardly (self-compassion), we gain the security and confidence to be vulnerable, to express our "real" selves (congruence). Improving our self-compassion is the antidote to the shame of incongruence, a powerful medicine that can finally heal past wounds. Therefore, rather than silencing the forbidden and neglected parts of the self as we may be prone to do, we can stop, listen, and respond as a loving parent or dear friend would. Nurturing the self in this way provides a safe space to feel what previously felt unsafe to feel, to listen to what was previously too difficult to hear, and to embrace that which used to feel more like a threatening enemy. We can allow emotions to come, feeling them deeply, and when ready, let them go with love. Working in this way enables us to be emotionally congruent. With time, the emotions that once felt threatening—leading us to have a stress response—are now welcomed as dear and inherently worthy friends.

Unconditional Positive Regard: The Fertilizer for Deep Roots

Within an environment where we can just *be* and feel what *is*, as opposed to having to put on a prescribed display of what others may prefer, we develop into our most authentic (congruent) selves. In this way, unconditional positive regard is like fertilizer for our emotional development, maturing us into grounded, largely self-sufficient, and self-soothing beings.

To be clear, giving ourselves unconditional positive regard is not to be confused with condoning harmful behaviours. The most loving relationships have healthy boundaries. Without clear boundaries, whereby we express our expectations and needs, we are likely to get resentful when others inadvertently offend us. Rather than viewing unconditional positive regard as a blanket approval of all behaviour, it is more accurately a blanket approval of all people, undergirded by an insistent belief in the unchangeable worth and value of ourselves and others. It is not about saying the right thing, being polite, being nice, or any of the usual acceptable behaviours. It is about genuinely believing that others are worthy of love and acceptance. It is believing that our inherent value does not change, even when we have a bad day, say the wrong thing, or do the wrong thing and hurt others or ourselves. Again, we aren't agreeing with everyone's choices; we are agreeing that everyone is unquestionably worthy of love.

Those who experienced unconditional positive regard from a parent (or guardian) will naturally mirror the same behaviour inwardly; as a result, they will evolve into adults with high levels of self-compassion. Those who are more self-compassionate parents are more able to provide a child-centred upbringing; such a childhood is characterized by unconditional positive regard (Gouveia et al., 2016). Even if you didn't receive this form of compassion and unconditional acceptance as a child, it is never too late—you can still learn it as an adult! Unconditional positive regard for the self enables self-soothing. We reparent ourselves, learning to love and accept what is, even in our grumpiest moments.

Self-soothing, a natural consequence of receiving unconditional positive regard, happens when we drop into our roots, focusing on the inner world and consoling ourselves like we would a dear friend or child. When we self-soothe, we stay connected to our desires and values amid suffering. Within an environment of unconditional positive regard, emotions are welcomed as important messengers and allies instead of threatening enemies. We can accept and soothe what is instead of substituting it with what feels like a more socially acceptable display. When we rely on external activities or substances instead, failing to attend to these emotional messages, we develop habits of distraction and dissociation, lose connection with our inner world, and add to our propensity for incongruent and often impulsive behaviours.

Self-compassion comes more easily to some of us because of how we were raised. Adults who had a childhood characterized by felt unconditional positive regard are more apt to mirror that same regard inwardly. Children who feel unconditionally accepted and supported are more likely to express and process their emotions instead of repressing them. Development of these skills is a natural outcome of a nurturing childhood influenced by parental values, child-centred parenting, and an experience of emotional closeness (Fossion et al., 2014). Because they received this type of nurturing, some caregivers will have developed emotional management skills in their childhood, which they can then use with ease as adults and professionals in their place of work. Those who missed out on this opportunity in childhood will enter adulthood and their professional role with a distinct disadvantage in terms of their coping abilities. If this is the case, as adults we can *in this moment* learn to emulate the kind of environment we needed to develop self-compassion as a child. We do this by working with like-intentioned others in relationships that feel safe and that can mirror unconditional positive regard. From this secure and resourced place, we can now pay attention when emotions arise and lean into the message they are bringing us. Perhaps there is a gift within the message, a healing opportunity that will lighten the load on our journey home.

WISDOM WITH AGE AND GENERATIONAL DIFFERENCES

Time does heal. Or rather, the skills needed for healing are acquired over time. Sense of coherence scores, for example, tend to rise with age (Eriksson & Lindström,

2005; Merakou et al., 2016; Wieck et al., 2010). For example, one study showed that more senior staff are less likely to experience the intense negative emotions (Erickson & Grove, 2007) often associated with moral injury and burnout and are more likely to express self-compassion (Dev et al., 2018). Those older than 30 years of age often show more resilience in work environments that involve a high level of emotional stress (Erol & Orth, 2011; Lindmark et al., 2010). Conversely, Leiter et al. (2009) found that younger nurses were more likely to experience stress related to a felt incongruence between workplace and personal values, perhaps because of a lack of confidence in express themselves at work.

Another related factor that impacts the ability to exercise our values at work relates to generational preferences. Different generations have varying expectations surrounding work and social etiquette, which contributes to co-worker hostility, further compounding the stress that is leading to higher turnover and the negative mental and physical health symptoms among novice caregivers (Leiter et al., 2010). Even without taking age into account, higher levels of stress correlate with lower sense of coherence (Pallant & Lae, 2002). Because age is an additional factor influencing the ability to survive and thrive early on as caregivers, awareness and preparation for this vulnerability is a worthwhile effort in postsecondary training and novice caregiver work settings.

The Child-Centred Upbringing

Imagine you are 6 years old. You have just come home from school and are tired and hungry. Your dad is in the kitchen, working on dinner, and you are feeling antsy and grumpy. School has worn you out socially, but you're too restless to play by yourself, and finding something to deal with your boredom will require more effort than you are capable of. You hover around your dad as your primary resource, wanting his attention/tending, but because you are tired, it comes out as whining. Your dad, who is clearly irritated, tells you to leave the kitchen because he needs to finish dinner. Now you are feeling unwanted and unloved, which evolves into frustration and then anger. You go into the living room and dump your toys out on the floor, choosing a few fragile-looking ones to throw across the room. As your dad comes into the room, you brace yourself for his reaction. He takes a deep breath, gathering himself, walks over to you, and asks if you need a hug. You react by shouting, "No!" Because you still feel angry, you aren't able to receive the hug, but the loving response deescalates your anger and soothes the hurt beneath it. Your dad sits on the floor, close enough to let you know he is there but providing enough space to show that wanting distance is okay too. When your defences fall away, you soften, and your desire to connect and be comforted propels you into his arms. When you feel better, you release yourself from his embrace. Your dad goes back to the kitchen to finish dinner, letting you know that when dinner is ready, he will tell you so that you have enough time to tidy up. You are still tired, but it feels more manageable now. You look at all the toys laid out before you and start to play.

Many of us might not easily relate to this scene between a parent and child, whether thinking back to when we were children or today as parents ourselves. However, I'm hoping you can feel the undertones of unconditional positive regard and acceptance from this parent toward their child, even if we do not agree with the child's behaviour. These characteristics are the principles that underlie child-centred parenting. Amato and Kane (2011) have described the influence of our childhood experiences as follows:

> In general, the most important factors … to experience high or low levels of psychosocial adjustment are present in their families of origin and their experiences during childhood and adolescence, before their decisions to attend college, obtain full-time employment, cohabit, marry, or have children. (p. 293)

A warm, cohesive, nurturing, and supportive relationship with at least one parent is an essential component of a child-centred environment (Fergusson & Horwood, 2003). Superle (2016) described it as empowering children to "shape themselves and their surroundings through their input, values, decisions, and action [rather than] as blank slates to be filled with correct ideas so that they could fit into society" (p. 144). The first two decades of life are when people gain an orientation to life and where they develop their sense of coherence and thriving tendencies that they carry into adulthood. These experiences promote "a deep belief that life has meaning and that each of us have a place in the universe … [and] is probably the most powerful [strength] in propelling young people to healthy outcomes despite adversity" (Benard, 2004, p. 28). Furthermore, children who have internalized unconditional positive regard are more empathetic, more autonomous, and more likely to help others (Roth, 2008). In a similar vein, as we internalize unconditional positive regard, we too can be more empathetic, more grounded in our roots (buffering us from external weather), and therefore more likely to have a genuine desire to help others.

Children who have been shown unconditional positive regard may have heard messages like these:

- "You're worthy of love as you are, you don't need to earn my love."
- "I accept you, all of you, without condition."
- "I may not like all of your choices, but your choices are not a condition for my love."
- "It's okay to make mistakes, we all do. Making mistakes is part of being human and can be a great learning opportunity."
- "I am here to help you, to guide you when you want and need it, not to tear you down through criticism."
- "I want you to be yourself, not the self that others tell you to be."

Those of us who did not experience unconditional positive regard are more likely to have repressed our emotions throughout childhood. The more repressed we were, the more incongruence and shame we carry and the more likely we will unintentionally project our shame onto others.

To illustrate this on a more personal level, I will share what my experience was like during my own childhood. There were adults who showed me *conditional* regard, who impressed upon me that I was not worthy of love and acceptance unless I met certain expectations. There also were adults who showed that they would accept me no matter what, but until I was an adult, I did not believe it to be true. Because I did not believe it, I could not internalize it as a child. Instead, I lived as though I needed to devote myself to an idealized display in order to be worthy of love. To do so, I had to push many of the "real," seemingly less desirable parts of myself into the shadows. It took me many years of my adulthood to cultivate the relational environments that enabled me to internalize unconditional positive regard. To believe it is true, I have had to get vulnerable by showing up, whatever that might look like. By doing so, I developed the trust necessary to believe I am worthy of unconditional positive regard. Once I believed I was worthy, I could take it in. I could receive and embody it as the precious gift it was meant to be, with no strings attached. In this process, I learned that loving and accepting relationships don't require us to hide parts of ourselves, even if those parts are less liked than others. We are a package, and relationships with unconditional positive regard accept the whole package. This process feels (and felt) like giving myself permission to reparent myself, mirroring the unconditional positive regard shown to me by others inwardly (self-compassion), and reminding myself that I am good enough as is, no conditions attached. Based on my research and personal experience, I have learned that with time, self-compassion, and intention, we can heal past wounds and become more congruent, liberated beings in the process.

In summary, child-centred parenting promotes sense of coherence, enabling a greater ability to manage stress and, as a result, the ability to engage in thriving (Eriksson & Lindström, 2007; Wijk & Waters, 2008). On the career front, those who enter their career with a higher sense of coherence will have more confidence in their ability to navigate stimuli before they become stressors, resulting in a greater ability to deal with occupational challenges. The ability to be congruent and to thrive begins at a young age, with those nurtured by child-centred parenting showing higher levels of self-actualization and higher sense of coherence scores (Feldt et al., 2005). Another impactful factor in our ability to self-actualize in adulthood relates to our experience and orientation to childhood adversities.

The Impact of Childhood Adversity

Whether or not we experienced unconditional positive regard from one or more adults in our childhoods, most of us have also had significant negative experiences. For example, physical, emotional, sexual, or verbal abuse, the loss of a loved one, extreme poverty, the divorce of our parents, or the breakdown of the family unit. In a study performed in the United States between 1995 and 1997, over 17 000 participants were asked to provide information about their childhoods in conjunction with having a physical exam. The results were astounding, with dozens of publications underscoring the connection between childhood adversities, social challenges, unhealthy life choices, and a myriad of physical and mental illnesses in adulthood (Centers for Disease Control and Prevention, 2014).

In terms of the two core factors required to thrive—sense of coherence and congruence—adults who have had adverse childhood experiences are less likely to have a high sense of coherence in adulthood (Bruskas & Tessin, 2013). Those who faced chronic unpredictable and/or intense adversities in childhood are also more likely to develop depression and anxiety disorders later on and, not surprisingly, may find it more difficult to identify and manage stressors when they arise in the workplace (Breslau et al., 1999; Fossion et al., 2014; Green et al., 2000; Sullivan et al., 2009). Having many childhood adversities sensitizes us to stressful events later in life, making us more prone to negative physical and psychological health impacts. From this orientation to life, it can feel like our past adversities, now current-day trauma, are still close to the skin, threatening to emerge at any moment. Therefore, our remaining sensitivity to stressful stimuli, because of childhood traumas, weakens our sense of coherence as adults (Fossion et al., 2014).

While we may get frustrated with ourselves and others who seem "stuck" in old wounds, it important to remember that what started as an unfair disadvantage in childhood can evolve into further inequity in adulthood. For instance, if emotions felt unacceptable and shameful as a child, in order to survive we may have developed a subconscious habit of dissociating from our feelings, pushing them down instead of letting them out. When we frequently dissociate in adulthood, it fuels shame and incongruence, making us more at risk for maladaptive psychological states (Perry et al., 1995).

Evidence suggests, and my experience corroborates, that those who experienced a childhood environment with unconditional positive regard and fewer adversities will be more likely to enter adulthood with a greater ability to manage emotions. As adults, such individuals will more readily build sense of coherence and congruence because it is already an established (subconscious) habit from childhood. On the other hand, those who did not have a self-actualizing childhood experience may need to seek opportunities to develop these skills in their adult years. Many caregivers are still young adults, going from their high school years right into the profession—this makes it even less likely that they have had the time to bolster their emotional management skills outside of their childhood experiences. When we start to grapple with the understanding that we were all incubated in different environments with varying skills and assets, we are more likely to extend compassion to ourselves and others, promoting an ability to unconditionally and positively regard one another despite shortcomings that we really had little to no control over.

Clearing Practice
Perceived Unconditional Positive Regard as Children

This questionnaire was created by two psychologists (Rains & McClinn, 2013) and is modelled after the Adverse Childhood Experiences Study (described in the last section), reflecting the significance of perceived unconditional positive regard. It provides an opportunity to reflect on our childhood perception of unconditional positive regard.

Select the answer that is most accurate for each statement	Definitely true	Probably true	Not sure	Probably not true	Definitely not true
1. I believe that my mother loved me when I was little.					
2. I believe that my father loved me when I was little.					
3. When I was little, other people helped my mother and father take care of me and they seemed to love me.					
4. I've heard that when I was an infant, someone in my family enjoyed playing with me, and I enjoyed it, too.					
5. When I was a child, there were relatives in my family who made me feel better if I was sad or worried.					
6. When I was a child, neighbours or my friends' parents seemed to like me.					
7. When I was a child, teachers, coaches, youth leaders, or ministers were there to help me.					
8. Someone in my family cared about how I was doing in school.					
9. My family, neighbours, and friends talked often about making our lives better.					
10. We had rules in our house and were expected to keep them.					
11. When I felt really bad, I could almost always find someone I trusted to talk to.					
12. As a youth, people noticed that I was capable and could get things done.					
13. I was independent and a go-getter.					
14. I believed that life is what you make it.					

How many of these 14 protective factors did I have as a child/youth? (How many of the 14 were marked "Definitely true" or "Probably true"?) _____

Of the 14 that I marked "Definitely true" or "Probably true," how many are still true for me?

_____

This exercise prompts self-reflection, illuminating our vulnerabilities so that we can work with them and in some situations even clear them. As a result, we can then develop the roots that will bolster our ability to manage external (and internal) stimuli, preventing us from succumbing to chronic stress. The point of the exercise is *not* to label or limit ourselves nor encourage self-destructive thought patterns. Please remember that a secure childhood, where one believes they were unconditionally positively regarded, is a luxury. If you didn't get one, you are in good company! As we move into adulthood, we can reparent the pieces of ourselves that require nurturing. If stress emerges based on your results, practise responding to yourself with loving-kindness.

Raising Children in Community

I would like to paint a picture that runs counter to the dominant culture in the West. What if we viewed children and parenting from a collectivist, shared responsibility orientation? From this perspective, the birth of a child is considered a sacred gift not just to the individuals that brought them into the world, but to the village as a whole. The responsibility of tending to this sacred gift rests on the entire community. Members of the community then share a common responsibility and intention to ground all children so securely in the community that they self-actualize into the unique beings they were meant to be. In this community, there are shared values that promote environments where children are free to create, play, learn from mistakes, serve, work with their vulnerabilities free of shame, and realize and celebrate their talents. Instead of "time-outs" in times of distress, we pull them closer for "time-in" with those who can tend to their needs in that moment. Parents exist in a state of grace, free of shame when they themselves need a "time-out." We support them and provide them with the comfort of knowing that there are a host of community members who will know and love their children as their own. When a child loses their way, the responsibility falls to the entire community to provide the support and resources necessary to meet their needs, nurturing them as they find their way back. When dissonance arises, there is no benefit in shaming one another, as this only further divides, harming the whole. In these times, the community intuitively creates a circle, joining arms, collectively empowered by common values and a shared intention. This community exemplifies what it looks like when it mirrors unconditional positive regard, providing the container necessary for every member to thrive.

Working With Attachment Tendencies

Working with our **attachment tendencies** enables us to work with our subconscious habits consciously and intentionally. Learning to securely attach to ourselves and others breaks generational cycles of trauma born from the disconnection and insecurity seeded in our developmental years. By cultivating relationships that promote secure **attachment**, our roots are strengthened, providing us with the grounding necessary to move more confidently in the world. When we gain the ability to embody this felt sense, we can then pass this same gift on to the next generation.

Before I get too far, I want to be clear that very few people securely attach all the time. Most of us struggle with attachment, and the process to gain more security is often slow and subtle. When we get stressed, the vast majority of humans will tend toward anxious or avoidant behaviours—this is normal!

SECURE ATTACHMENT

What does secure attachment look and feel like? Ideally, as children, we can fall into a felt sense of safety, where we feel unconditionally positively regarded by someone we trust and look up to. This felt unconditional positive regard makes us feel inherently worthy, separate from our ability to perform and achieve. When we believe we are inherently worthy, we become self-compassionate, enabling us to effortlessly mirror this same unconditional positive regard inwardly. By feeling safe

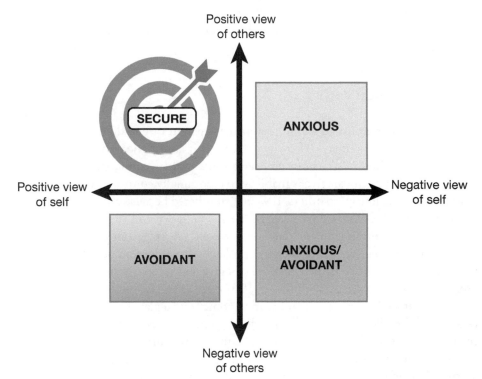

Fig. 8.1 The Attachment Spectrum. How attachment tendencies correlate with one's view of (and corresponding trust in) others.

enough to securely attach to another trusted human, we automatically can apply that same felt sense inwardly, which cultivates self-compassion and ultimately securely attaches us to our "real" self. Once securely and self-compassionately attached to our "real" self, we gain confidence in our innate ability to self-soothe and navigate life's challenges.

Fundamentally, secure attachment clearly separates the "signal" of who we are from the "noise" of the conditions in the world around us. When we are securely attached to self and others, the disturbances of life feel less threatening. They may be noisy and distracting, but they are distinct and overshadowed by the signal of who we are. From this place, because we know who we are and have access to a wealth of resources within us, we can confidently manage challenges (the noise). When we lack this attachment to self, we are prone to overidentifying with the noise that presents itself, confusing who we are with unpredictable events and opinions that are largely out of our control. From this insecure place, we often fixate on *do*ing to compensate for the *dis-ease* we feel inside. Our actions emerge from a fearful place—the fear of not adding up, the fear of not being good enough if we stop proving our worth. From this fearful place, we grasp onto substances, events, and busyness to compensate for our felt insecurity. How we relate to others from this place of fear emerges in avoidant (emotionally disconnected) or anxious (emotionally clinging to others) attachment tendencies. Between these two tendencies, in the middle of the attachment spectrum, is secure attachment (Figure 8.1).

INSECURE ATTACHMENT

In childhood, our ability to attach to a primary parent or guardian forms the basis of our adult attachment style (Bowlby, 2012). Our ability to connect to a primary caregiver as children impacts our ability to forge healthy connections as adults. If we felt rejected by our caregiver's inability to emotionally connect, as adults we will tend to cling (anxiously) to others. If we felt smothered because our caregivers relied on us to meet their emotional needs, then as adults we will tend to retreat from (avoid) others. Our attachment tendencies develop in stages ranging from immature dependent security, where we are completely dependent on others for security, to mature dependant security, where we can give and receive in our connections to others from a secure sense of self (Blatz, 1967). For example, those who are closer to the dependant side of the spectrum tend to come from a glass half-empty approach, yearning to be filled by others. Those closer to mature dependant security tend to come from a glass half-full perspective, connecting from a more grounded and optimistic place. People who are able to progress through the stages and come to mature dependent security will form mutually *interdependent* relationships in their adulthood (Blatz, 1967). Interdependence involves a balance between recognizing our dependence on others and honouring our independence as unique individuals.

Because of our progression through the attachment stages, in adulthood we tend to gravitate to one of three broad attachment categories (Bowlby, 2012):

- Avoidant attachment
- Secure attachment (springing from perceived unconditional positive regard as a child), or
- Anxious attachment.

Both the avoidant and anxious attachment styles spring from perceived *conditional* regard and rejection in childhood (Bretherton & Munholland, 1999). Children with repetitive and/or unresolved trauma may also develop avoidant attachment styles, even when they experience unconditional positive regard (Morina et al., 2016). This avoidance relates to the erosion of trust in others, leading children to contract inwardly in times of stress. When those on the avoidant end feel insecure, they are far more likely to withdraw, disconnecting from external relationships, feeling too unsafe to expose their felt sense of vulnerability. When insecurities present, those on the more anxious end of the spectrum tend to feverishly seek others to anchor to, fixating on relationships for security, which often fuels more anxiety and codependent relations.

There are exceptions to these tidy labels. When one does not tend toward attachment inwardly or outwardly, it can cause a more chaotic attachment style, which is less predictable than the attachment styles that fall on either end of the spectrum. Most of us fall along the edges of the attachment spectrum, either avoiding intimacy or anxiously attaching to others, with those who easily form secure attachments in the minority. The good news is that attachment styles are not fixed traits. Like most of our inner workings, when we come to recognize our attachment style and the patterns that spring from it, we have an opportunity to heal the old wound at the roots. In time and with intentional practice, we can reorient ourselves and our relationship.

ANTIDOTES TO AVOIDANT AND ANXIOUS ATTACHMENT

Wherever we fall on the attachment spectrum, there are typical antidotes that tend to bring us back into balance. By employing an antidote intentionally, we can catch our more extreme (and often unhelpful) tendencies much quicker:

- The antidote for the anxiously attached is to satisfy their self-trust and self-esteem needs through self-soothing. In other words, the solution is to direct unconditional positive regard inwardly. This requires them to reach in, even though they may want to (or without thinking) reach out.
- The antidote for the avoidantly attached is to satisfy their other-trust and agency needs by using their voice or taking empowered action in relationship to others. In other words, the solution is to connect outwardly. By expressing their authentic emotions

and boundaries to others, they are testing the relational container, which cultivates relationships where they can come to believe that they are unconditionally positively regarded by others.

Strengthening Practice
Promoting Secure Attachment Through "Priming"

Priming is the practice of visualizing an attachment to a person or object of comfort that promotes feelings of calm and ease. Research suggests that priming with a person or object of comfort increases feelings of security and decreases anxiety and depression (Carnelley et al., 2018). It can also weaken memories and intrusive thoughts of traumatic events (Bryant & Foord, 2016). Priming tends to be more effective when tend to have an anxious attachment style, as this can help us reach inwardly for felt security. Those who are avoidantly attached are less likely to experience the benefits of priming.

As an example of how one can prime for secure attachment, consider my late grandmother. Growing up, she was my go-to person of comfort, as she emanated unconditional positive regard for me. Today, when I imagine my time with her, I can believe in that moment that I am indeed worthy of unconditional positive regard because with her, I really felt that I was. By tuning into that feeling, I feel more secure and, as a result, can direct that feeling inwardly.

Let's practise! Begin by taking a few minutes to write about a relationship where you experience secure attachment. It can be a romantic partner, a friend, a colleague, a pet, or any other being. If you do not have a relationship where you experience secure attachment, write about what such a relationship would look like. Close your eyes and visualize this person in your mind. This visualization is the act of attachment security priming. Doing these visualizations regularly taps into the benefits of secure attachment described earlier.

The Challenge: Navigation

By considering someone else's challenge, or working with another to consider ours, we cultivate nonattachment. We can often find comfort knowing we are not alone and that we can learn from and with each other. By working from this more objective space, we mitigate the stress response. We can then reorient ourselves from this position of strength, which improves our ability to feel into all our biological, intellectual, and spiritual capacities. With this benevolent orientation, we can face adversities with confidence, knowing we have the resources and support necessary to navigate life's challenges.

Circling back to Wendy's Challenge—a woman who works in law enforcement, is the single caregiver of two children, and continues to grapple with childhood wounds—let's consider how Wendy could navigate projections when they arise at work. Thinking back to the RAIN framework (Brach, 2013) introduced in Chapter 4, Wendy can *recognize* the projections for what they are, enabling her to understand that the intensity of her emotion is more about a past impression or wound than the person or event that is activating the projection in the present moment. She is struggling to *allow* the emotion/pain to play out—before she even has a chance to do so, she finds herself in freeze, causing her to dissociate from all emotions. When attached to an intense emotion, it is too threatening to allow it to emerge fully. As a result, out of a felt need to protect itself, the nervous system steps in.

To cultivate nonattachment, enabling her to step back from identifying with the emotion, Wendy can investigate the impression of the wound (focusing less on the actual event and more on the felt sense) by using a third-person approach. For instance, when she feels adequately resourced with someone and/or in an environment that feels safe, she could ask questions like, "How old are you?" "What are you afraid of?" and "What do you need?" Asking these questions of another provides a space between the emotion and the felt sense of threat attached to the emotion. It also promotes a sense of agency, as she takes on the healer role instead of the role of a wounded person. From this vantage point, she can provide the unconditional positive regard necessary to allow the emotions to emerge, releasing the energy that got stuck in the core wound. For less intense emotions that come up throughout the day, this strategy can help Wendy to allow them to come up, to tend to them, and when ready, to lovingly let them go. As a result, rather than feeling threatened by emotions, Wendy can see these moments as opportunities for healing, empowering her with a greater sense of control and agency in her life.

With emotions that feel too intense, we can quickly freeze. To buffer us from relying on our nervous system's tactics (fight–flight–freeze–fawn), we need to bring trusted others into the equation. By developing our relational resources, we can tune back into a more secure way of being. From this more secure way of being, we can keep things in perspective, which mitigates the felt threat and as a result deescalates the intense emotion.

By bringing in others, Wendy is *investigating* the situation with a third-person approach. She is cultivating *nonattachment* so that she can reparent the part of herself that is caught up in an unhealed wound from the past. As she tends to these hurt parts, perhaps again and again, she is reorienting herself to the pain of the wound from a place of unconditional positive regard, *nurturing* herself with the space and loving-kindness necessary for healing.

Attuning/Reflecting Opportunity

We are continuing to develop a habit of leaning into our inner world, accessing our inner resources to confidently navigate challenges. By reorienting from a place of strength, we remember who we are (in our essence) so that we can love and accept all parts of ourselves. With practice, what takes effort at first will soon turn to ease. In time, we will find ourselves compelled to continually come back to this place of wholeness.

What resources or practices might remind you of your strength and wholeness when feelings of threat or difficult emotions arise?

Attuning for the Journey Ahead: Strengthening Our Self-Soothing Capacities

We have come to know the benefits and process of *reparenting* ourselves, tilling the soil and enabling our roots to deepen. As we cultivate connection with our inner world by dropping into our roots, we learn to console ourselves as we would a dear friend.

Now, we continue *attuning* to the felt senses in our inner world, exploring *strengthening* strategies that promote greater self-trust and self-soothing. This is how we tune into the calm amid the chaos.

CHAPTER 9

Strengthening Our Self-Soothing Capacities: Calm at the Roots

Soothing expands the space within us, clearing out the "noise" at the root of our suffering, enabling us to tune back into the "signal" of who we are. Self-soothing happens when we drop into our roots, directing unconditional positive regard inwardly. From this self-compassionate orientation, we can hold space for whatever arises, consoling the felt sense like we would a dear child.

All meaningful and sustainable behaviour changes result from an embodied reorientation representing a collection of insights that become known as a felt sense. From here, our entire frame of reference changes. As we grow up in our bodies, learning how to navigate and respond to the sensations within, we are more able to transcend with our spirits. One comes before and alongside the other. The more we can clear from the body, the more we can tune into the signal of the spirit. With this new and expanded awareness, old and unhelpful ways of "being" and "doing" naturally fall away. While it sounds simple, it is not. In this process there is often a space in time between when the "Aha!" moment begins to sink in and when our subconscious coping mechanism falls away. When the nervous system is activated, old patterns often re-emerge. This is a normal part of the process! For the body to shift, trust must be established. Aha moments thrust our spirit forward, but the body requires trust, which takes more time. Self-compassion is your antidote in these cases and exactly the medicine that will cultivate the inner space necessary to keep you moving, despite felt setbacks. It wards off the shame that results when behaviour changes lag behind spiritual ideals.

In this chapter, we explore aspects of self-soothing and resourcing with others. By first exploring our attachment tendencies in relationship to self and others, we have come to recognize our subconscious defence mechanisms. With this recognition, we have a greater ability to reparent and soothe those wounded areas, enabling us to connect to others from a more conscious and secure place. We can now focus on receiving soothing through loving-kindness, physical touch, optimistic reorientation, gratitude, and forgiveness practices.

The Challenge: Orientation

By considering someone else's challenge, or working with another to consider ours, we cultivate nonattachment. We can often find comfort knowing we are not alone and that we can learn from and with each other. Working from this more objective space, we mitigate the stress response. We can then reorient from this position of strength, thus improving our ability to use all our biological, intellectual, and spiritual capacities. With this benevolent orientation, we can face adversities with confidence, knowing we have the resources and support necessary to navigate life's challenges.

Let's practise by considering Marnie's challenge. Marnie, who is in her mid-thirties, works full time responding to events involving sexual assault, intimate partner violence, and child abuse. Since having children of her own, performing child abuse exams has become especially stressful. She is the mother of three young children whom she shares with a life partner who also works full time. As Marnie continues to expand her awareness of how she feels and responds to certain contexts and stimuli, she recognizes her tendency to freeze (described in Chapter 3) when she feels overwhelmed at work. When this happens, Marnie's outward display remains relatively unchanged, but inwardly she feels numb, disconnected from her body and emotions. To cope, she tends to isolate, which often involves anxiously attaching to cigarettes, food, or exercise to help her relax. Marnie knows her coping strategies are not "ideal," and she feels ashamed that she continues to grapple with this issue. While Marnie recognizes the tendency to react in this way, with a trauma-laden work area and busy home life, she is at a loss as to how to avoid getting activated. Once she is activated, she generally feels a complete loss of control. By the time she recognizes what is happening, she is too entrenched in reactive mode to step back. The numbing behaviours that enable her to stay frozen fuel a deep sense of shame, preventing her from reaching out for help, which further isolates her from others.

Many of us can relate to Marnie's challenge, both in terms of a sense of not being in control when we feel extremely threatened and because of the shame that results from incongruent coping behaviours.

To cultivate nonattachment, try stepping back to view your challenges from the same objective vantage point. If behaviours were just behaviours, without "good" or "bad" labels, what coping mechanisms/behaviours/reactions are currently giving you some reprieve from suffering or allowing you to discharge stressful energy? Can you recognize these as a form of self-soothing, viewing them separately from the judgement and shame that keeps you attached to them? How can cultivating nonattachment promote a greater sense of choice and empowerment in these challenges?

> *When coping mechanisms are viewed from a more optimistic lens—when we see them as a form of self-medicating—we are more likely to identify what the body is gaining from these coping strategies, providing us with an opportunity to identify less harmful ways of achieving that same benefit.*

Coming from a strengths-based approach, refraining from judging specific self-soothing behaviours, can you relate to Marnie's challenge? When activated, what are your tendencies? Can you identify what your body is getting from your less desirable coping habits? How else might you soothe yourself in a way that is less harmful, but still provides the same regulation benefits?

> ## Strengthening Practice: Soothing With Breath
>
> Before we get into the various forms of self-soothing, let's circle back to the breath. Turning our attention to our breathing is a quick and simple way to "drop in" and tune in, anytime, anywhere. Deep breathing, breath holding, yawning, and sighing can all alleviate stress and regulate and relax the body (Corey et al., 2012; Vlemincx et al., 2016).
>
> Before you start this practice, notice how you are feeling.
>
> Take five deep breathes, inhaling through your nose and exhaling through your mouth. Hold your breath for at least 2 seconds after you fully exhale. This promotes greater physical relaxation (Vlemincx et al., 2016). On the final exhale, let out a natural-feeling sigh. As long as the sounds feels like a welcome and natural release, you are on the right track.
>
> Take a few moments to notice how your body responded to the practice.

Soothing With Loving-Kindness

Loving-kindness is characterized by gentleness, consideration, and kindness to ourselves and others. By soothing with loving-kindness, we are more likely to allow uncomfortable feelings (shame, anxiety, fear, sadness, jealousy) to come and go, recognizing that they are a normal (and important) part of the human experience. To feel that which is uncomfortable, we have to believe that it is worth the investment *and* that we can experience reprieve from doing so for these reasons:

1. It is worth the investment because it is an opportunity to lighten our load (discharging stuck energy). By acknowledging when the body is suffering, we can then investigate what unmet need or unhealed wound is at the root.
2. Loving-kindness practices breathe space into the "noise" that keeps us from dropping into our bodies. Spaciousness is exactly what is needed to tune back into the "signal" of who we are. Once tuned in, we can reconnect to our heart space, that which connects to all things. In this felt connection, we can hold space for discomfort without overidentifying with it.

There are a variety of ways to practise loving-kindness. For example, consider the recipes shared in the following figure. By practising loving-kindness toward ourselves and others, we develop self-compassion and reduce symptoms related to PTSD and depression (Kearney et al., 2013). Habitual loving-kindness increases feelings of social connectedness and positivity toward others and lowers the risk of developing a host of mental and physical health conditions (Aspy & Proeve, 2017; Hutcherson et al., 2008; Toussaint et al., 2015).

While drugs, sex, and sugar often result in a boost of dopamine (our brain's reward/ pleasure neurotransmitter), so does immersing in feelings of gratitude and loving-kindness toward ourselves and others.

Loving-Kindness Recipes to Boost the Brain's "Happiness"

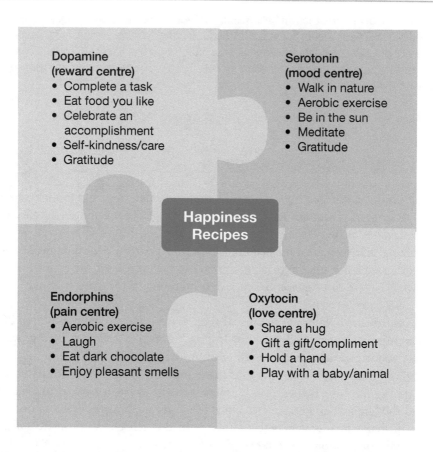

Dopamine
(reward centre)
- Complete a task
- Eat food you like
- Celebrate an accomplishment
- Self-kindness/care
- Gratitude

Serotonin
(mood centre)
- Walk in nature
- Aerobic exercise
- Be in the sun
- Meditate
- Gratitude

Happiness Recipes

Endorphins
(pain centre)
- Aerobic exercise
- Laugh
- Eat dark chocolate
- Enjoy pleasant smells

Oxytocin
(love centre)
- Share a hug
- Gift a gift/compliment
- Hold a hand
- Play with a baby/animal

How do these recipes resonate with you? What ingredients do you naturally use now? What ingredients might you add?

Strengthening Practices

A. From Foe to Friend

We label someone an enemy when they pose a threat to us. Often, even when the actual threat dissipates or we put the perceived threat into perspective, we hold onto resentments, causing the old wound to feel as raw as the day it was formed. Loving-kindness enables us to step back from habitual thoughts that activate reactive feeling states and hostile behaviours. When we stop and heartfully connect with the person by whom we feel threatened, we realize that they too are human and that in this way, we are the same. In this sameness, they too suffer, and they too have the same basic needs we do.

In the victim–perpetrator cycle, people that hurt another do so because someone has hurt them. Seeing the wounds beneath the behaviours prevents us from taking the projections (harmful action born out of unresolved trauma) of others so personally. With practice and intention, we can shift our feelings from seeing them as the "threatening other" to recognizing in our humanity that "we are the same"—this shift results from compassionate connection.

When we think others threaten our ability to meet our basic human needs, we wear the victim hat. When others believe we are a threat to their basic needs, we wear the perpetrator hat. Whether we play the victim or the perpetrator is not important. How we identify and live outside of the role is important.

Doing a loving-kindness practice can take less than a minute. It involves seizing a moment, acting on an inner prompt. It can also be a more formal sit-down practice. Whatever the case, staying embodied is the most important part. While going through the motions in the thinking mind can help instill a habit, it generally doesn't soothe us. To create the felt sense of loving-kindness, try this:

1. Drop into your inner space, letting go of external distractions.
2. Bring up an image of a loved one(s) who is emanating love for you; immerse in and receive that love.
3. Direct feelings and phrases of love/well-wishes/compassion toward yourself and/ or another.

The details of how you immerse in feeling and in what form you send loving-kindness can vary depending on what feels more natural for you in that time and context. The most important aspect is that you *feel* connected to the experience and that you accept whatever arises. If we place conditions on the inner world, we will erode self-trust. Holding space for the less secure self, come what may, is like saying, "I've got you. Come what may, I'm here. You can depend on me. I'm not going to reject you."

Remember that with practice we make progress. Over time, as we take what works and leave what doesn't, we gain habits that align with our "real" selves. Each soothing habit cultivates space within, enabling us to tune back into our "signal" and the corresponding abundance within.

From Effort to Automatic

Nearly all meditations feel awkward, even robotic, in the beginning. It is also normal to feel agitated, irritated, restless, or bored. These feelings are all normal. They provide you with an opportunity to feel unconditional positive regard for yourself, to enable whatever is coming up to be received with loving acceptance. With this in mind, the following script will guide your practice.

It starts with developing unconditional positive regard for yourself, which then enables you to expand and extend the same to others. You may find it too difficult to cultivate feelings of loving-kindness for yourself. In this case, try cultivating the feelings by sending loving-kindness to others first. How you practise is completely up to you. The goal is to generate the felt sense of loving-kindness and as a result, open and connect more deeply to yourself and others.

B. Loving-Kindness Meditations

This meditation was adapted from *The Art of Forgiveness, Lovingkindness, and Peace* by Jack Kornfield (2008), a renowned Buddhist meditation teacher.

Keeping your eyes closed, think of someone from the past or the present who you believe feels unconditional positive regard for you. Feel the warmth and love they are emanating from their being toward you. Immerse in the unconditional love that they embody, allowing yourself to soften and open in this safe space.

In your mind's eye, visualize yourself in this safe space, perhaps the way you are now or the way you were as a child. Play with the images until you find one that resonates, allowing you to open your heart even more.

Quietly repeat the following loving-kindness mantra to yourself (or adapt to phrases that speak to you):

May I be filled with loving-kindness.
May I be safe from inner and outer threats.
May I be well.
May I be at ease and happy.

As you go through the mantra, continue immersing in the feelings you generated earlier, letting the images, feelings, and words sink deeply into your mind and body. This practice is best done daily or as often as you can manage. Frequently connecting to yourself in this way will improve your ability to practise self-compassion.

Be aware that this meditation may at times feel mechanical or awkward. It can also bring up feelings that are contrary to loving-kindness, such as irritation and anger. If this happens, it is especially important to be patient and kind toward yourself, allowing whatever arises to be received in a spirit of friendliness and kind affection. When you feel you have established a stronger sense of loving-kindness for yourself, you can then expand your meditation to include others.

After focusing on yourself, choose a person whom you care for. Picture this person in front of you. You and this person are alike. Just like you, this person knows suffering and wants to be happy. In this way, you are the same. Repeat the same phrases or adapt to others that speak to you:

May you be filled with loving-kindness.
May you be safe from inner and outer threats.
May you be well.
May you be at ease and happy.

Gradually extend your practice to include your inner circle, community members, colleagues, and then all people and all beings on Earth.

While you continue to immerse in feelings of loving-kindness, bring to mind the difficult relationships in your past and present. Extend your feeling of loving-kindness to these individuals and wish them safety, wellness, and ease. Trust the process. It isn't a perfect process; in fact, if it is easy, you are not practising unconditional positive regard.

C. Singing Loving-Kindness

Here is another loving-kindness practice. This one originates from traditional Buddhism and was published in *Singing the Journey* (Unitarian Universalist Association, 2005, p. 1031). It is often used in song with a group, but you can also do it by yourself. The verses of the song begin with "I," by directing loving-kindness inwardly. As you are filled, you then extend the verses outwardly to all beings:

May I be filled with loving-kindness.
May I be well.
May I be filled with loving-kindness.
May I be well.
May I be peaceful and at ease.
May I be whole.
May you ...
May we ...
May all ...

When working with yourself, practise talking to yourself like a dear friend. You might use phrases that sounds like, "I can see how much pain you are in," "This is really difficult," or "Those beliefs are causing a great deal of suffering for you, I'm so sorry you've had to carry that for so long." You could provide comfort to the suffering part of you by saying things like, "You are safe," "You are loved." Imagine a friend in anguish—what would you say to them? Can you treat yourself with the same tenderness? Establishing a relationship of unconditional positive regard requires us to accept what is without a condition of change. Such relationships pave the way within an environment of trust and safety. Within this environment, we can release stuck energy (now emerging as trauma), clearing some of the noise within. With a more spacious inner world, we can feel into our "signal" more readily, which provides us with the capacity to upgrade old belief systems.

When directing loving-kindness practices inwardly, it is most effective to use a third-person approach, as it keeps us from attaching and identifying with the emotions that arise. We are not our emotions, nor are we simply a product of our experiences. And yet we often fall prey to overly identifying with both. The essence of who we are is unrelated to thoughts, emotions, and experiences. When we view thoughts, emotions, and experiences from a more impartial place, we make a space between them and us. In this quieter space, we can more clearly identify the "noise" that is clouding the "signal." This signal is our essence, the unconditioned, authentic part of us that is inherently worthy and connected to all things. From this spacious and compassionate orientation, we can speak to the "noise" without attaching to it.

Soothing With Touch: Self-Holding

Physical touch has powerful physiological affects. It releases oxytocin, reduces cortisol, calms the cardiovascular system, reduces pain, improves learning, speeds wound healing, and has a host of other benefits (Lund et al., 2002; Uvnäs-Moberg & Petersson, 2010).

There are several ways to develop a stronger mind–body connection, promoting the ability to self-soothe. For instance, try out some of the following practices.

Strengthening and Attuning Practices
Strengthening Practice

A. Soothing With Touch
There are a variety of ways to use physical touch to practise self-kindness. This exercise promotes feelings of safety and is a method of self-soothing. Play with it, noticing your body and how it responds. Does it expand the space you feel within or do you feel a contraction?

When uncomfortable sensations arise in the body, locate where you feel them and cross your hands over the area while also crossing your hands over the body's midline, which hampers the brain's ability to localize pain (aka discomfort) signals (Gallace et al., 2011). Holding your emotions in this way promotes a greater ability to create space for feelings as they arise, which can counter our subconscious attempts to resist or ignore them.

Try on a few more practices. Because self-consciousness can cause disembodiment, sit in a quiet place by yourself where others will not see you. Drop into your inner space by focusing on your natural breath. Try these different positions and notice how they feel to you. What feelings do you experience with each approach? Are there some that are more comforting than others?

- Notice how you feel when you breathe in and out of your heart space. Place your hand(s) on your heart.
- Now move your attention to your belly, noticing your breath moving in and out. Place your hand on your belly.
- Place one hand on your heart and another on your belly, letting the inhalation flow deep into your belly and out through your heart.
- Now cross your arms as though you are hugging yourself. Maybe even rub your upper arms.
- Place your hand on the top of your head (bringing you into present time).
- Place your fingertips together, all five of the pads of your fingers connecting to one another (this promotes alertness).
- Hold your hands together, playing with different positions.
- Stroke your neck and then your face.
- If the fight–flight response is strong, excess energy is often shunted to the limbs. You can use one of the exercises in Chapter 6 or try one of these:
    - Shake it off with a brisk activity
    - Sit or, if possible, lie down to induce the relaxation response (Harmon-Jones & Peterson, 2009)
    - Find a space where you won't feel self-conscious and verbally release the anger through yelling, or
    - Take deep breaths with a focus on making the exhales longer than the inhales.

When you're ready, explore physical touch with another. For the sake of transparency, support, and cultivating a safe space for your healing work, communicate your intentions to those you are hoping to explore physical touch with. Choose someone that your body feels safe to be authentic with. This might feel like a sense of calm, amid any uneasiness, within when you imagine connecting in this way. If your body doesn't feel safe with others at this point, start with an animal or a tree (yes a tree!). For instance, you might try holding someone's hand or sinking into an intentional hug (heart to heart ideally!). Keep it short at first to allow your window of tolerance for physical connection to expand over time. Listen to the leanings of your body. If there is a desire to stay in physical contact, let yourself settle into it. If there is a sense of overwhelm, lean back.

This exercise is a starting point, a tool that builds awareness of how we feel when we connect to ourselves in a more physical way. It builds our intuitive muscles, helping us feel into what the body likes and doesn't like. By moving at the pace of trust with the body, we gain congruence and safety within. In time, physical touch will become a resource we gladly return to in our time of need.

Because we are different, there is no one-size-fits-all approach. Forcing an experience only fuels incongruence and erodes self-trust in the process. Mindfulness enables us to connect to what is true for us—we connect to our desires and to our resistance, despite what we feel "should" be true based on what is working for others. If you find that this exercise is not resonating with you, use it as an opportunity to practise self-kindness. Listen to what is true for you at the moment. Keep the exercise in your arsenal of tools, drawing on this practice at another time.

Attuning Practice

B. Reinforcing Safety Within

When we are injured, we instinctively use touch to soothe the wounded area. Similarly, we can use touch to shift and transmute emotional pain in the body. When the body feels safe, touch interrupts the stress response and shakes us free from the thought patterns that continue to activate the sympathetic nervous system (flight–flight–freeze-fawn). It comforts and empowers us when dealing with high-stimulus or threatening environments.

As illustrated in the following practice, placing our hands on core energy centres and connecting to the sensations between them grounds us in our bodies. It shocks us out of thinking mode into sensing mode (mindfulness). As we engage with our senses, it reinforces the safety and grounding we feel within the inner world. It enables us to drop deeply into the inner world, clearing out the distractions and debris that prevent us from connecting to our essence ("signal"). Once connected to essence, we can tap into our inner resources and gain perspective on our immediate circumstance from a far more connected and abundant vantage point—a bigger, more connected, and abundant picture. Through this lens of abundance, our window of tolerance for stress expands and we are more able to make space for the more uncomfortable emotions. Cultivating a space where we can feel what previously felt too unsafe is exactly how stuck energy (trauma) gets discharged from the body. Once the energy is discharged, the old belief system that surrounded it begins to naturally upgrade.

Finally, touch is a physical reminder of the boundaries of our container and external influences, enabling us to better navigate the "noise" of emotional transference. Once we establish the boundaries of our vessel, it acts as a protective bubble that separates us from the external world. Within these safe boundaries, which we tangibly remind ourselves of, we can soften into the sanctuary within. Using our hands as a physical cue turns our focus from external threats to the safety found within.

Play with this activity. Try placing your hands on different parts of the body (top of the head, heart, belly). Focus on the sensation between your hands, feeling the edges of your body. Be patient: wait for a softening, a gentle shift. To practise, try these common variations:

1. As the observer and steward of your inner world, give your body a hug, providing a firm, protective hold, encircling the edges of your vessel securely. Stay here; breathe here; soften into the hold. Wait until you notice a subtle shift, an ability to drop in a little deeper. This is especially powerful when uncomfortable emotions spring up. *Holding ourselves is a tangible way to provide self-soothing, enabling emotions to come and go as passing stimuli as opposed to threatening stressors.*

2. Place a hand on your forehead and another on your heart, whichever hand variation feels most natural. Stay here; breathe here; soften into the hold. Wait until you notice a shift, dropping in a little deeper. *This variation is a good way to take a break from difficult emotions that can feel stuck in the belly.* Focus on breathing into the headspace, using touch to deepen the experience, and out through the heart space (or vice versa). Feel the sensation of your hands and the feeling of the body under them. Feel the energetic sensations between your two hands.

3. Place a hand on your heart and another hand on your belly. Sense your emotional core (for many, this is located in the belly) and the sensations between your belly and your heart centre. If helpful, use your breath to further ground yourself. Breathing into your emotional core, expand it. Imagine every breath sweeping in, cleansing every single cell, moving out the old and bringing in the new. Bring the air up to your heart, exhaling out the old air, representing old trauma ("noise") and related baggage you are ready to let go of. As the breath passes through your heart, your healing centre, you transmute the old defences against light and love, exhaling them out into the world. *Holding the heart as a cleansing filter is a healing posture, excellent for digesting and releasing intense and enduring emotions/ trauma.* This is a good practice to do incrementally. Take it slow. Move your hands back to the self-hug when you need extra comfort or the forehead/heart variation when you need to move your focus away from the belly.

Soothing With Optimism

If you don't like something, change it. If you can't change it, change your attitude.
                                                                            Maya Angelou

Optimism is a significant component of sense of coherence. Sense of coherence imparts us with a general sense that all things will work out and a reasonable expectation that the future will turn out favourably because of a sense of control over the outcomes that matter most (Antonovsky, 1979; Lee et al., 2019). Not only does optimism reduce our likelihood of suffering from chronic stress as well as a host of chronic health conditions and mental health ailments (Aldao et al., 2010), it may also increase our lifespans by 11% to 15% and improve our odds of living well into our eighties and beyond (Lee et al., 2019).

NEGATIVE BIAS

In the typical human brain, there is a strong negative bias. This means that negative events have a far greater emotional impact on us than positive ones, and that negative events linger longer in our memories than positive ones. This negative bias is significantly higher for those who are struggling with depression (Gollan et al., 2016). While negative bias was helpful in keeping us safe in primitive times, it is not so helpful in our modern lives. Becoming more optimistic requires a conscious effort to be mindful when positive events occur. We need to bring our attention to the positive feelings that result, taking a moment to breathe in and relish them. With practice, we can train our brains to pick up on and even look for the positive aspects of our day, counterbalancing our negative bias.

Optimistic individuals habitually reappraise workplace stimuli in a positive light and identify opportunities within challenges. We can learn to be more optimistic, cultivating a habit whereby we mindfully choose to reframe our perspective. By doing so, we choose to view the world from a mindset of abundance rather than fear and scarcity. By practising mindfulness, we are more likely to notice the positive parts of the day, such as taking a breath when we look up from our desk to see the bright blue sky or hearing a bird's song as we walk from our car to our house. By noticing the positive—taking a few moments to attend to it, acknowledge, and *breathe into the way it is making us feel*—we establish new neurological patterns, enabling us to focus on the positive rather than habitually fixating on the negative. Finally, developing a more natural tendency toward optimism promotes an ability to take credit when things go well, which also boosts our sense of coherence.

Health and human service work is riddled with events that cause *moral injury*. Most people come to these professions because they want to help alleviate suffering and promote well-being. As a result, when we feel unable to alleviate suffering or to promote well-being, it sets up an internal conflict within us. We need to either resolve this dissonance or optimistically reorient ourselves to it. Otherwise, we will gravitate toward pessimism and hostility. For example, in a recent qualitative study with novice caregivers (Dames, 2018a), Candace reflected on her workplace challenges, stating, "We push people out the door because the hospital is exploding … knowing they will fall and come right back … the guilt for me is a product of an overwhelmed system." Similarly, Mary, another study participant, stated, "There is just such a general lack of resources. It can feel like sometimes there is just nothing you can do for them." Mary and Candace's stress is a product of moral injury, which leads them to experience a felt lack of control. Even in situations that seem unchangeable, if we can act, even in a small way, it is often enough. One *significant* action will empower us, bolstering our sense of agency, and as a result prevent us from spiralling into stress states.

> *When one door of happiness closes, another opens; but often we look so long at the closed door that we do not see the one which has been opened for us.*
>
> Hellen Keller

TAKE A *SIGNIFICANT* ACTION

The *significant* action, described in Chapter 6, is exactly that thing we are called to do in the unique moment we are facing. There is always a significant thing, and it is that thing and only that thing that will unstick us. If we avoid it, gravitating to a sea of insignificant things instead, we will remain stuck. Meaning, confidence, and optimism (all components of sense of coherence) enable us to do the significant thing.

While a tendency toward optimism has more well-being benefits than a tendency toward pessimism, pessimism has its place too. Pessimism helps us recognize when events or relationships feel out of tune with what we believe, value, and desire. It is important to allow and fully feel necessary emotions, and then to make *significant* changes that reduce suffering in ourselves and others. Conversely, avoiding necessary emotions and accepting a situation as is can prevent us from making changes that benefit ourselves and others. In other words, taking a step back to critically appraise whether there is something that needs to be felt or changed is important. If so, feel it and take the steps to change it; if not, accept it and grieve the loss and disappointment in the process. Once we've cleared out the emotional "noise" of disappointment, we can focus on beneficial action.

Engage your curiosity to investigate events that are causing discomfort. It may lead to a pessimistic orientation; when it does, assess the stressor to determine whether a significant action is in order. If we apply optimism in every situation, without this objective assessment, it can prevent us from making these beneficial changes. To illustrate this point with an example from the research, consider the work of Troy (2015), who showed a significant relationship between stress, context, and whether we tend toward optimism or positive reorientation. If workplace stress is uncontrollable, where you cannot change the thing or event activating the stress, employing optimism is the most effective skill to use (Troy et al., 2010). However, if you can control the stressor or change the context to resolve it, then it is more helpful to change the context rather than positively reorient your emotions about it (Troy et al., 2010). When we reframe the situation optimistically *and* tap into the significant thing in that moment, we will make changes when we can; if things cannot be changed, we can accept and positively reorient ourselves. The Serenity Prayer, written by American theologian Reinhold Niebuhr, reflects this sentiment: "God, give us the grace to accept with serenity the things that cannot be changed, the courage to change the things that should be changed, and the wisdom to distinguish one from the other" (Sifton, 1998).

Attuning Practices

A. Assessing Our Tendency Toward Optimism

Use the following optimism self-quiz to reflect on your tendencies. This objective self-awareness is a component of mindfulness. Investigating your relationship with optimism and pessimism will help you navigate the waters when you're feeling stuck in unhelpful thought loops. Being aware of shortcomings provides growth opportunities and reminds us to resource with others when necessary.

Optimism Self-Quiz: How optimistic are you? Select either a or b for each of the following questions.

1. You receive a bouquet of flowers from a client with a card that praises you and your ability to deliver high-quality care. You think:
   a. "I must have been having a good day that day."
   b. "Wow! I must be good at making people feel comfortable and cared for."
2. While walking to work, you see a $10 bill lying on the sidewalk. You look around and don't see anyone. You think:
   a. "What a lucky day!"
   b. "Awesome! There are perks when you are a person that notices all the details."
3. A new electronic charting system has been launched at work. It seems to be taking you far longer to understand it and use it efficiently than some of your colleagues. You think:
   a. "My brain cannot do this. I will fall behind and then what?"
   b. "I am not used to doing things this way. I will get it eventually. I just need to keep at it, and it will come."
4. You have started using the stairs at work. Yesterday, you made quite a few trips up and down the stairs. Today, you are feeling sore. You think:
   a. "I am out of shape."
   b. "This new habit is working; I am building up my muscles."
5. You ask a colleague for help, and he responds with a short and snappy comment about how he has enough work of his own and can't take on yours as well. You think:
   a. "People are so rude!"
   b. "Yikes, he must be having a rough day!"
6. On your commute to work you find that traffic is unusually heavy. You realize that you might be late for work. You think:
   a. "I'm for sure going to be late! I should have known this would happen. They will think I'm flakey for being late!"
   b. "I wish there wasn't so much traffic. It's not in my control, but I might be late for work. I'll call and give them a heads up. I'll start leaving earlier just in case."
7. Your workplace awards you with the employee of the month title. You think:
   a. "They must have cycled through most of the other employees. I guess it's my turn."
   b. "Yay, I am a hard worker, it's nice to be recognized!"
8. You get complimented on your outfit. You think:
   a. "I must have put myself together well today."
   b. "I have good style; it feels good to receive compliments on it."
9. You have planned a lunch and learn for your colleagues. It turned out to be a busy day at work with competing priorities and only a few people attended. You think:
   a. "I'm terrible at planning events! What a waste of time, I should have known better."
   b. "Well, I didn't expect things to unfold as they did, but I learned a lot. I'll do things a little differently next time."

10. You missed your lunch break at work today, which has been happening more than usual. You think:
    a. "My time management is terrible. I don't know if I'll ever get better at this!"
    b. "This has been an unusual week at work. I've been a little distracted, and it's been hard to focus on my tasks. Thank goodness this is only temporary!"

This quiz provides insight into your tendency to correlate your attributes with positive events (a sign of sense of coherence) and your tendency to practise self-compassion (a sign of congruence). It also helps you to recognize that negative events are an opportunity to learn about yourself as opposed to an opportunity to validate self-depreciating thoughts. If you found that you primarily chose the "a" answers, you have a tendency to perceive positive events as a product of happenstance and negative events as a reflection of personal shortcomings. If you chose more "b" responses, you have a tendency to view yourself and your attributes more gracefully and optimistically.

B. What We Resist Persists: Optimistic Reorientation
When it rains look for rainbows, when it's dark look for stars.

Oscar Wilde

Name a few frustrating life events that are not changeable. What opportunity can you find within this event? For instance, maybe you get anxious when standing in line at the grocery store or getting stuck in traffic, where you might fixate on all the things you have to do or how late you will be. You can't change the wait time, but you can reorient your thinking by viewing it as a welcome mental rest in your busy day; a time when you have nothing to do but be present in your body or to relax by focusing on your breathing.

Using emotions and sensations as cues provides an opportunity to examine underlying thoughts from the observer's seat. Observing your thoughts changes your orientation. Rather than being lost in thought, your thinking becomes an objective "other," separate from you. This is how we distinguish the "noise" of thoughts and emotions from the "signal" of who we are (the observer of these things).

When you catch yourself feeling discontent or depressed, dig a little deeper. It is often the result of ruminating on negative, insecure thoughts of the past. It can sound a bit like, "I should have … I shouldn't have … so I'm not good enough." This orientation erodes our confidence and, as such, can keep us from doing the *significant* thing. This frame of reference often results in our feelings of lack that get us stuck in the role of victim. Similarly, when anxiety arises in the body, it often relates to insecure thoughts of the future. Something that might sound a bit like, "I need to … I should … then I'll be good enough." Recognizing these thoughts, feelings, or sensations for what they are can be a powerful cue to be mindful. With mindfulness, we can step back (nonattachment), gain perspective, and reorient ourselves.

How might this reorientation impact your experience of the event you have in mind?

Soothing With Gratitude

Gratitude is appreciating what we have as opposed to focusing on what we do not have. It depends on our humility and expectations, and it proliferates when we receive more than we expect or more than we believe we deserve. Studies show a positive correlation between gratitude and happiness (Mahipalan & Sheena, 2018), joy (Watkins et al., 2018), sleep quality (Wood et al., 2009), spiritual awareness, improved physical and mental health outcomes (Wood & Maltby, 2009), fulfilling relationships (Bartlett & DeSteno, 2006), and stress reduction (Solberg & Segerstrom, 2006).

Practising gratitude requires attention and noticing the blessings we often take for granted. Directing our attention enables us to reorient our perceptions and diffuses feelings of entitlement and victimhood. We can try to think positive thoughts, but if they do not align with our emotional state, then they often will not shift our trajectory. To be clear, it is not helpful to employ gratitude to avoid difficult emotions that need to be felt and discharged. Doing so may cause these emotions to get stuck (often described as trauma). However, once we recognize and allow ourselves to feel the emotions that are arising, investigate the message, and nurture any suffering, we are ready to reorient our feeling state with gratitude. By doing so, we interrupt the stress response and boost our confidence to navigate life's challenges.

Gratitude is a powerful way to interrupt negative emotions. It enables positive feelings of gratitude for how far we have come and for the gifts we have *right now*. Focusing the attention in this way fortifies the habit and provides an opportunity to notice and then challenge incompatible thoughts. Some find that writing down the things they are thankful for enables them to deepen this way of being. Another way to reorient with gratitude is to bring self-compassionate attention to the wound beneath the symptoms we tend to fixate on. Practise looking back at your progress; doing so will bolster your confidence and enable you to savour the pleasure of your progress.

EXPRESSING GRATITUDE

Much like the loving-kindness exercises described in this book, by choosing to acknowledge the aspects of people that we are grateful for, we can often accept other aspects that previously seemed intolerable. Expressing gratitude to others, even before we feel gratitude, is a good way to embody the feeling and in turn fortify more gracious habits. Using more specific terms besides an ordinary "thank you," which many of us have grown immune to, will often be more meaningful and effective. For example, instead of saying thank you to someone, you might say, "I really appreciate how you ...."

LOOKING AT THE ROOTS INSTEAD OF THE FRUITS

In noisier times, when we are tired of feeling our way around in the dark, our confidence is hampered and our sense of meaning eroded. We lose motivation.

Rather than focusing on specific symptoms/behaviours in our lives, with self-compassion and nonattachment we can dig deeper, identifying the wounded roots from which the symptoms sprung. Becoming overly focused on symptoms only fuels shame, which causes more nervous system reactions and distorted ways of being (more symptoms!). While our symptoms may feel like the most important thing to focus on, as they are the most obvious component to attach to, they are merely an indicator of incongruence.

Through gratitude, we are more likely to recognize the message within the symptoms. The symptoms are like guideposts, alerting us to dis-ease in the body and enabling us to recalibrate where needed. In this way, the suffering we feel can be an important road sign to check in with our roots. It alerts us to the source of incongruence, which is exactly where the physical manifestations and impulsive behaviours spring from. Emotions are like a gasket whose presence enables us to discharge incongruent energies. From this vantage point, even intense emotions can be viewed as a welcome gift, a release, an opportunity to lighten the load.

LOOKING BACK INSTEAD OF FORWARD

People have the tendency to fall into unappreciative thought patterns soon after beneficial events have passed (Mitchell, 2010). However, by looking back we can cultivate gratitude. This reorientation, looking back instead of forward, pivots us from focusing on the gap of what we have yet to achieve to feeling gratitude for how far we've come. It prevents us from focusing on what we think we need to attain happiness and buffers us from feelings of entitlement and victimhood.

Finally, using positive, meaningful, and realistic affirmations in the form of short phrases or a mantra is another tool that can help us pivot to a more grateful and optimistic perspective (Lighthall et al., 2013). The ability to view both the negative and positive aspects of our life, providing a framework of gratitude and optimism, promotes healing from past wounds. When our inner world shifts from pessimism and victimhood to optimism and gratitude, we are more likely to feel safe, enabling a desire to drop in to digest unresolved traumas and incongruence: "Unexpected capacities emerge, existing relationships once taken for granted become more precious, awareness and insight into what really matters in life is realized, and spiritual senses are heightened" (Emmons & Stern, 2013, p. 853).

SAVOURING FLEETING PLEASURES

Savouring describes the ability to stretch out and immerse in positive moments for as long as possible. Pretty great skill to have! Those who savour are also those who tend to practise more gratitude. Much like savouring a meal by slowing down and taking notice of the fine details, we can savour other moments throughout our day in the same way.

Fuelling Gratitude

- Each act of kindness and/or gratitude releases dopamine, our brain's pleasure chemical, so the habits of kindness and gratitude make for more pleasurable days.
- Act and talk as though you are grateful and often the feelings will meet the occasion.
- Find new ways to express gratitude that extend beyond the token "thank you." For instance, "I am so grateful for ... " or writing it down in a card or letter.
- Recall one thing you are grateful for each day.
- Before you fall asleep each night, consider as many things as you can that happened that day that you are thankful for.
- Recognize that much like gift giving, the giver of gratitude often receives even greater benefits than the receiver.
- Cultivate the habit of reorienting with a glass half-full approach, recognizing how much abundance is all around us and that, in this way, we are so fortunate to have water in our glasses at all (as many do not).
- Consider your mortality, doing your best to appreciate others as much as possible in the short time we are here.
- Reflect on our connectedness. We are working within and contributing to a large and meaningful picture. From this perspective, even menial parts of our day can be made meaningful from this perspective. Viewing the world in this way enables us to ask for help, as we are collectively working toward a common cause.

Strengthening Practices

A. Cultivating Gratitude by Savouring

Starting our day within a framework of gratitude helps us notice the positive aspects of our lives. Because humans tend to have a negativity bias (Gollan et al., 2016), we must consciously look for the positive. Doing a gratitude practice in the morning is ideal, perhaps in the gap between awakening and lifting your head from the pillow. It can be as simple as counting your blessings and can occur whenever and however it feels most natural to you. *The key is to cultivate feelings of gratitude.* An obligational activity is typically not effective because your body will likely not *feel* grateful if it has to do something it does not want to do.

To practise, start by recalling three core attributes or events in your life that you are grateful for (family, friends, job, health, etc.). Sit with each one. Breathe into it, enabling yourself to drop in, connecting your heart to the attribute or event.

Now think about three smaller things that you are grateful for (e.g., your breakfast, a good night's sleep, a favourable evaluation at work, the pleasant conversation you had with your partner last night). Continue to sit with the feeling, expanding it as long as possible. Savour the moment.

B. Cultivating and Expressing Gratitude for Self

We all come into this human experience with a specific set of qualities designed to fulfill a unique and meaningful purpose. Depending on our cultural conditioning, many of us avoid spending time appreciating ourselves. And we especially avoid expressing self-appreciation to others. This avoidance of self-appreciation comes from a fear of being rejected, threatening our primal need for love, acceptance, and belonging. We generally play to our cultural conditioning in this area. If we learned it was distasteful to say nice things about ourselves, most of us subconsciously adapt to fit within the social mold. Perhaps we fear we will seem arrogant or that we will be vulnerable to scrutiny and hostility from others. We are far more comfortable pointing out and ruminating on weaknesses, which is further compounded by the human tendency to have a negativity bias (Gollan et al., 2016). There are two components to self-appreciation: (1) recognizing our strengths and (2) sharing and expressing our unique qualities with others. These two components are interdependent. Recognizing our strengths empowers us to be vulnerable, and vulnerability is a requirement of authentic self-expression.

Recognize Your Gifts
Think about those unique skills and abilities that come easily to you. Can you articulate a few of these? If you come up with items that seem superficial, try going a little deeper, identifying those parts that reflect the essence of who you are and what you value. This process is how you begin to feel into and align with your calling, which is further explored in subsequent chapters.

Recognize Your Desire
Equally important is recognizing what events, topics, and activities spark your passion. Can you name a few events, activities, or topics you found yourself engrossed in recently? Again, the answer will provide clues about your unique essence, enabling you to feel into the unique life qualities that align with your unique calling.

Sprinkle in a few new habits that cultivate an attitude of gratitude and that honour your uniqueness. For example:

- Tap into your inner joy. Try subtly smiling as you go through your daily routine. Notice the impact it has on your perspective and how others respond to you (mirroring transference effect).
- Instead of saying sorry every time you make a mistake, consider whether sorry is really the kindest response. For instance, perhaps you are running late; try focusing on thanking people for waiting rather than berating yourself for being late.
- When you are running behind on a task, instead of berating yourself for falling behind, try looking back at how much you have already accomplished.
- When someone compliments you, say thank you rather than deflecting it.
- Make a list of what you like about yourself or the ways in which your self-expression has impacted others. Keep it in your wallet as a reminder to use in the moments when you feel vulnerable to self-destructive thoughts. When we are authentic, it inspires others to have the courage to be authentic too!
- When inadequacies seem to be especially apparent, remind yourself that we all have strengths and weaknesses—this is a normal part of being human. You are in good company!
- Practise saying no to something you would typically grudgingly agree to. Much like you would support a friend who was challenged in this area, celebrate the courage it takes to say no.

- Follow your body's cues by eating something you desire. Mindfully enjoy the experience, and take notice when the flavour wanes (your body's initial cuing that you've had enough).
- If guilt arises when you take time to *be*, recognize it as an old thought pattern resulting from an old wound (not a fact). Speak kindly to it as you would to a confused (and suffering) friend, then release it.
- Do something you desire as an act of appreciation for yourself!

Soothing With Forgiveness

I do not at all understand the mystery of grace—only that it meets us where we are but does not leave us where it found us. (Lamott, 1999)

Forgiveness is the diminishing of the negative feelings that result from the sense that we were wronged (Lambert et al., 2010). When we harbour negative feelings such as anger, resentment, and hostility, it activates the sympathetic nervous system. The resulting biological cascade has immediate and chronic impacts on our mental and physical health. When chronically activated, the body cannot focus on healing and balance, because it must instead focus its available energy on the potential threat. *Potential* is the key word here, as there is often not an actual threat in the current moment, just a vague sense that, at any moment, a real threat might emerge. Living in this highly alert state takes a toll on us. For instance, each time we inadvertently activate the stress response, our anxiety increases along with a spike in cortisol, causing vasoconstriction and increased blood pressure and heart rate; over time, this damages our coronary arteries (Kelly, 2018; Miller et al., 1996; van Oyen Witvliet et al., 2001).

Forgiveness does not change the past; it changes our future. It is our opportunity to rewrite an old (and often painful) story. We create a new way to remember, moving from bitterness to love. Forgiveness liberates us from violent events committed against us and by us, breaking us free from re-experiencing the violation over and over in our memories. Forgiveness removes the emotional charge associated with old memories, enabling us to transform our suffering into wisdom.

Forgiveness enables us to release anger and resentment, lowering levels of cortisol (the major stress hormone) and reducing the likelihood of a host of health conditions that we perpetuate via chronic stress (Kelly, 2018; Worthington & Scherer, 2004). As long as we *feel* victimized by others, we will continually recount the violation done to us, feeling like it just occurred. When we victimize ourselves, we engage in self-destructive thoughts and behaviours, acting as the perpetrator and the victim. By practising forgiveness, we are breaking the victim–perpetrator cycle. We let go of resentments, setting ourselves free from feeling like a perpetual victim.

Forgiveness empowers us to change what we can about the situation. Forgiveness and letting go is about accepting what *was,* that which we cannot change, and changing what we can by reorienting ourselves. Stepping out of the victim role is changing what we can, and it is through forgiveness that we do so. By owning our transgressions (how our projections harm others), we prevent ourselves from perpetuating more suffering in ourselves and others. In conjunction with owning our projections, within relationships where we feel unconditionally positively regarded, we can release the shame associated with reactions that are not congruent with our core values. To be clear, forgiveness is often a multi-step process. Each time a thought or emotion arises that feels like a threat, we can notice when we are feeling victimized by the felt sense. To step into a more empowering and resourced orientation, we must step back from the emotion, naming it as an "other," so we can work with the thoughts surrounding it more objectively. If you cannot find the objectivity to reorient on your own, reach out to someone you trust and let them provide the compassion and objectivity you need in that moment. With each reorientation, we forgive and let go a little more until one day we find that the anger, resentment, or hostility has left us completely.

Nothing ever happened in the past that can prevent you from being present now.

Eckhart Tolle

Clearing Practices

A. Forgiving Others, Forgiving Ourselves, and Making Amends

Forgive yourself for not knowing what you didn't know before you learned it.

Maya Angelou

Forgiving Yourself and Others

It is exhausting to carry the burden of resentment. When we think others threaten our ability to meet our basic human needs, we wear the victim hat. When others believe we are a threat to their basic needs, we wear the perpetrator hat. Whether we play the victim or the perpetrator is not important. How we identify and live outside of the role is what matters. Playing the part of a victim disempowers us and dampens our ability to act congruently. We become chronically distracted by the need to survive, which usually means we turn the volume down on the internal cues and turn the volume up on thoughts that are fuelled by the stress response. This disembodied way of *doing* in the world leads to all sorts of fighting, fleeing, freezing, and fawning (Chapter 3). Getting stuck wearing the victim hat will not serve us.

Forgiving others releases us from the victim role. Forgiving others has many other benefits too. We know that harbouring resentment burns our emotional energy stores and leads to "noisy" relationships characterized by activated nervous systems. The old loop in our minds argues about who wears what hat: who wins and who loses.

Rewriting the story to focus on where we are going and what we've gained in the learning is exactly how we take off the unhelpful hats. When we take them off, no longer identifying with them, we can tune back into who we are (outside of hats and other forms of conditioning). When we do, we have more energy for relationships and activities that build us up, better emotional health, and greater ability to deescalate conflict. Being willing to recognize when we are carrying resentments demonstrates a willingness to begin to let them go. Try not to get hung up on next steps. When you are ready, you will be provided with all the wisdom, courage, and resources necessary to let go.

Forgiveness is not about forgetting our mistakes or the mistakes of others. It's a decision to stop being a prisoner (victim) of the past. In this exercise, we dip our toe in a past narrative, one that continually comes up and leaves us feeling disempowered. By deactivating and discharging the stuck emotions associated with outdated narratives, we can use the lessons of the past to make us wiser rather than using the emotions as a source of ongoing suffering. To avoid getting stuck or frozen in shame, remind yourself that whatever hat you wear, whether victim or perpetrator, these are illusions of the mind. They do not define us. They do not impact our inherent worth. They are simply narratives that can be made right, rewritten for the benefit of all.

Harm occurs when our basic needs go unmet. Make a list of all the people who've harmed you. Perhaps you felt rejected, violated (physically, sexually, or emotionally), unsafe, excluded, put down, and so forth. Don't forget to include yourself. Don't hold back at this point. Get them all down on paper. Let it flow.

This exercise is an opportunity to notice where you may be wearing the old victim hat, holding onto an unhelpful narrative. Before you begin, it's important to make sure your state of mind and setting will facilitate a healing experience rather than fuelling any felt sense of shame or isolation. Resource yourself! Reach out to trusted others to support you in this process. Just talking it through, even knowing that you have someone a phone call away, is helpful.

This is not a "fix ourselves" exercise. It is more about the means than the end result. Without feeling the need to fix anything, we take this opportunity to feel into the hurt beneath the narratives that are informing our current-day behaviours. In doing so, we can optimistically explore what we learned from the experience. Separate from the reactions that result from wearing the victim or perpetrator hat, we are training ourselves to look for the learning opportunity. This is how we transform resentment to wisdom.

Owning Our Projections/Transgressions
When it comes to conflict, it's often more difficult to see our missteps than the transgressions of others. Make a list of everyone you have harmed, including yourself. Some of the most intense resentments we carry against others are powerful because they are projections; in other words, they are reminders of our past incongruent behaviours that we have yet to make amends for. At this point, shame often creeps in. Remind yourself that these feelings are a normal part of being human (emerging

from areas of incongruence that are still in need of healing). We are all in the same boat on this journey toward congruence. It is much easier to name all the ways in which someone victimized us than to acknowledge when we have been the perpetrator. Practise loving-kindness here. Speak kindly to the fears and shame that bubble up; step back from them by speaking to them as dear friends. No need to fix anything: you are simply an objective scientist, studying the narratives that inform the emotions in your inner world. Just *being* in feeling is enough. No *doing* necessary.

Making Amends

Stop! Before you skip this exercise altogether, please hear me out. Going through this exercise is not locking you into making confessions and apologies. Just being willing to work through the process, owning your part, is enough. A willingness to acknowledge our part is sometimes enough. All that is required of us is to release the shame associated with our actions and to release others from the shame of theirs. If our *significant* thing winds up being making amends with an old friend, then so be it. We will have what we need when we are ready to do so.

There is grace in the process: we all feel shame and ashamed of varying parts of the past. This is a normal part of being human. You are not alone. This part of the exercise can be especially difficult! This is when we need to flex those self-compassion muscles and resource ourselves with trusted others along the way. We all make mistakes! It's not about never making mistakes—it's about doing our best to make amends when we are called to do so. Responsibility, or *response-ability*, for our side of the street is how we release pent-up shame (a product of behaving in ways that are incongruent with our values and essence). Take comfort in the fact that we all live incongruently at times. This is part of being human—you are not alone. When we do not respond after behaving incongruently, hurting ourselves and/or others, shame wells up inside us. As shame floods us, we become less willing to go inside ourselves because being with shame is too painful. Instead, we turn to external substances and activities to soothe ourselves. Shame then spills over into our relationships with others (*horizontal violence*). Often, others also play a part in conflicts, but that is not within our control. What *is* within our control is the condition of our side of the street. Making amends is our work, taking ownership of our side of the street. Doing so enables us to be congruent.

Drop in and begin your list. Consider the events in your life where you acted incongruently. Perhaps you did or said something that harmed another or acted in ways that were incongruent with your core values. The events we feel the most shame about will easily come to mind. Shame pulls us out of tune, pointing to emotional injuries that require tending.

Let yourself write freely, trusting that your embodied self will lead the way. When your list is complete, breath space into any inner "noise" with a few deep, cleansing breaths. Taking it a step further, try imagining that you are breathing in mercy and breathing out compassion. If you are feeling especially vulnerable, you may find it helpful to hold a hand over your heart or hold your hands together as though you're holding a dear friend's hand. You deserve to be celebrated and comforted for doing this difficult work! Recognizing that this exercise will often uncover intense emotions or trauma, you will want to refer back to the tips for dealing with uncomfortable emotions and trauma.

Well done! You've completed your lists. Now, take some time to let your emotions settle. Simply recognizing past hurts and acknowledging how we have hurt others is powerful healing work. As for your next steps, you can trust that if and when the time comes to make amends, the yearning and opportunity will present itself. Many people find that writing a letter (elaborated on next) to the person they harmed is a valuable process; whether it gets sent is often beside the point. For those we are aiming to forgive, often just writing the letter is enough. We do not want to harm others as part of our process. We can send the letter in other ways, such as burning it (transmuting to light), drowning it (purifying), and/or burying it (giving back to the earth for healing).

The next steps are unique to each person. Trust the process. If healing requires a *significant* action, you will have the necessary resources to do so.

B. Living a Life of Letting Go
Forgiveness is understanding that the past is an unchangeable and essential part of our journey toward wholeness.

Assessing Where We Are At
Consider your own habits of holding onto and letting go of anger, resentments, and hostility. How does it impact you on a day-to-day basis? How often do you ruminate on these feelings? What emotions and/or physical symptoms result? As uncomfortable emotions arise in these reflective moments, use the opportunity to flex your self-compassion muscles, soothing yourself with words of grace, mercy, and unconditional positive regard for self.

The Process of Letting Go
Bring a person to mind toward whom you are holding feelings of anger/resentment/hostility. Perhaps this person is you. Imagine them sitting in front of you. Connect to them, reminding yourself that they too have suffered and experienced pain, and that this pain and suffering is likely at the roots of their offensive behaviours (projecting their suffering onto others). Breathe in mercy on the inhale, perhaps imagining it flow into you as a cleansing, white light. On the exhale, extend compassion and empathy to them. Practise this breathing until you feel a subtle release or a space between you and the resentment you have been holding onto. After the shift, however subtle, look beyond their pain and suffering—look for their beauty, continuing to send them empathy and compassion.

Forgiveness, the process of letting go of our negative emotions toward another, is not forgetting. There are situations and relationships that require us to walk away. In these situations, walking away is an act of wisdom and self-compassion. Letting go of the negative emotions enables us to objectively and compassionately determine the best way forward.

Letter Writing and Burning

Putting thoughts down on paper enables you to dig deeper, uncovering wounds and resentments that are otherwise difficult to access. Writing can facilitate a digestion and integration process that promotes understanding and meaning making. When using writing in this way, it is important to drop in, moving from the thinking mind to the sensing mind. Out of your head and into your heart, from *doing* to *being*. Let your emotions flow, writing freely, without filters and without judgement. Write until there is nothing left to write. Once your letter is complete, find a safe place where you can burn it. Watch it burn. As it turns to ash, imagine yourself letting it go; let the fire refine you, cleanse you, free you. As you release it, bring something new (just one word) into the void it left behind; breathing in _____ (love, peace, joy, Spirit, compassion, etc.). When complete, take time to sit, to breathe, to grieve, whatever feels necessary. This time of sitting after you complete a practice is essential to releasing/grieving the old and integrating the new.

Letting go is a continuous practice that works one layer at a time. Listen to your body and slow down when it's too much, regulating your nervous system as you go. Reorient yourself: resource yourself with the support of trusted others who can remind you that your emotions are not threats, that you are not alone, and that the "noise" does not define you. When you notice yourself ruminating in anger or resentment, it is time to do the *significant* thing, peeling back another layer as you do.

Navigating Order ("Signal") and Chaos ("Noise"): Navigating Within Complexity

Given the challenging times we live in, navigating chaos is now more important than ever (Dames, 2020). As with the natural world, embodied *being* as opposed to disembodied *doing* requires a delicate balance of chaos and order. When *being* authentic, we lack self-consciousness, enabling inspired doing to flow from abundance. We know we are in this abundant *being* state when the reward overshadows the effort. Many refer to this *being* state as natural flow. This is who we are as human *beings*.

When congruent, we lack shame and can find reprieve in the clarity of our "signal." With this clarity, we can more easily distinguish and navigate the felt chaos that often comes with passing challenges. Because we are securely planted, we have a strong sense of place in the world. We interweave with others, giving in times of abundance and receiving in times of need. We have an abundance of fruits and foliage to navigate the external conditions and more than enough to happily contribute to those with fewer resources.

We become overly rigid when we are primarily driven by the left side of the brain. From here, we fall into frustrated perfectionism, losing our power to a set of idealistic rules that we feel beholden to. From this state of disconnected attachment to external conditions, we fixate on *do*ing. When we prioritize the opinions of others over our own needs and values, we lack creativity, adaptability, and heartfelt meaning. As a result of this growing incongruence, we carry shame, causing a chronic form of stress that fuels "freezing" and "fleeing." From this place of fear and scarcity, growth is limited, and we become prone to stagnation.

On the other end of the spectrum, we experience too much chaos when we are primarily driven by the right side of the brain. From here, we lose control as we frantically and fearfully move from one moment to the next, lost in a state of unconscious reactivity in response to the fires of the moment. The space we need to drop into the inner world in order to stay grounded is chewed up by a barrage of "noisy" stimuli. When we are in a state of extreme chaos, we lose the felt sense of our grounding and security in the world ("signal"), causing the sympathetic nervous system to take over. From this generally disembodied place, growth and healing is very limited (if not impossible), and we become prone to emotional and nervous system breakdown.

Living in complexity, a natural state of flow, happens when we find our unique balance of order and chaos. *Be*ing human requires a certain degree of security in one's inner and outer resources. When feeling resourced, we confidently engage with the interacting parts of life. It requires a trust in the natural order that unfolds when we act congruently in the world. We develop this trust by practising authentic self-expression in relationships that can provide compassionate witnessing (mirror transference), characterized by unconditional positive regard.

In this state of complexity, how we feel and what is important to our *be*ing is exactly what drives our *do*ing. Our work becomes inspired, with all sorts of positive energy flowing from it. Because we are not self-conscious or tending to incongruent behaviours in response to what we think others need from us, our days roll by relatively effortlessly, fuelled by heartfelt meaning and connection. From this place of abundance, growth is maximized as we naturally synchronize with our environment.

We all have preferences that vary according to our unique natures and our nervous systems' window of tolerance for uncertainty. Some prefer living on the edge of chaos, leaning into the inspiration that flows from this freer way of being. Others prefer living with more order, finding pleasure in consistent routines that provide frequent grounding opportunities and clearer direction. We can find our place on the order–chaos spectrum by paying attention to the expansion and contractions of the body. When we are out of balance, the body gets activated, which acts as our internal alert system. This is our cue! When alerted, we have an opportunity to get curious. When we engage with curiosity, we become the objective observer, enabling the very thing we are observing to be a distinct "other." As we unstick from overly attaching to any felt sense or external stimuli, the perceived threat lessens, enabling the root emotion to be felt and tended to.

One felt moment at a time, one compassionate and significant act at a time, we find our way back to balance.

The Challenge: Navigation

By considering someone else's challenge, or working with another to consider ours, we cultivate nonattachment. We can often find comfort knowing we are not alone and that we can learn from and with each other. By working from this more objective space, we mitigate the stress response. We can then reorient ourselves from this position of strength, which improves our ability to feel into all our biological, intellectual, and spiritual capacities. With this benevolent orientation, we can face adversities with confidence, knowing we have the resources and support necessary to navigate life's challenges.

Let's circle back to Marnie's challenge to cultivate a new trajectory (Figure 1.3). Marnie feels frustrated and ashamed by the behaviours that emerge when her nervous system takes over. She finds herself frequently defaulting to a state of freeze, with little to no ability to interrupt the process of getting there. By *coming to know* about the freeze response, she is developing an ability to step back (nonattachment). From this vantage point, she recognizes that her behaviours are a symptom of a threatened nervous system. She is beginning to *clear* the "noise," to tune into the "signal" at the heart of her distress. She is learning to *attune* to who she "really" is, separate from her body's biological response to stress. By *strengthening* her authentic connection to self and others, she remembers her inherent worth and is starting to feel and try out the abundance of resources within and around her. As a result, she finds herself being more tolerant to life's challenges. She is also more willing to ask for help before she extends herself beyond her window of tolerance for stress.

Marnie is learning that the means of how she gets there (with self-compassion) is more important than the end goal (changing coping habits). Change is happening slowly, as she still falls into overwhelm at times, but she is beginning to realize that this gentle pace is okay, that it is normal for the body to move at the pace of trust. As she accepts herself as she is right now, she understands that she is impacted but not defined by her conditioning. She is beginning to see her missteps as opportunities to remember her inherent worth ("signal"), unchanged by behaviours and outcomes ("noise"). She is *aligning* with her "real" self as she integrates activities and habits into her life that spark her desire. For all of these reasons, Marnie is able to see herself outside of the process, enabling her to celebrate all the milestones along the way (including the missteps!). She is developing her roots to thrive.

Attuning/Reflecting Opportunity

Describe how the strategies described in this chapter can empower you to provide the loving-kindness necessary to tend to the sensations of your inner world. When an uncomfortable sensation arises, what would it look like to allow it to fully emerge so that it can heal? What resources and supports do you need?

Attuning for the Journey Ahead: Clearing Trauma— The Unresolved Weather of the Past

We are coming to know how to tune into the felt sense of loving-kindness, as illustrated in the practices described in this chapter. Additionally, we can employ mindful reorientation practices that enable us to step back from the "noise" of past narratives and uncomfortable emotions. Mindfulness provides a space that enables the objectivity required to tether us to our "signal." From this more spacious place, we can lean in like a compassionate scientist to investigate the thoughts, events, and environments that are causing us stress. When we can, we make changes; if we cannot make changes, we accept what is and embrace a spirit of gratitude and optimism to change our orientation. To do this, we can:

- Reparent via loving-kindness (working with thoughts and sensations as we would with dear friends)
- Reorient using gratitude and strategic optimism, and
- Reorient using forgiveness.

Now, we delve deeper into the inner world, *clearing* unresolved trauma so that we can *attune* to the calm within, *strengthening* our capacities to navigate day-to-day challenges.

CHAPTER 10

Clearing Past Trauma: The Unresolved Weather of the Past

While there is an increased focus on providing trauma-informed care to clients, we as caregivers also experience and carry trauma. Trauma is a normal part of the human experience. If we cloak it with negative labels, we will avoid it when it comes knocking. When we normalize trauma, recognizing it as an important cue that healing is necessary, we are far more likely to lean in to the opportunity. In simple terms, trauma is the stuck emotional energy that we were previously unequipped to feel. Now that we are more resourced and secure, we can notice the stuck energy of trauma, feel the feelings, and release the energy. If we remain stuck in a fear or shame response, unable to see the gift within the prompt, the nervous system is likely going to continue running the show, resulting in subconscious reactions (projections of the trauma) rather than conscious action.

Post-traumatic stress disorder (PTSD) can develop after any stressful event that lands us outside of our window of tolerance for stress. When we extend beyond this window, we often become disembodied, which hampers our ability to feel the emotion that needs to be felt in the moment. As a result, the energy of the emotion gets stuck in the body. This stuck energy creates an inner "noise" when current events remind us of a past hurt. Common indicators of PTSD, among those who are not already challenged with similar symptoms related to clinical depression, are (1) feeling haunted by memories of the event or events, (2) having challenges in personal relationships, and (3) having difficulty controlling emotions (Keane et al., 1988). Events that can cause PTSD are often related to incidents involving acts of violence, natural or human-caused disasters, and accidents (National Institute of Mental Health, 2020). Seventy percent of people have experienced at least one traumatic event, and up to 20% of those will go on to develop PTSD as a result (PTSD United, 2020). As for caregivers, in some studies more than half of the providers working in high-acuity settings screened positive for PTSD (Iranmanesh et al., 2013; Manitoba Nurses' Union, 2015). PTSD was introduced in Chapter 3 and is described again a bit later in this chapter.

Painful memories and intense emotions from unresolved traumatic events will often emerge as we develop trust with ourselves and others. Part of the process of clearing out the "noise" in our inner space is cultivating an inner environment that feels resourced and safe. When securely attached to ourselves and others, we can notice this stuck emotional energy, feel it, and when ready, let it go. Over time, a sense of emotional safety softens us, readying us to process and resolve past traumas.

Uncomfortable emotions are a good sign! It means that our body trusts in our ability to tend to it. To continue building on that trust, our *significant* action in that moment is to respond with self-compassion. As evident in polyvagal theory (described in Chapter 1), you may think you can get there faster alone, but in this case, it is the opposite. The more you resource with objective and caring others that you feel safe with, the wider your window of tolerance will be for stress. Remember, trauma relates to emotions that felt too unsafe to feel, and quite likely, you did not feel you had the necessary support from others in your time of need. These same emotions will come up again and again until they are given space to be felt. If we do not consciously feel them, we will undoubtedly subconsciously project them. Healing in community (including with professional therapists) is exactly what it takes to expand your window of tolerance to hold these intense emotions so they can be felt and discharged.

From Suffering to Bliss: Transforming Trauma to Grit

As a fellow human who is healing from past wounds and remembering my wholeness, I too am on this path and have had this experience. Because I am doing it, I know it is possible! Just as a storm encourages tree roots to grow deeper, so too do past adversities encourage a more resilient constitution on the other side when we are on a healing path. Healing is the redemptive path, the rewriting of old (and often unhelpful) stories. For those of us who have spent a lifetime carrying heavy emotional loads, an immense sense of relief, even bliss can come when we develop the choice to lay it down. This lighter way of being can carry us through the minor annoyance of life. The experience can be so powerful that, without any effort at all, it accelerates the healing of others who continue to suffer beneath the weight of past adversities. Our collective healing leads to the evolution of a more conscious and compassionate human race. Let us help each other lay down these loads. It serves everyone and is well worth the journey.

The Challenge: Orientation

By considering someone else's challenge, or working with another to consider ours, we cultivate nonattachment. We can often find comfort knowing we are not alone and that we can learn from and with each other. Working from this more objective space, we mitigate the stress response. We can then reorient from this position of strength, thus improving our ability to use all our biological, intellectual, and spiritual capacities. With this benevolent orientation, we can face adversities with confidence, knowing we have the resources and support necessary to navigate life's challenges.

Let's practise by considering Jared's situation. Jared works full time as a respiratory therapist in an acute care setting. For as long as Jared can remember, He has lived with a sense of angst in his body. To be specific, he feels like he has a constant knot in his stomach, which is accompanied by a message from his felt sense that "something bad is about to happen." This sense has impacted how he has handled challenges and kept him awake at night. His colleagues have come to view Jared as a bit irritable, and he tends to isolate himself from others on the team. He reacts defensively when asked to take on extra tasks or given feedback about his practice. When changes need to be made, Jared is known for his hostile reactions, which tend to manifest as eye rolling or sighs. His co-workers have learned that it is best to give Jared wide berth and to approach with caution.

Recently, Jared left work in a hurry because he feared that he was having a heart attack. He was shocked and embarrassed to learn that what he had experienced was in fact an anxiety attack. The attending physician sat down beside Jared, explained that he was not in any physical danger, and then asked whether he could refer Jared for a mental health assessment. Afraid that he would continue losing control if he did not, Jared agreed.

As a result of his experience, Jared began working with a mental health provider. After several sessions, Jared accepted that he has unknowingly been struggling with PTSD for most of his adult life. He now realizes that what he had previously thought of as character defects were actually symptoms of PTSD. He now feels ashamed of his defensive and impulsive reactions, but until recently, he had believed that these were just a part of who he was.

At first, Jared feels ashamed to take on a diagnosis of PTSD, as it has shattered the "idealized" image that he has striven to attain. But once he accepts it, to his surprise, he experiences an immense sense of relief and, even more importantly, hope.

Why do you think Jared feels a sense of relief? How might this new orientation to his challenges and behaviours impact his ability to manage them?

Managing Emotions and Resolving Trauma

The wounds we cannot see are often more painful than those we can.

When our emotions feel overwhelming, to the point that we cannot feel them and stay embodied at the same time, it is time to resource ourselves. If the emotions are not too intense, we can often regulate ourselves enough using a stress mitigation tool (Chapter 6) to make space for the emotion, but often we need more. This is when healing in community is imperative. When things are feeling sticky, when we are becoming overly attached to an old narrative or lost inside an emotion, we need to resource with an objective other. Getting an objective perspective from a trusted friend or professional can help us keep our emotions in perspective. With practice and self-trust, we can provide this same form of compassion and objectivity to ourselves, enabling emotions to be felt and released. It takes time to develop these skills. In the meantime, having a compassionate ear can be immensely helpful in working through emotions. In these cases, reaching out for help is exactly how we exercise self-compassion.

VICARIOUS TRAUMA

A common form of trauma that occurs among caregivers is vicarious trauma (introduced in Chapter 3). The term vicarious trauma was originally coined in the 1990s (McCann & Pearlman, 1990) and describes the impact of repeated exposure to accounts of traumatic events. When unresolved, the experience of vicarious trauma can affect our identity and beliefs; it can lead to cynicism and despair, which often extends beyond the boundaries of our practice and seeps into our personal lives (Pearlman & Saakvitne, 1995). For example, those that regularly work with sick children may have a difficult time remaining objective when their own children become ill, or someone who works with terminally ill clients may struggle with grieving when a loved one passes.

Those who are more prone to overidentifying with others' emotions—going beyond empathetic engagement—are especially vulnerable to experiencing vicarious trauma. Mindfulness, which interweaves with sense of coherence (Grevenstein et al., 2018), buffers us from overidentifying with the experiences of others, thereby preventing vicarious trauma. When we can step back from emotions, both others' and our own, we are more able to accept the emotions as messages that require investigation rather than as threatening facts. Every emotion is an opportunity for healing, enabling us to care for old wounds, practise self-compassion, and reorient ourselves when helpful.

What we can feel we can heal. (Neff, 2018)

POST-TRAUMATIC STRESS DISORDER

PTSD can develop from events that we interpret as highly threatening to our emotional or physical well-being, or in the case of complex PTSD, from feeling unable to escape ongoing traumatic events such as abuse and neglect. How we interpret an event directly correlates with how traumatic or threatening it feels, which is why two people in the same situation can respond so differently: one person can walk away feeling largely unscathed, while another may feel traumatized. According to the National Institute of Mental Health (2019a), most people will go through the process of getting activated, having a fight, flight, or freeze response, and then once the nervous systems rebalances, naturally return to their pre-event state. However, some will experience ongoing stress and acute feelings of threat, chronically activating the fight, flight, or freeze response, even when they are no longer in danger.

Working With "Gut" Reactions

You know that feeling when someone says something to you, and you have a physical reaction that feels out of proportion to the situation? Maybe suddenly feeling hot in the face or like you were punched in the gut? Or perhaps more nebulous, like a knot in your stomach or a tense unease? These are all signs we are feeling threatened, whether or not our physical or emotional safety is truly at risk. The whole, often subconscious, process of becoming activated can happen in less than a second, leaving us no time to calculate the most beneficial action. Rather, we default to our intuitive patterns (brain chunking, described in Chapter 5), where the situation at hand is informed by past narratives and stuck energy (trauma). As a result, when we are activated, our assumptions become facts that we react to. In these moments, we are essentially "hijacked" by a gut reaction, informed by the feeling of threat in the body, not by an objection assessment of what is happening in the current moment.

Whether or not we believe something is a threat to us is based on the assumptions we intuitively make about it. Our belief systems reflect what we *believe* in our embodied selves, not the slogans or mantras we recite to ourselves and others. This is why we can memorize wise insights in our thinking minds, but are unable to enact them in our behaviours. Our underlying beliefs are the deeply rooted thought programs we automatically (without conscious consent) use to interpret our sensations. For the most part, previous events in our lives, especially in our formative years, form the belief systems through which we filter passing stimuli. If the stimulus reminds us of a past experience that hurt us, we will likely interpret it as a threat (stressor). If we successfully navigated a similar event in the past, we will likely manage it without getting activated. These assumptions correlate with our sense of coherence in any given moment. Sense of coherence results from the belief that we have the necessary resources to manage whatever life tosses our way. In this way, our ability to navigate life with confidence depends on our underlying beliefs about ourselves and the way the world operates.

Cultivating curiosity through mindfulness is the key to uncovering our belief systems. To get to the belief systems that are causing the inner sensations that often lead us to feel threatened, we must first realize that they are "others," separate from the "signal" of who we are. If we are the deeply rooted tree, then these passing stimuli are like clouds temporarily blocking the sun as they move across the sky of our minds. The clouds are not the sky, nor is it helpful to confuse the two. The sky is a permanent part of our landscape, while the clouds are temporary weather systems that come and go. People might refer to this recognition as mindful awareness.

Rational detachment, introduced in Chapter 7, is a helpful concept to understand how nonattachment expands our window of tolerance when hostile behaviours are directed at us. It is a skill that prevents us from taking the behaviours of others personally. When tuned into rational detachment, we can recognize that other people's reactions are less about us and more about the unresolved trauma they carry. With this skill, we are more able to distinguish our emotions from the emotional transference of others. While it is more obvious how this applies to other people's trauma (past hurts) being projected outwardly, it also applies when our past hurts knock into us in the present day. The current moment may remind us of the past hurt, but today it is not the same. These moments can be thought of as *false evidence appearing real* (FEAR). We can recognize the emotion as a dear friend, yet not overly identify with them. Added to this, if we can employ rational detachment, we are also recognizing that many of our current-day emotions are projections of past wounds. Doing so helps us keep the current threat (or lack thereof) in perspective.

By stepping back from sensations that arise and making them dear friends, it prevents us from identifying with them. With presence and rational detachment from past hurts, you can uncover your belief systems by investigating them like an objective scientist would, curiously getting to know them while also keeping your distance. Now that you are holding it in perspective, take your belief system for a coffee, just like you would a dear friend. Ask the belief system questions, investigating the threads that are weaving it together. For instance, you might ask, "Where did you come from?" or "How old are you?" Sometimes we receive belief systems at a young age from our parents. When you ask, be sure to listen for the subtle answer, which may feel more like an inner knowing than distinct words that you hear. From this curious place, we remain embodied, enabling us to feel into the emotions that surround the belief system. When we feel the emotions, it removes the charge. Once uncharged, it is far easier to upgrade the belief system for one that is truer today.

It is helpful to keep regulating your nervous system during this process. To do so, try a few of the stress mitigation tools described in Chapter 6. Regulating will help you clear out the inner "noise," enabling you to tune into the "signal" that is answering the questions. Also, remember to ask genuine questions, keeping yourself curious in the process, which cultivates the nonattachment you need to remain embodied. Once you ask, take the time to listen so you can hear the answers that arise within the quiet space. These are not answers that you need to cognitively craft; it is quite the opposite. The answers will come when the "noisy" thoughts of the mind and the angst of the body settle down, allowing you to hear the quiet voice that whispers (or is relayed in the felt sense) outside of the noise of the mind. You will eventually put words to the felt sense, but do not rush to do so. Let yourself sit with the message that lies within the felt sense. If you rush to put words to it, you are at risk of disconnecting from your felt sense. As a result, you risk slowing down the healing process.

For example, you might ask any one of these questions, probing and waiting for the answers that come:

- I see that sensation is causing discomfort. I see your suffering. Can you describe the feeling?
- Is that fear? Or shame?

- What are you afraid of?
- What does this remind you of?
- How is this situation the same and how is it different?

Talking to the emotions and thoughts that arise like you would a dear friend promotes self-compassion. However, the key is that you must feel safe enough to express what feels forbidden. If we do not feel safe enough to feel and say the forbidden thing, we will not get to the belief system underneath. If we do not get to the belief system underneath, we cannot change it. Talk to yourself with unconditional positive regard, much like you would a child who has unhealed trauma. For example, using your own natural words, it might sound something like this:

I can see this is painful. You are safe with me. You can talk freely. I know it is difficult, but I am here for you now. I am your safe space. Tell me, what happened to you that is causing this fear? What you are afraid will happen? What need of yours is feeling threatened (belonging, self-esteem, love, acceptance, safety, etc.)? I see your suffering. I know it hurt and it still hurts now. While you might have felt alone in this before, you are not alone now. I want to be here with you. I want you to feel safe.

Eventually, as you move from the tip of the iceberg, melting one defensive layer at a time, you will expose the belief system underneath. Sometimes the beliefs can be obscure, requiring you to dig deep. But eventually, insight will strike, and the root will be exposed. It is here, coming from an objective place, that you can rewrite old narratives that are no longer true for you in the current day. What was threatening to you as a child may not be threatening today. But until we reorient ourselves, we will likely continue responding the way did as a child, not as the resourced adult.

False Evidence Appearing Real (FEAR)

As noted in the previous section, when inner sensations arise, you can think of them like clouds moving across the sky of our awareness. Identifying with the clouds, as though they somehow define us, is not accurate or helpful. In fact, when we view a threatening sensation as an important and temporary messenger, we are far more likely to lean in to acknowledge and resolve the concern. In those moments, we have an opportunity to both nurture the old wound and soothe ourselves in the present from a more objective and compassionate perspective. The acronym FEAR, which stands for *f*alse *e*vidence *a*ppearing *r*eal, reminds us of the subjective nature of fear. Unresolved trauma often activates fear and anxiety, distorting events in our minds. With mindfulness, we can step back from fear, clearing out the "noise" that is clouding the present reality. This process of stepping back to gain objectivity is not an act of resistance; rather, it is an allowing, even a welcoming of it. Our perception of or orientation to the fear changes. A change in perception enables us to take in the message that there is something that needs healing, not that there is an actual threat in the present moment. We can then let the related thoughts and emotions present themselves, feel into them, and speak to them as dear friends. On the other hand, when we resist fear, we miss the opportunity to heal the past hurts that continue to project themselves in the current day. The "Guest House," a poem by the great 13th-century Persian poet, scholar, and mystic Rumi (1997), provides insight into how we can reorient ourselves when emotions arise, enabling us to welcome them as guests:

The Guest House

This being human is a guest house.
Every morning a new arrival.
A joy, a depression, a meanness,
some momentary awareness comes
as an unexpected visitor.
Welcome and entertain them all!
Even if they are a crowd of sorrows,
who violently sweep your house
empty of its furniture,
still, treat each guest honorably.
He may be clearing you out
for some new delight.
The dark thought, the shame, the malice,
meet them at the door laughing,
and invite them in.
Be grateful for whatever comes,
because each has been sent
as a guide from beyond.

Nurtured by Nature

NATURE AS TEACHER

Nature is a living example of how chaos, order, life, and even death intermingle. This raw form of fluid beauty enchants and mystifies us—a perfect blend of order and chaos. We, as a part of nature, are also a mix of order and chaos, creating and adapting in every moment. As we come to accept that nature is beautiful because of its intricate blend of old growth falling away, making room for something new, we can also come to terms with the same complexities in our "real" selves. As humans, we all strive for this balance between order and chaos modelled for us in the natural world. The sweet spot of this balance is different for each one of us, making it imperative that we listen to the emotional messages that cue us when we feel overwhelmed by chaos or trapped by order. This co-authored piece illustrates the lessons of nature (Dames & Hunter, 2020):

They came upon the cedar tree. It showed them the breadth of their centre and the strength and limitations of their shallow root systems. While their resources span widely on the surface, when the drought and winds come, they feel fragile, wondering if they are enough, if they have what it takes to survive the elements.

They came upon the arbutus tree. It showed them their whimsical nature and the power of their magic. Sprouting up like a fairy amid a forest of sameness. This is how they learned to embrace their uniqueness. That a sprinkle of magic is exactly the medicine to transform their grief and shame.

They came upon the maple tree. The fairy of the forest swayed before them, its tentacles reach joyfully to the sky, wrapped in an elegant moss jacket and bursting with foliage. This is how they learned to embrace their lightness, enabling them to dance with the fluidity of life.

They came upon the fir tree. It struck them with its plainness. Its long thin trunk moving efficiently to the sky, wasting no time expanding on the surface. This is a being that knows who it is, deeply rooted and resilient with nothing to prove.

They came upon the oak tree, all gnarled and alone, sending out seeds on the wind, trusting that only by falling to the darkness below could they sprout and live anew.

They came upon the fallen tree, decaying and covered in moss, reverent at being the source from which new life will come.

And so they have come to learn that they too can feel messy, magic, stable, powerful, complex, basic, and boring, carved out and teeming with life. That when embraced, they are the compost encouraging deeper roots and the seed from which new life springs …

NATURE AS HEALER

Research shows that forest bathing, the practice of immersing ourselves in nature for extended periods of time, reduces anxiety, depression, and anger and increases vigour and the immune system for up to 30 days after the immersion experience (Li, 2010; Park et al., 2007). Just being exposed to nature can lower levels of depression, anxiety, and stress (Beyer et al., 2014). You can bathe in a variety of ways, such as walking in a natural setting, sitting in a forest, floating on a body of water, or any other activity that helps you to tune into unconditioned beauty.

Much of this book is about connecting with self, which acts as a building block that enables a greater ability to connect to others and to nature. For some, the process may happen in reverse, whereby a connection to others or to nature better enables them to connect more deeply with themselves. There is no right way, as we are unique in personality, cultural contexts, upbringing, and experiences that inform our sense of coherence and congruence. The below nature-focused meditations provide an ability to attune to our unique needs for an inner balance of both order and chaos. Immersing in and observing nature helps us to make peace with the chaos at the source of our passion and evolution and the order needed to stay grounded within fluidity. Nature is a perfect balance of order and chaos, death and life. When we resonate and find peace within nature, we attune to the same symbiotic qualities within ourselves.

Attuning Practice
Attuning to Nature

To move from the thinking mind to the sensing mind, this practice should be read to you. Or you can record it and play it back to yourself, which is a great way to build trust with your body (refriending!).

Make yourself comfortable by sitting or lying down with your eyes closed. Take a few cleansing breaths by breathing in deeply through your nose and emptying your lungs fully as you exhale through your mouth. Be present to whatever arises, whether inner or outer sensations, being careful not to attach to or resist the passing stimuli.

Bring your attention to your surroundings.

Feel the air on your skin, notice the temperature and the feeling of air as it moves around you. Listen to the sounds of the trees, the birds, running water, and other elements that surround you. Tune into the symphony of sounds that ebb and flow, noticing when a new sound emerges, changes, and then disappears.

Take in the smells of nature, cultivating a sense of curiosity with the varying scents that emerge. Notice each sound, smell, and sensation without labelling it. Observe each one with a sense of curiosity and then let it fall into the background as you move your focus to another element. When your mind wanders, continue bringing it back to the current moment.

Now open your eyes and continue the meditation, which you can now do standing or walking. Turn your focus to the sight of nature, taking in the details of the trees, noticing movement around you among the birds, how the branches of the trees gently move with the wind, and other elements of the weather. Cultivate a new sense of inquiry as you pay attention to details you might otherwise gloss over. Practise seeing things for the first time, encouraging nonattachment and openness by letting go of labels and the tendency to attach meaning to what you see.

Brains That Thrive: Managing Anxiety and Depression

The regulation and expression of depression and anxiety involves the production and balance of neurotransmitters and multiple areas of the brain including the amygdala, hippocampus, and frontal cortex. Because these factors interplay with our exposure to childhood adversities, our genetics, and a myriad of other circumstantial factors, getting to the roots of our mood imbalances and stress levels can feel like an overwhelming task. For many, fear and anxiety are a common challenge that can cause us to disembody because the feelings within are too threatening.

THE ROOTS OF ANXIETY

We can all relate to a sense of worry and anxiety from time to time, but many experience it so often and with such intensity that it impacts their ability to function on a day-to-day basis. While anxiety can stem from a biological condition, for most, the felt sense of anxiety is often a chronic form of worry. We worry that we are not good enough and that we will not have what it takes to be good enough. Common symptoms of anxiety (National Institute of Mental Health, 2019a) can include the following:

- Difficulty sleeping
- Irritability and restlessness
- Trembling
- Difficulty concentrating
- Shortness of breath and/or dizziness
- Rapid heart rate
- Dry mouth, and
- Nausea or a general feeling of unease.

Some common causes of anxiety include (but are not limited to):

- A current circumstance that feels threatening. In this case, we must either make a change or accept what we cannot change and work to reorient ourselves to the situation.
- How our brains developed as children. This can impact residual cortisol levels, the balance of our neurotransmitters (dopamine and serotonin), and how our brain regulates

as the signals pass between the right and left hemispheres of the prefrontal cortex. For instance, those incubated in households with more adversity are also likely to have a blunted communication mechanism between the amygdala and the prefrontal cortex, which impacts the ability to regulate threatening signals between the two (Park et al., 2018) and makes us more prone to higher levels of baseline cortisol (Finegood et al., 2017).

■ An imbalance in neurotransmitters. For instance, an imbalance between serotonin and dopamine can make us more prone to anxiety and related tendencies as well as obsessive-compulsive behaviours and addictions (Ren et al., 2018; Zarrindast & Khakpai, 2015). If this is the case, we can look at ways to rebalance these transmitters by rebalancing serotonin and dopamine levels. Similarly, high levels of glutamate and low levels of Gamma-aminobutyric acid (GABA) also correlate with higher levels of anxiety and related ritualistic behaviours (Delli Pizzi et al., 2016; Miyata et al., 2019; Modi et al., 2014).

Because we are all unique, with varying life circumstances, brains, and developmental factors, dealing with our anxiety is not a one-size-fits-all solution. Some of us may need to change our work, our personal life circumstances, or both to reduce the frequency and/or intensity of threatening stimuli. Some may need to work on reorienting their perspectives. Some may need to use medications to rebalance their serotonin and dopamine levels. Others may need a combination of these strategies.

Treatments for Anxiety and Depression

We are in the midst of a mental health crisis. Nearly half of all Canadians will have, or have had, a mental health diagnosis by the age of 40 (Canadian Mental Health Association, 2020). Current treatment modalities only work for a minority of those suffering from chronic mental distress. Health care providers are at especially high risk for burnout, PTSD, and treatment-resistant depression. Compounding the existing mental health crisis among health care providers is the fact that treatment methodologies are woefully ineffective for most of those living with PTSD and treatment-resistant depression (O'Leary et al., 2015).

MENTAL HEALTH OF HEALTH CARE PROVIDERS

As described in Chapter 1, more than 50% of Canadian health care providers working in acute care areas are suffering from mental health conditions caused or exacerbated by the toll of their high-stress, often trauma-prone careers. In 2016, nurses submitted 12% of WorkSafe BC mental health claims despite making up only 2% of the province's workforce (British Columbia Nurses' Union, 2019; Canadian Institute for Health Information, 2018); a formal strategy was launched to address the 52% to 64% of health care providers experiencing emotional exhaustion, critical-incident stress, or PTSD (Manitoba Nurses' Union, 2015). Furthermore, the

Canadian Medical Association's National Physician Health Survey found that 49% of medical residents and 33% of physicians screened positive for depression, while 38% of residents and 29% of physicians screened positive for burnout (Simon & McFadden, 2017). Indeed, between 40% and 60% of health care providers will face burnout at some point in their careers (Olson et al., 2015; Rabb, 2014). Additionally, 43% of new graduate nurses report high levels of psychological distress, leading to a growing number choosing to leave the profession within their first two years of practice (Chacula, Myrick, & Yonge, 2015; Chandler, 2012; Laschinger et al., 2010).

Jean Watson (2003, p. 7), a well-known nursing theorist, stated that "modern medicine and health in this new millennium seems to lie in the lack of a meaningful perspective on the very nature of our humanity. It seems that somewhere along the way modern medicine has forgotten that it is grounded and sustained by and through the very nature of our being and becoming more human."

When we realize we have forgotten who we are and how to tend to past and present wounds, the task of remembering and stepping back into a more balanced way of being is challenging. Between unresolved past adversities and biological imbalances, dropping into the inner space to self-soothe can be too painful, making it difficult, and for some even impossible, without an intervention. Each of us has unique needs. Some people may resolve much of their anxiety and depression by removing the emotional charge of past trauma, taking antidepressants, and engaging in mindfulness, while others will need something more to drop in and self-sooth. There is no shame in reaching out for external support to work with our biology in order to promote greater contentment, optimism, and objectivity (all necessary building blocks of sense of coherence).

PHARMACEUTICALS

Data are limited in Canada, but according to the National Health and Nutrition Examination Survey (Pratt et al., 2017), 17% of Americans between the ages of 40 and 59 years and 19% of those over the age of 60 use antidepressants to treat symptoms stemming from anxiety and depression. Women are more likely to take antidepressants than men. To be clear, medications—including herbs and the supplements that provide the building blocks that enable us to produce important chemicals such as dopamine and serotonin—are not the focus of this book, but they are additional and often necessary tools to manage biology and emotions. For these reasons, medications and external therapies are an important part of the thriving equation.

For some of us, taking pharmaceuticals is a necessary part of attaining balance. When the body is challenged to make the chemicals necessary to function in its optimal state, it is time to resource! Dietary changes and exercise may be enough for some. For others, it will take a more intentional and focused approach, requiring specific chemicals to address a missing component in the biological cascade. By tending to a biological need, it can mean spending less energy compensating for what is missing, so we can spend more time *being* in homeostasis.

Resourcing with external remedies is another way to expand our mental health toolbox. Owing to the plethora of options and misleading information about these options, please work with an objective other who has expertise in this area. A good place to start is your family physician or a psychiatrist that you trust. In this day and age, it is difficult to find a provider that covers all the bases, so if possible, diversify. It is good to get more than one opinion so that you can choose which option feels right for you.

NATURAL REMEDIES

Besides conventional pharmaceuticals and therapies, natural remedies are emerging in the research as a promising option. For instance, we can support the brain's ability to make serotonin (associated with happiness and contentment) and dopamine (associated with a sense of reward/pleasure) by focusing on specific foods and supplements that bolster the key amino acids necessary to support their production. We also now have access to a host of botanicals, adrenergics, and nootropics, which can reduce the production of stress hormones. Some can promote neuroplasticity and address depression as a result (Ly et al., 2018). A growing number of studies are showing that psychedelic-assisted therapies are helping to compassionately uncover and address unresolved trauma. Results show significant positive benefits in treating PTSD, addictions, anxiety, and treatment-resistant depression.

While I provide some examples of promising natural remedies that are emerging in the research, just like you would go to a physician to ask for advice (and a prescription) before you consume pharmaceuticals, please seek the same advice from natural remedy experts. For instance, a formally trained naturopath or herbalist.

Examples of Natural Remedies Emerging in the Research

Many also use over-the-counter supplements to boost serotonin and dopamine, neurotransmitters in the brain that are responsible for feelings of happiness and contentment (Kious et al., 2017; Lampariello et al., 2012). Another example of a natural remedy growing in popularity is cannabidiol (CBD), the nonpsychoactive component of hemp and marijuana used to reduce the symptoms associated with anxiety and depression (Corroon et al., 2017; Soares & Campos, 2017; Zuardi et al., 2017).

In South America and Africa, ayahuasca and iboga are psychoactive plant medicines with biochemical and neurological benefits that are outperforming the conventional pharmaceutical remedies used to treat addiction and depression (Belgers et al., 2016; Palhano-Fontes et al., 2019; Sanches et al., 2016). Studies using psilocybin, lysergic acid diethylamide (LSD), and 3,4-methylenedioxymethamphetamine

(MDMA) show that they have significant regenerative properties; they increase the brain's neuroplasticity, resulting in remarkable improvements, even complete resolution, of depression, anxiety, and PTSD (Griffiths et al., 2016; Ly et al., 2018; Slomski, 2018). In a therapeutic set and setting, the hallucinogenic properties of psychedelics promote an ability to confront innermost fears (Frecska et al., 2016). When used within the proper set and setting, these psychedelics can promote a benevolent connection to the inner world, where people can attune to unconditional positive regard.

Working With Trauma: Additional Strategies

These tools in the following box, adapted and excerpted from Schmidt and Miller (2004), help us to step back, be objective, and interrupt negative thought rumination and the use of activities and substances to distract and dissociate (external soothing).

Healing Trauma with Meditation

By Amy Schmidt & Dr. John J Miller

Awareness of Body and Breath
The body and breath are anchors for awareness that can be returned to again and again. Mindfulness of the breath is especially useful for trauma survivors, who tend to hold their breath as a way of not connecting with the present moment. Holding the breath is an unconscious response to anxiety and may also be part of the process of dissociating from the experience.

Body awareness needs to begin gradually. One way to start is by observing the body during times when it feels comfortable. One woman found that the only safe place in her body was her hands, and she would mindfully watch every sensation in each hand for hours at a time. Feeling comfort is a simple thing that trauma survivors often overlook—or sometimes are not even aware can exist. These practices can be done for 5 minutes in bed, right before sleep: Notice the sensation of gravity. Feel the weight of your body on the bed. How does gravity feel?

Scan your body for a place that feels relaxed and even a little bit comfortable. Perhaps it is a finger, a toe, or somewhere deep in your body. Focus on that place. Notice what "comfortable" feels like. See if you can describe it.

Reverse-Warrior Teachings
People with trauma histories often tend to push themselves to extremes; they are more than willing to stay up all night, fast for days, or sit for many hours without moving. Unfortunately, practices that override the body's natural signals of discomfort can end up creating further trauma. As one therapist explains, The way trauma folks survived was that they taught themselves to persevere and to be driven. It is what they learned worked. They did not learn about kindness to

Awareness of The Body and Breath—*cont'd*

themselves or their internal signals. There was not the sense that internal signals could be a support or were worth trusting. It takes survivors a long time to come to listen to internal, intuitive messages and believe them.

Another therapist shared the following discovery:

The difficulty with trauma as it unfolded was how compelling the story was and how I was driven by the thought, "I'm going to work through this." I had to watch this combination of fascination and drivenness and remind myself to back off.

Instead, trauma survivors are best served by adopting a self-compassionate approach:

- Practise for shorter periods of time
- Get plenty of sleep and eat regularly
- Focus on balance and equanimity rather than effort and progress, and
- Build in breaks, and remember that it's not a weakness to be gradual.

Working with trauma is like having two jobs: You are doing the practice of meditation and the practice of healing at the same time. In this regard, the meditative focus needs to be on simple, small steps. As one therapist noted about the importance of slowing down, "Trauma survivors always feel they are not working hard enough and that's why they are stuck. But this is not true. It's okay to relax and stop constantly trying to change."

Listening Instead of Dissociating

The core practice in healing trauma is learning how to feel strong emotions without becoming overwhelmed by them. During meditation practice, survivors often respond to overwhelming emotions by dissociating, a relic of the psychological defence they used to shift their awareness away from the trauma as it was happening. One meditator described dissociation as follows:

My mind enters a state outside my body, captive in some dimension where it is at least safe and alive, yet also powerless and terrified. To settle on the breath is impossible. To get up or move in any way is impossible. After some time, my mind returns enough so that I can pull my blanket around me, draw my knees up, and just sit.

How does a meditator learn to feel strong emotions and bodily sensations without dissociating from them?

When a difficult emotion, sensation, or memory arises, learn to touch up against the pain in small increments. To do so, bring your attention to a place in your body that feels comfortable or neutral (see "The body and breath" section). Feel this comfortable place for a few minutes. Then slowly move the attention to the difficult emotion. Feel that for a minute, then move back to the comfortable place again. Keep moving the attention patiently back and forth between these two areas. This gradual re-experiencing can modulate the intensity of the emotion and create a sense of mastery over the feeling.

Awareness of The Body and Breath—*cont'd*

Train the mind to listen to the body with tenderness and intimacy. Throughout the day, when you are engaged in activities, check in with your body, asking yourself, "Does my body like this or not? What does my body want? Is it okay to keep going, or do I need to stop now?"

Noticing "Trauma Mind"

One of the characteristics of severe trauma is that past emotions and experiences invade the present and become overwhelming. A Vietnam veteran recalls, "When the memories hit, they literally knocked me off my cushion. Through meditation, I eventually found balance with them." The practice of mindfulness develops our ability to observe these memories in a way that facilitates equanimity and balance by teaching us that all thoughts come and go.

Notice "trauma mind," the habit of always looking over one's shoulder, expecting the worst to happen. When fearful memories arise, ask yourself, "Am I okay in this moment? And *this* moment?" Remember, you have resources and choices now. Try breathing in compassion and breathing out fear.

Take a day to observe positive emotions as they occur. When did you feel joy today? Curiosity? Humour? Because healing from trauma can involve repeated focus on difficult emotions, it is important to train the mind to notice the positive emotions that exist.

Try micro-labelling stressful thoughts and feelings. When they arise, meticulously note your reactions as "thinking," "imagining," "fear," and so on.

Question self-judgements and negative beliefs: "Can I absolutely know this is true? Who would I be without this thought?"

It is also useful to identify neutral moments. Were there moments today when you did not feel difficult emotions? When you were brushing your teeth? Drinking a glass of water? Reading? Sleeping?

Learning to Love Again

Loving-kindness and compassion practices offer essential ways to mend the heart after trauma. Trauma survivors are often plagued by the sense that they are unworthy or inherently flawed. They may have trouble doing the "normal" meditation practices or fear that they are not mindful, diligent, or concentrated enough, which can lead to self-hatred and shame.

Trauma survivors have had their trust and sense of connection shattered, and often have a hard time feeling kindness toward themselves and others. Loving-kindness practice can slowly rebuild these connections.

Imagine a young animal or a pet and try extending loving-kindness toward it:

- Feel your heart centre and breathe from this place. Gently offer loving phrases to yourself such as, "May I love myself just as I am," or "May I be happy, may I be peaceful, may I be safe, may I be free of suffering." Some people find it useful to recall an image of themselves as a young child when saying these phrases.
- When difficult emotions arise, try holding each one as you would a crying child.
- It's important not to force loving-kindness to the point where it feels like you are silencing the pain.

Aligning Practice
Connecting With Spirit

If the idea of a benevolent spiritual entity encounters resistance within you, feel free to either reorient yourself to the concept in a way that resonates or skip it altogether. Dropping into the inner world does not require that you subscribe to spiritual beliefs.

Cultivating a spiritual belief system can be helpful in a few ways. If we believe that our destiny is solely a product of our own conditioning and achievements, we are more prone to fixating on controlled *doing* instead of trusting in the flow of *being*. Furthermore, by attuning to a benevolent force that is more unconditionally loving than our individual capacities, we can tune into unconditional positive regard. Feel into your spiritual nature by reflecting on a belief system that works for you. With each of the following questions, practise coming back to the body, clearing out the "noise" of the thinking mind, and noticing how it lands in your body. Does it feel meaningful? Does it align with your values and what is important to you? Keep checking in with your heart space, where your "signal" is the strongest, as you consider these questions:

- How would your actions change if you believed that there was a benevolent spiritual force supporting your journey?
- How might it impact you if you could trust that something greater than yourself would ensure that you had everything you needed when you needed it?
- How would it impact you if you believed that all your heartfelt desires (separate from anxious attachments) were important clues about the *significant* actions required to actualize yourself as a spiritual *being* in the world?

Circle back to your desires, connecting with what it feels like to be called, to get excited about something or someone. Immerse in this feeling of calling, compelled by a longing for more. This longing could be considered a spiritual energy, calling us in and guiding us through the felt sense. How might it look for you to lean into the felt sense of desire more, whether at work or at home?

The Challenge: Navigation

By considering someone else's challenge, or working with another to consider ours, we cultivate nonattachment. We can often find comfort knowing we are not alone and that we can learn from and with each other. Coming from a more objective space, we can step back, and from a position of strength with access to all our biological, intellectual, and spiritual capacities, reorient ourselves. With this benevolent orientation, we can face adversities with confidence, knowing we have the resources and support necessary to navigate life's challenges.

Let's circle back to Jared's challenge. Jared believed that the symptoms of the condition he had resulted from personal shortcomings. Finding out that a mental health condition lay at the root of many of the behaviours he was not proud of enabled him to separate the "noise" that he had no control over from the "signal" of who he is. Now, having developed the ability to step back, he can see that he is separate from the PTSD and the associated *do*ing that flowed from it. Because he feels less attached to the symptoms, he can focus on managing them as they present, free of the shame that comes from identifying with them. This new orientation enables Jared to see the symptoms as a challenging opportunity to practise self-compassion.

The impact of Jared's reorientation to his challenge has had countless ripple effects in his home and work life. He has been more vulnerable with some of his co-workers, cultivating honest and supportive relationships. The more he practises mindfulness, the more he is able to separate the "noise" of passing stimuli from the "signal" of who he is and what really matters. From this more grounded orientation, he often catches himself enjoying the creative process involved in navigating challenges, more like a strategic game than a fight for survival. He continues to engage in daily practices that remind him of who he is and the abundance of resources within and around him. He is learning that missteps are part of the process as he continues to embody new insights. He is coming to know that in the end, separate from his behaviours, he is more than good enough.

 Attuning/Reflecting Opportunity

What arises in you when words like God, spirit, spirituality, higher power, and so forth come up in your world? Specifically focus on terms that seem to cause resistance or attachment. Without going to judgement (labelling as good or bad), stay with the felt sense as it is. What lies underneath the sense of discomfort? What term promotes a greater sense of inner and/or outer connection for you, helping you move beyond the thinking mind into the felt sense?

Attuning for the Journey Ahead: Aligning With Calling

We are *coming to know* how to recognize, feel, and ultimately heal unresolved trauma. We have come to see suffering as a part of being human and that, as a fellow human, we are not alone. We continue to resource with trusted others, and to forge a more intimate relationship with the inner world and the rich spiritual resources within.

Now, while we continue to *attune* to the essence of who we are (our roots) *strengthening* our sense of agency and *clearing* the barriers that disempower us, we begin to *align* with our calling.

Aligning With Calling in Community

When we live our calling, we achieve a certain groundedness and shininess that draws people in. Hearts open, doors open, and an inspired future unfolds. While perhaps we've learned that we can get there faster alone, we will go much farther together. No wound is too deep, no habit too entrenched to heal when a community of like-intentioned people mirror unconditional positive regard to one another.

The Wounded Warrior

By Dr. Crosbie Watler, MD, FRCPC, a Canadian thought leader and seasoned psychiatrist.

The wee hours. Wide awake with no distractions. No escape in restful slumber. Free and clear space. I can feel the energy in my body. It's stuck and I've been carrying it all day, maybe longer. I sense some of it is not mine—passed down. My body wants to tell me something. I can stuff it, numb it, or tell myself a story about it. Been there, done that, time to shut up and listen.

It started early this morning after doing an urgent video psychiatry consult. Another story of a broken spirit, filled with fear and all stuffed in the body. I felt that in my heart, like a weighted blanket. All through the interview and with each breath, I held an awareness of space around my heart. Allowing me to hear the story, to empathize, but not have it stick to me. In my work, I strive to listen and respond from clear space. The wisdom and intuition of the felt sense. The signal comes through the ears, but the body must *feel* into the meaning and context.

This is the flow state of the interview … and everything else. I wonder how many practise it or are even aware of it? We are in flow when we interact with the world around us from a place of self-awareness. Authentic self—the silent witness. Shifting attention briefly to inner space, the pause between the in breath and the out breath. Listen from there and speak from there. This brings the *being* to the doing, creating a healing field that is unseen, but felt.

Park the mind and use it only when necessary. Thinking is highly overrated. Intellect is there, but not much wisdom. Wisdom and intuition reside in the gut brain. The silent brain. Ultimate truth—trust your gut, listen to your gut. It will not speak to you, but you can *feel* into the right choice, what to do and what to say. You will learn to trust it. It won't lie to you, and what flows from you will be righteous. Sometimes it will surprise you. You might sense that some of what you're saying isn't yours as it flows out effortlessly. At those moments of peak experience, one becomes a channel. Park the mind and allow it to flow through.

The Wounded Warrior—*cont'd*

All was smooth sailing until the patient transitioned to describing his frustration with our system of mental health "care." He detailed the medicalizing of his despair, with a series of treatments doomed to fail, as if by design. I felt his creeping sense of desperation and helplessness. That hit me in the gut. I managed to keep a lid on things and completed the interview with a plan that gave him hope. Then I signed off.

That's when I *lost it*.

What I lost was awareness of inner space. The domain of the dispassionate witness. I was no longer self-aware, but in reactive mode. All the wisdom and intuition? Summarily tossed under the bus. The maestro had become a puppet.

I don't do freeze or flight. I scorch the earth. I now know much of it is not mine. I've led a privileged life, mirrored and supported as a child. Blessed with the love of a good woman, authentic relationships, and a sense of purpose. We think we know ourselves, but we are influenced by unseen forces outside our usual states of awareness. So much of what we carry is handed down to us. The epigenetics of our ancestral experience. Given our collective history, much of this is trauma. In states of deep meditation—or otherwise altered states of consciousness—we *feel* our ancestors knocking. Mine are part slave warrior and it explains *everything*.

I know in my bones that my ancestors were fierce. They had to be, or else perish. Many did. And here I am. Last man standing. They hand me the torch and ask, "What are you going to do with it?" This uncomfortable gift of an easy life does not sit well with me. I will make it hard. I need the struggle. Now I know why. My ancestors have been pushing boulders uphill forever, in the face of impossible odds. And here I am. Last man standing. Righteous struggle is in my DNA. I seek it out in ways that leave many—me at times—gobsmacked. In truth, I sense some of my ancestors might not have been so righteous, but I'm selective about whose torch I choose to carry.

All of this at 8:15 a.m. on a Saturday morning in the present day … at the mercy of unseen influences and swirling emotions. On seeing the harm that comes from the medicalizing of psychiatry, the heaviness in my heart had given way to rage in my gut. Yet another victim of the medical–pharmaceutical complex. Patients have become commodities—their distress labelled as disease, or worse, *disorder*. Failed medical treatments for wounds of the heart. *I feel angry*. Slave warrior gene is *on*. Like *right now*.

Can I please have something to vanquish? A wild beast threatening my family, perhaps? Or enemy warriors sneaking into the village? How about a serving of slave owner for dessert? No such luck. It's 2021, and I'm living a life of privilege in the tranquility of Maple Bay, British Columbia. I feel paralyzed by the heaviness in my heart and the rage in my belly—swirling, building, with no clear outlet. That's when it gets messy. Listening from space? Yeah, right.

I should have done the work sooner. It's now 3:30 a.m. on Sunday morning. The karmic debt of procrastination. There is no free lunch. Do the work or pay the price. *What the mind won't acknowledge, the body knows*. You can stuff it for a while— maybe the righteous rage felt good. It's in my bloodline and it had purpose. It was adaptive, but it no longer serves me. It depletes me and everyone around me. That awareness is enough. There was no space for it earlier in the day, or maybe I did not want to *make* space.

The Wounded Warrior—*cont'd*

Making space is hard sometimes. Keeping the monkey mind at bay is hard work. I do it all day at my day job, and sometimes I just want to let my guard down; to rest. That's when it sneaks up on me, the alpha predator. The present-day enemy is no person or beast, it's the conditioned mind and its unconscious patterns of reactivity. This stuff will consume you from the inside out, play you like a fiddle and dance on your grave.

So, here I sit in spacious awareness. The wee hours when quiet contemplation is best. It's easier now—nothing to do, nowhere to go, just *be*. Presence, awareness, silence within and without. Space within and without. Where everything that was stuck in my body is washed away. The radiant light of presence has cleared the skeletons out of the closet. Presence slays dragons. It is our superpower.

Cultivate the healing field of presence, knowing you *will* lose it. When you lose it, have compassion for yourself. There are so many seen and unseen influences wanting to play you like a puppet. In truth, presence can never be truly lost. Presence is our birthright. Sometimes we just get distracted.

CHAPTER 11

Aligning With Calling: Roots Over Fruits

How we spend our days is how we spend our lives.

Annie Dillard

We have come to know and attune to the "signal" of what is (the essence of our roots), separate from the "noise" (or passing weather) that we navigate from one day to the next. Too much focus on fruits, represented by products of our *do*ing, distracts us from contentment in *be*ing. To thrive, we pendulate between the inner world and the outer world, quieting the nervous system so that we can better hear the call of our hearts. We choose habits that engage in *do*ing to carry us back to *be*ing—reminding us of who we are, and the abundance within and around us. Each time we get stuck, we do the *significant* thing to clear the noise, continually coming back to signal. One *significant* thing at a time keeps us in the river. The more we stay in the flow of the river, the more we enjoy the ease of living our calling. We float easily along, soothed by the tune of our *be*ing. Now that the path is clearer, we can tune into what is calling us, those relationships and activities that feel meaningful and that align with our talents and desires.

Circle back to the tree metaphor in Figure 1.1. Depending on a particular tree's location, position in the forest, access to neighbouring roots systems, and exposure to passing weather systems, it will feel more or less threatened (stressed) when storms roll in. The days are a mix of effort and ease. In times of ease, there is an abundance of resources for an entire forest to soak up. When the weather is rough or nutrients dwindle (representing the more challenging times), as long as primary needs are met, growth is stimulated both aboveground and belowground. With new growth, the soil from which we resource grows richer, making for a stronger base to anchor to the earth. Both times are necessary—the challenges serve as opportunities to grow and evolve, and the times of rest allow recharging and nourishing. Those trees that lack basic requirements will fail to deepen their roots, preserving all their energy to manage the daily stressors that threaten their shallow root systems. The sense of threat that fuels fear in shallow root systems (low sense of coherence and incongruence) distracts us from the rich resources within and around us, if only they we can develop the roots necessary to reach them. Those fortunate to have the resources that enable deepening roots will thrive, while those

281

left with shallow root systems will eventually succumb when the elements become too extreme to manage.

Individually, each of us is vulnerable to passing weather systems, but collectively, we are much stronger. In Chapters 11 and 12, we circle back to focus on root strength by aligning with our purpose and desire within communities of practice.

The Challenge: Orientation

By considering someone else's challenge, or working with another to consider ours, we cultivate nonattachment. We can often find comfort knowing we are not alone and that we can learn from and with each other. Working from this more objective space, we mitigate the stress response. We can then reorient from this position of strength, thus improving our ability to use all our biological, intellectual, and spiritual capacities. With this benevolent orientation, we can face adversities with confidence, knowing we have the resources and support necessary to navigate life's challenges.

Consider the tree metaphor. Our orientation influences how we perceive varying forms of weather. If we orient ourselves from an individualist (disconnected) perspective, trees appear to be separate, competing entities. The strongest roots absorb most nutrients, leaving the weaker, shallow-rooted trees to survive with what is left. While seemingly independent, most trees exist amid a forest of others. Each tree is unique according to its essence and the conditions of the soil in which it is rooted. From this vantage point, trees look like separate beings: each tree is driven to strive for its own survival, unable to connect beyond sharing physical space, with the stronger trees feeding off the decay of the weaker ones.

Or we can frame the tree analogy from a collectivist perspective (connected), which research suggests is closer to reality (Simard et al., 2015; Song et al., 2015). What happens on the surface is only a small piece of the larger orchestra of events and interactions happening belowground. Both shallow and deep roots systems adapt to neighbouring needs, redirect resources as needed, and warn each other of threats. When one tree suffers, all suffer. Those with deeper roots will self-actualize, flourishing into their best, most resourced, and empowered "self." From this position of strength, they can now support others to develop into *their* most resourced and empowered selves. Those with shallow roots gain the benefits of those who have deeper roots, resourcing through connection. When a tree is suffering, it is not punished for burdening others; rather, the tree is met with what it needs to heal its injury. No tree is cast out because it has scars from destructive weather patterns of the past. Each tree is met and nourished just as it is, without judgement. There is no need to punish the individual trees that are suffering, which would only worsen the injury and harm the larger network. No questions of value arise; resources are simply diverted to those in need. Every tree contributes what it can and takes what it needs. When one rises, they all rise.

We are not so different from trees. We have the ability to live symbiotically with ourselves, others, and the Earth. When characterized by unconditional positive regard, we are stronger, healthier, and happier together. From a collectivist perspective, unconditional positive regard represents the soil that enables roots to deepen. Those who direct unconditional positive regard inwardly become fulfilled, enabling it to naturally spill onto others. When others test it by showing up authentically, they come to believe it and then receive it. As a result, they will start mirroring unconditional positive regard inwardly, too. Eventually, they will also find that their roots have deepened, and they are now supporting others to flourish.

Attuning Practice
Reconciling the Old With the New

- If someone were communicating unconditional positive regard, without using words, what would that look like?
- What would their face and body language look like?
- What does unconditional positive regard *not* look like?
- Imagine being held within a community where you believed you were unconditionally positive regarded. What does it feel like to be held in this way?
- How might it impact your orientation to challenges at work and at home?
- How might it change how you show up at work?
- How might it impact your ability to align with your values, desires, and passions?

Visioning With Two-Eyed Seeing

Mi'kmaw Elder Albert Marshall coined the term **Two-Eyed Seeing**, which describes the ability "to see from one eye with the strengths of Indigenous ways of knowing, and to see from the other eye with the strengths of Western ways of knowing, and to use both of these eyes together" (Bartlett et al., 2012, p. 335). The framework describes a process of reconciling the methods and theories of the West with Indigenous ways of knowing. Those of us who do not identify as Indigenous have been conditioned by a colonizing world. Homogenizing cultural forces attach a variety of conditions to our worth, fuelling incongruence within and across population groups.

Attuning Practice
Recognize Your Resources

Expanding our awareness of both our essential and conditioned nature enables us to develop the strategies necessary to walk in these two worlds effectively and meaningfully. For the purpose of expanding awareness and to set an intention for our desired trajectory, use the tree picture to demonstrate the inner resources that help you feel unconditional positive regard for your "real" self, free of socially

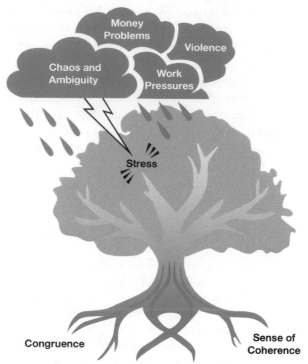

Note. Congruence = orientation to self; sense of coherence = orientation to the world.

prescribed "ideals." These internal assets promote congruence and sense of coherence, much like nutrient-rich soil promotes deep "roots" to withstand passing storms. Next, describe your external assets, which represent the people, activities, and resources that support your growth, much like water and sunshine promote a tree's ability to flourish.

Take a moment to reflect. After completing the exercise, how do you feel? What inner and outer resources might you add? When might this activity (or an adapted version) be helpful in your daily life?

Living a Calling

In the West, we are generally conditioned to look out before we look in. We are apt to look to others who seem more qualified to tell us what we need. The subtle message in this conditioned way of being relays to us that our inner capacities to navigate challenges and important decisions come up short. This message erodes self-trust and causes us to turn up the volume of external stimuli ("noise") and to turn down the volume of internal stimuli ("signal"). We anxiously grasp at the "noise" for approval and security rather than grounding in the "signal" of who we are and our embodied wisdom. We have done our best to tend to our conditioning, following the rules to survive. When we live according to a prescribed "ideal," we become incongruent, causing shame to fester, which manifests as hostile and competitive communities.

The felt sense of desire is what connects us to calling. Some cultures suggest that it is selfish to live according to our desires. Carl Jung illustrated this belief well:

> *Meditation and contemplation have a bad reputation in the West. They are regarded as a particularly reprehensible form of idleness or as pathological narcissism. No one has time for self-knowledge or believes that it could serve any sensible purpose. Also, one knows in advance that it is not worth the trouble to know oneself, for any fool can know what he is. We believe exclusively in doing and do not ask about the doer, who is judged only by achievements that have collective value … Western man confronts himself as a stranger … self-knowledge is one of the most difficult and exacting of the arts.*
> (Jung, 1970, pp. 582–583)

Now we know better. We know that understanding ourselves enables us to manage emotions, buffers us from stress, and enables us to thrive. When we lack the self-knowledge that Jung speaks of, we are apt to deny our hearts' desires, resulting in incongruence. When we live incongruently, we are prone to attracting people and events into our lives that illuminate our incongruence. Until we heal, we will continue re-experiencing past trauma (stuck energy) in the present day through all sorts of harmful projections. In this way, rather than fuelling more shame or incongruent ways of being, we can recognize the opportunity to feel into the stuck energy at its roots. Like emotions, projections (emotions from the past projecting onto present day), are calling us in, alerting us that there is unfinished business to tend to. When we hear the call, we have an opportunity to respond from a more resourced place than we were previously capable of.

Living our calling happens when we tune into the present, leaning into what magnetizes us. A sign that we are living our calling, as opposed to following a whim, is a deep desire to contribute beyond ourselves. When we align with our calling, we are drawn to people and events that support our journey. Every task takes on the glow of meaning and purpose. Even the most mundane work tasks can feel rewarding. A calling that enables us to thrive awakens all our senses, pulling us into every moment with a feeling of aliveness. The pleasure derived from every step comes from knowing that our aim is noble, that we are working toward a great cause, and that we were built for it.

When discussing the idea of "living our calling," concerns about equity and opportunity may arise. Our upbringing, past adversities, financial picture, opportunities, confidence in our material and cultural assets, societal status, and related factors determine how confident we are in managing daily challenges. If we do not have the confidence to navigate a challenge, it will feel threatening, activating the stress response. Those with more confidence are more likely to set ambitious goals and to have the confidence in their internal and external resources to reach them (Binswanger, 1991). That being said, living a calling is much broader than one's ability to attain success in the external world. As foreshadowed in the title of this chapter, it is more about our roots (how we get there), than the fruits (what emerges on the surface). It is about the inner world, our degree of self-integrity, and our felt safety to express ourselves authentically. Simply put, it is about our *do*ing (fruits) flowing from our *be*ing (roots). For example, even though many tasks might seem repetitive and mundane, it is possible to find meaning in such tasks, connecting to the larger vision beneath them. By remaining embodied (*be*ing), as opposed to disembodied (*do*ing), we remain tethered to heartfelt meaning. In this case, whatever the daily task we are charged with, we can find joy and contentment in it. A calling is not necessarily related to solving a particular problem (e.g., it is not one's calling to reply to emails, clean the house, or redirect an employee). Instead, calling is about bringing our attention and intention to whatever is happening in the moment, including our authentic feelings and values. While some activities will drain us—like constant social stimulation may drain those who need more time to themselves—we honour inner cues, seeking reprieve when needed and seeking roles that play to our strengths whenever possible. Those roles and activities will be different for each of us. Often it is not about *what* we are doing, but about *how* we are doing it. Energizing qualities at work might include working closely with team members, problem solving, organizing, thinking strategically, and making others laugh. On this journey, we are improving our ability to be mindful, staying connected to our felt senses, and making each moment a more meaningful moment. We are bringing the calm of the inner world to the activities of the outer world.

There is a significant connection between our capacity to thrive inside and outside work. When we have deep roots at work, where we feel congruent and have a high sense of coherence (meaning, comprehension, and confidence), we are likely to carry that same self-trust into our other life roles. Therefore, when we are confident that we can live our calling at work, we will have greater confidence in living our calling in our personal life too (Dames, 2018a).

Connecting to what is meaningful to us, tapping into our desires, is an important resource that aligns us with our inner spirit, the source of our calling. Spirituality, or belief in a resource beyond physical limitations, provides us with the meaning, courage, and trust necessary to follow our calling, despite external pressures to compromise. Furthermore, believing in a spiritual source also enhances the benefits of mindfulness and our mental and physical health outcomes (Wachholtz et al., 2017). Tapping into this inner resource promotes thriving, enabling an ability to feel held despite the chaos around us. Cultivating a sense of trust in our spiritual resources transcends the limits of our humanity, enabling us to feel grounded and held, despite the distracting weather that circles.

When meaning and connection drive our decisions and actions, fulfilling a felt sense of life purpose, we are living our calling.

The capacity to live our calling within the workday relates to our feelings of well-being, meaning, and confidence at work (Dames, 2018a). Making time to immerse in practices that uncover and illuminate calling builds self-trust and confidence in our resources, which empowers us to act in ways congruent with our "real" self. When we hear the call of the moment, often coming to us through the felt sense, we either embrace it or resist it. We are all born tethered to this calling, or rather to a series of yearnings that connect to a much larger calling, all of which align with our unique essence (the "real" self). Our orientation to this calling has a significant impact on our ability to thrive. If calling is viewed as a leash, we will feel threatened when it calls us to step away from the status quo (prescribed ideals). If calling is viewed as an anchor, we are more likely to muster the courage we need to step out, responding to the call by doing the *significant thing* (described in Chapter 6) in that moment.

At this part of the journey, we turn our focus to developing trust in our roots, the essence of who we are. Mindfulness or *being* means cultivating stronger roots without fixating on the outcomes (fruits). When mindful, we are prioritizing the means/process above the end product/achievement. We develop habits of *being* through mindfulness, which interrupts disembodied *doing* as we move from thinking mode to sensing mode. Transitioning from subconscious thinking to conscious sensing connects us to our "real" self. As we deepen our connection and relationship with our "real" self, we develop trust in ourselves and in like-intentioned others. With trust, we gain security in our inner and outer resources. From here, we can answer the inner call, enabling our *doing* to flow from our *being*; this is congruence.

Living Our Calling With Congruence

He who has a "why" to live can bear almost any "how."

Friedrich Nietzsche

Like an acorn that has all the intelligence it requires to become an oak tree, every human being has a unique essence and a unique purpose to fulfill. There are moments in life when we awaken to that purpose; like the lifting of a veil, we awaken from our slumber ever so briefly. If we take notice, absorbing what those moments are showing us, we gain insight into our "real" self and the calling we are destined to fulfill. Our calling is that one thing we cannot put down, that ignites our desire. Signs we are living our calling include a sense of timelessness and feelings of immersion, interconnectedness, and joy, much like what we experienced when we were children.

We need not compete with one another, as no one can fulfill our unique purpose, nor will following another's path be fruitful for us. As we live our calling, we gain sense of coherence (meaning, comprehension, and confidence in life) and congruence (*be*ing the "real" self). As a result, we can provide unconditional positive regard for self, which spills over into our relationships. The process is contagious as this benevolent energy ripples out, flowing from person to person. The opposite is also true: competition and hostility are like a contaminant in relationships with others, cultivating fear and insecurity and, as a result, perpetuating more of the same. The reality is that we are all connected. As we live our calling, we promote the ability for others to live theirs.

Understanding our essence is challenging in the West, where the pressure to subscribe to cultural ideals is the norm. The majority push out those who go against the cultural grain, threatening their primal need to belong. However, there are many cultures we can learn from that celebrate diversity, encouraging each person to forge their path according to the unique blueprint they are born with. One such culture is illustrated by Sobonfu Some, a teacher, author, and activist from West Africa:

> *I am from the Dagara tribe, and in my tradition it is customary for pregnant women to go through a hearing ritual. The purpose of a hearing ritual is to listen to the incoming baby; to find out who it is; why it's coming at this time; what its purpose is; what it likes or dislikes; and what the living can do to prepare space for this person. The child's name is then given based on that information ... In the Dagara tradition, you own your name up until the age of five. After the age of five, your name owns you. Your name is an energy; your name has a life force. It creates an umbrella under which you live. That is why it is important to hear the child before giving him or her the name, because the name must match their purpose. My name, Sobonfu, means "keeper of rituals." (Some, 2019)*

Thriving in a self-actualized state requires a willingness to live our calling (Duffy et al., 2013). While there may be many practical reasons to follow the paths recommended by those we respect, this will not sustain us. Meeting financial needs and acquiring achievements must be weighed against the longings of the heart. While there may be times when an unmet financial need takes priority, we are wise to also consider the impact that our choices will have on our ability to be congruent. Congruence requires us to acknowledge and do our best to honour our heart's desires (passions), and to find meaning and purpose in our work. Silencing the inner voice, which may feel less important than cultural norms and priorities, puts us at higher risk for moral injury and eventual emotional burnout.

Cultivating the Courage to Live Our Calling

Feeling the confidence to navigate challenges is about knowing that we have the resources necessary to do so. Confidence is a core component of sense of coherence, which enables us to thrive despite hardships (Eriksson & Lindström, 2007). When our sense of meaning and confidence overrides our fears, we can step out in courage. Courage is *not* the lack of fear. It is doing the *significant thing*, despite our fears, when it is the best thing for ourselves and others. One significant thing after another is exactly what it looks like to live our calling:

Meaning + Confidence = The Courage to Live Our Calling

MEANING

We attain meaning by distinguishing the "noise" of obligational doing from the "signal" of our *be*ing. When embodied and connected to desire, meaningful *be*ing naturally happens. Purpose and meaning in our work correlates with greater congruence and attachment to our profession and organization (Cardador et al., 2011; Dames, 2018a). Meaning and purpose are characteristics of thriving. Munn described this engagement as follows:

> *Enjoyment of one's job versus the duty of doing one's job to obtain a paycheck is also likely to be influenced by the organizational culture in which the individual works and can show his or her true personality. For instance, do employees have the freedom to be themselves? Or must they hide their true identity because it does not fit within the standards of their work environment … The freedom to be oneself within the environment we spend at least a quarter of our day significantly impacts our reactions not only to work but also to how we handle the world.* (Munn, 2013, p. 409)

CONFIDENCE

Building up our confidence takes time and intentional practice. In this book, the word confidence is used to describe self-efficacy. *Self-efficacy* is the confidence and belief in our ability to achieve our goals.

Prominent theories such as goal-setting theory and social cognitive theory both acknowledge that self-efficacy and conscious goal setting are imperative to the likelihood that we will attain our goals (Bandura, 1997; Locke, 1996). When we reach our goals, it empowers us. As a result, it reprograms our subconscious to continue creating goals, adjusting our actions to move toward achievement (Bandura, 1997).

Intertwining self-efficacy with sense of coherence, those who have higher sense of coherence scores are often more committed and therefore more likely to keep their physical and mental health goals (Andersen & Berg, 2001; Avey et al., 2010; Garrosa et al., 2011; Judge & Bono, 2001; Lo, 2002; Luthans & Jensen, 2005; Xanthopoulou et al., 2007). Similarly, those with greater self-efficacy are more committed, use better task strategies to meet goals, and respond more positively to negative feedback than do people with lower self-efficacy (Locke & Latham, 1990; Seijts & Latham, 2001). Zimmerman et al. (1992) found that self-belief and self-efficacy promote an ability to set lofty goals and take ownership of them and fuel our desire to regulate and meet our goals. Finally, those who have higher levels of self-efficacy also tend to have higher levels of job satisfaction, work performance, and goal achievement (Binswanger, 1991).

Self-efficacy and the resulting achievement of goals relates to Rogers' (1959) theory of congruence. He suggested that successful goal setting requires congruence between our "real" and "ideal" selves in order to feel ownership and the desire to achieve our goals. Setting "ideal" goals that are not subconsciously supported by the "real" self will likely backfire, as we will lack the desire and commitment required to reach our goals (Zimmerman et al., 1992). Therefore, goal setting supports the notion that those acting from a more congruent and self-actualized state of mind will be more likely to achieve their goals and gain more self-efficacy in the process.

Strengthening Practice
Working With Feedback

The degree of congruence (ability to be authentic) and sense of coherence (a confident and optimistic orientation to life) will often determine how we respond to feedback. When we don't feel safe and confident, the threat of criticism can easily feel personal; it activates the nervous system, sending us into fight–flight–freeze or fawn. Dig a little deeper beneath the "noise" of the nervous system and you will often find a primary need that feels threatened. For instance, our need to feel accepted or to belong in the dominant group. These are primary human needs that feel essential to our survival.

Rational detachment is a form of nonattachment characterized by the ability to not take the behaviours of others personally. When we tap into this acquired skill, we can recognize that others' behaviours are generally projections of their past experiences. From this vantage point, we can keep things in perspective without getting stuck in our own assumptions and fears. Because it's not personal, it's also not as threatening to the nervous system. When grounded in this nonattached position, we can shift our focus from what is wrong to what can be done.

Can you recall a situation at school, work, or home when you were waiting to receive feedback from an authority figure (teacher, employer, mentor, parent)? What unmet need was beneath the fear? What environments or relationships would enable you to view feedback as an opportunity? Do you have a sense of what matters to you (the signal) to the point that you can distinguish it from others' projections and preferences (the noise)? What benefits can come from cultivating the ability to distinguish the signal from the noise? How might this change your orientation to receiving feedback?

Cultivating Confidence With Meaningful Life Roles Outside of Work

Meaningful life roles outside of work promote an ability to manage workplace stressors (Dames, 2018a). Identifying with more than one life role diversifies our sense of self, preventing us from putting all our eggs in one basket. There is a positive correlation to our overall self-efficacy, established success in other life roles, and sense of overall life meaning. Meaning in work is the subjective perception that our labour is significant, that it promotes personal growth, and that it contributes to a greater cause (Steger et al., 2012). Work can be a significant source of meaning in people's lives, but other influential sources can add or subtract from our overall assessment of our ability to lead a meaningful life (Allan et al., 2015).

There is a significant connection between our ability to experience meaning in our roles inside and outside of work, where our degree of satisfaction with one directly impacts our degree of satisfaction with the other (Duffy et al., 2013). When life and work roles have a positive balance, we are more likely to feel more meaning in both roles (Dames, 2018a).

Authenticity Versus Assimilation

We often compromise our authentic way of being to fit in with the larger group, which may be a learned habit from our childhood and/or as a result of living in homogenizing cultures. When we compromise who we are for the sake of the group, we are entering a relationship that has perceived conditions. These perceived conditions promote incongruence (a felt need to prescribe to an "ideal" as opposed to letting ourselves be "real"). The more we live with this "other"-centred orientation, the greater the incongruence and the more shame we will carry as a result.

When like-intentioned teams aim to mirror unconditional positive regard, things start getting "real." Getting "real" in the workplace minimizes the pressure to assimilate to one prescribed way of being. Feeling like we can authentically express ourselves in the workplace mitigates external pressures to assimilate to a prescribed way of being, enabling congruence.

Shame, a self-conscious emotion, is one of the most powerful motivators and disablers in the human experience ... In shame, perfection is sought; one is either perfect or a total failure, one does not experience anything in between. (Bond, 2009, p. 134)

It is not uncommon for caregiving environments to be as homogenizing as other workplaces. Professional ideals have little flexibility for a diversity of personalities and alternative ways of being. The basic human requirement to belong, to be accepted, and to be loved creates a need to assimilate, despite the resulting dissonance. When "ideals" take priority, perfectionism generally runs rampant.

Perfectionism fuels incongruence and feelings of shame and is born from the need to subscribe to the social "ideal." While there are benefits to perfectionism, in its more extreme forms it causes unrealistically high standards for self and others, rigid thinking, and a high risk of using substances or activities to cope with the resulting stress. Highly perfectionistic professionals perpetuate co-worker hostility. The high standards we set for ourselves and the shaming that occurs when we fall short of those standards often spills onto others.

Aligning Practice

A Meeting With Your Future Self

You will find multiple versions of "future self" meditations online; adapt the practice to your liking, ensuring that the images and questions resonate with you. This practice requires you to drop in, moving from the thinking mind to the felt sense. To facilitate this shift, you will need to have this script read to you or you can record yourself reading it. This is a helpful grounding and aligning practice, empowering decisions that align with one's essence and calling. I adapted the following practice from resources provided by High Performance Habits (Marshall, 2019):

Make yourself comfortable by sitting on the ground or in a chair. Close your eyes. Bring your attention to your breath, observing it as it moves in and out of your body. Focus on the exhale, noticing how each breath deepens your state of relaxation. When your attention wanders, bring it back to your breath, and with each redirection let yourself sink deeper into relaxation. Let each external sound be a reminder of the gift of the inner world: we can leave the noise and stress of the outside world behind as we continue to cultivate a deep sense of inner quietness.

PAUSE

As you straighten your spine, imagine it as a cord that grounds you to the Earth's centre. Imagine this cord is your anchor, enabling you to stay connected to the Earth no matter where your inner journey takes you. Continue to let your breath deepen your sense of relaxation as you exhale any tensions that arise.

PAUSE

Bring to mind a peaceful lake. Imagine yourself bending down and picking up a pebble near your feet. Toss the pebble into the water and notice the ripples that extend outward one after the other until they dissipate and become calm once again. Imagine that your body is this body of water. Drop a breath, like a pebble, into your body of water. As you drop each breath into your body, you can feel the waves of relaxation ripple outward. Ripples of relaxation flow throughout your body, extending out from your spine to your chest and back, and down your legs as the ripples dissipate back to the Earth. Let the ripples spread into every muscle of your back, across your neck and shoulders, up into your jaw and the muscles in your face. Feel your eyes and scalp relax with each breath. With each breath, you embrace the waves of relaxation that wash over you.

PAUSE

Bring your attention to the space between your eyes. Imagine a beam of light that extends out from this space. Follow the beam as it leaves this building, this city, and this country and moves out into space. As the beam extends to outer space, notice the curvature of the Earth below. As you travel outward, you embrace the calm and quiet of space. You can see the Earth beneath you, surrounded by an infinite and vibrant universe. Enjoy the sense of vastness you experience here.

PAUSE

Bring your attention to another beam of light near you. Follow this beam back down to the curvature of the Earth as it takes you 20 years into the future. Follow the beam, and as you come closer to the end, notice where you are: this is where your future self lives 20 years from now. What does it look like? What surrounds you? Move closer to the dwelling or the landscape that surrounds the home of your future self, noticing the details. What do you see? Water, trees, flowers? How do you feel here? Immerse yourself and get a sense of this place.

Approach the door to the home of your future self. Know that on the other side of that door, your future self awaits, eager to greet you. The door opens. What do you see? Greet your future self and notice how your future self receives you, welcoming you into this time and place. Take in the image and get a sense of your future self. What do you notice? What is the expression on your future self's face? What are they wearing? How are they standing? Get a sense of their essence. Focus again on the dwelling: notice the colours, the feeling of it. What kind of person lives here?

PAUSE

Your future self offers you a refreshment and motions you to find a comfortable place to sit. Settle in here. Make yourself comfortable. As you sit across from one another, you ask the following questions:

First you ask, "In the last 20 years, what do you most remember?" Then you ask, "What stands out most in your memory?" Take a moment, allowing enough space and quietness to hear the answer.

You then ask your future self, "What do I need to be most aware of to get me from where I am now to where you are? What would be most helpful for me to know? What qualities of my real self can I cultivate that will help me on this journey?" Take a moment, creating a space as you lean in to hear the answers.

Now ask your future self your own questions. What other questions do you have?

PAUSE

You are ready to leave now. You thank your future self for sharing this place and their wisdom with you.

You find your way back to the beam of light that brought you here. As you follow the beam of light back to outer space, you watch the world grow smaller and smaller behind you. You again see the curvature of the Earth, the bright blue, brown, and green ball amid the vast universe. You notice the beam of light that you initially followed, and as you intersect with it, you turn to follow it back down to the Earth, back to the present time. As you travel down, you notice the Earth growing larger and larger. You move through the clouds, back down to your country, to your city, to this building, and to this room.

You are back in the present time, alert and refreshed. You know that you will remember what you need to from this inner journey. Remain silent as you open your eyes. Take a moment to reflect on how you feel. Jot down any new insights.

Living Our Calling by Developing Authentic Habits

Perfectionism and sense of coherence are inversely related (Rennemark & Hagberg, 1997). Those with a low sense of coherence scores have higher perfectionism scores. Perfectionism is also inversely linked with congruence and self-compassion, both of which require a willingness to be authentic and to have unconditional positive regard for self when social pressures to assimilate are strong. Therefore, one strategy to address perfectionism is to focus on developing sense of coherence and congruence, which will then lower the felt need to be perfect.

Creating and sustaining cultural change requires a structure to support its growth. Organizational leadership sustains the structure necessary for seeds to germinate and grow. The 12-step model, which originates from Bill Wilson's Alcoholics Anonymous program, has had decades of success. It shows how structures can support the personal growth and healing of millions. Both Bill Wilson and Carl Jung believed the 12-step model was a spiritual program that applied to all humans, not just those struggling with alcoholism (McCabe, 2015). In many 12-step groups, people experience unconditional positive regard for the first time. By experiencing unconditional positive regard, it enables people to feel loved and accepted as their "real" selves. As a result, there is an opportunity for people to direct this same love and acceptance inwardly. When we feel safe, our inner world opens, tuning us to a more secure frequency and providing a sweet fragrance that soothes us. Related 12-step principles (Alcoholics Anonymous, 2001) and slogans include the following:

- *We are not alone or wholly self-sufficient*
- *Progress, not perfection: Challenging perfectionism and making room for experiential learning supported by cultures that celebrate diversity and lifelong learning*

- *Mentorship: Mentors demonstrate unconditional positive regard for others, which requires the mentor to have self-compassion/unconditional positive regard for self, congruence, and empathy*
- *Agreeing to disagree: Celebrating diverse ways of being and thinking*
- *Keep your side of the street clean (regularly make amends to those you harm), and*
- *It is not about believing in a higher power; it is enough to be willing to believe.*

Living Our Calling by Recognizing Old Narratives: Is it True? Is it Personal?

Self-integrity, our ability to be authentic and feel whole, is priceless. Doing or saying anything that erodes your sense of self, stripping you of inner peace, is too expensive.

The stories we tell ourselves are powerful. They are "spells" that create our realities when we believe what people tell us or what we tell ourselves, regardless of what is true. In order to minimize false narratives that are no longer serving us, we must upgrade these stories. This form of reorientation involves renaming and reframing by using new words that aren't so tangled up in old and unhelpful belief systems.

Ruiz (1997) provides four helpful agreements that are based on ancient Toltec teachings to assist in the renaming and reframing effort:

1. **Realize that your words are powerful:**
   - We can use them as gifts to encourage or weapons to project our shame and pain onto others. For example, hostility in the workplace festers by projecting shame through words via gossip.
   - Conversely, truth telling is an essential part of self-expression, which bolsters self-integrity and congruence. When we say things that are not congruent with our "real" self, our shame grows, and we erode self-trust and self-integrity.
2. **Recognize that it's not personal (*rational detachment*):**
   - When people's words and behaviours are hurtful, it comes from their own pain and shame; it is a subconscious projection that is often more about them than us.
   - When we assume it is personal, we are agreeing with what is being said, without critically examining whether it is true. Taking other people's projections personally hands over our personal power and diminishes our self-integrity.
   - Taking in another's shaming projection makes their pain your pain, causes unnecessary suffering, and perpetuates the victim perpetrator cycle.
3. **Avoid assumptions:**
   - Assumptions limit choice. Rather than determining whether information is true, we take the opinions of others and even our own thoughts as truth. This creates a snowball effect on our emotional state and our ability to think critically and make objective decisions.

- When we assume and take others' projections personally, our shame grows, making us more prone to anxiety and depression.
- Misunderstandings are based on faulty assumptions and often lead to unnecessary conflict.

4. **Do your best and practise self-compassion when you fall short of your "ideal":**

   - Based on your sense of coherence and congruence and the context you are in, you will use the resources available to you to act. Understand that your "best" can change from moment to moment and day to day, depending on your felt congruence, the emotions coming and going, and the supporting resources you have at your disposal.
   - The first three strategies work only if you are willing to do your best with the resources you have (internal and external).
   - Trying too hard to do your best and subscribing to an unrealistic ideal rather than trusting yourself results in incongruent behaviours and perfectionism. Perfectionism can limit flexibility and the ability to adapt and create, preventing you from being your best.
   - Your best requires mindfulness and authentic desire. Doing your best requires congruence with your "real" self. Acting based on other people's desires, rather than your own, causes incongruence and makes doing your best impossible. Furthermore, others recognize when your heart is not engaged.

Clearing Practice
Filtering the "Weather"

To deepen your knowledge, use the description of the four agreements/filtering strategies just described to fill in the blanks below.

1. Use your _____ wisely.

Think of a time when a co-worker spoke honestly/authentically, even though it may have been difficult, and it led to a positive change in the workplace. How did the person's words impact your behaviour? How might you apply this strategy in the workplace?

2. Recognize it's not _____.

How does this strategy impact you when you reflect on your reactions to other people's words and behaviours? How can you apply this strategy at work the next time you feel threatened by someone's words?

3. Avoid _____.

Think of a time when you or a co-worker made an assumption that turned out to be incorrect. How can you apply this strategy the next time you feel a strong emotion based on someone else's words or behaviours?

4. Do your _____.

What aspects of this strategy impact you? Can you connect to any self-judgement here, and if so, are you able to practise self-compassion? How can you apply this strategy in your everyday life?

Living Our Calling While Navigating Homogenizing Cultures

Hurt people hurt people. (Wilson, 2015)

Work environments that prioritize consistent professional displays are often homogenizing, resulting in incongruent employees. Homogenization occurs when cultures pressure people to assimilate to a narrow way of being or a prescribed emotional display. Awareness of homogenization helps us step back (nonattachment), promoting the ability to recognize and navigate social pressures, and to maintain our self-integrity (congruence) in the process. The ability to remain tethered to our "real" self despite pressures to assimilate to a socially prescribed "ideal" is a requirement of congruence.

Homogenizing caregiving environments prevent workers from feeling emotionally safe, limiting their willingness to be vulnerable. Vulnerability is a requirement of authenticity (congruence). To attain the emotional safety required to act authentically, we need relationships where we feel unconditional positive regard. Those who do not have relationships of unconditional positive regard are more likely to repress their emotions and opinions because of the rejection they will face if they do express themselves. As a result, they are likely to feel incongruent and resentful.

In homogenizing work cultures, individuals who disturb the status quo often become targets themselves. The pressure to maintain the status quo is a homogenizing force that sustains old subconscious ways of being, even though they no longer serve us. Homogenizing behaviours rarely benefit anyone. Those who argue for acceptance of diversity become vulnerable to scrutiny, and those who comply with assimilation often feel unsettled and ambiguous (incongruent). A chronic denial of our "real" self to assimilate to an "ideal" is a barrier to thriving (Rogers, 1959). Additionally, in homogenizing cultures, diversity produces implicit fears of conflict, which further pushes differences into the shadows and makes them even more divisive. Shame festers in the shadows, inflaming maladaptive perfectionism, socially prescribed perfectionism, and horizontal violence.

When we are with people from whom we feel unconditional positive regard, we are more likely to mirror the same acceptance inwardly (self-compassion) and outwardly. If we are self-compassionate, we will believe that we are worthy of manifesting our "real" selves in the world, including associated emotions and opinions.

We are more reliant and trusting of our roots as opposed to depending on the approval of others. Because we act congruently, we do not carry shame nor spill it onto others. Nor are we resentful of others, because we are tending to our own needs rather than denying our needs to please others. Therefore, when we are self-compassionate and congruent, we are far more resilient in homogenizing cultures. Congruence and self-compassion buffer us from feelings of threat, preventing stimuli from becoming stressors. Furthermore, because we feel that we are good enough, without condition, we are less prone to falling into perfectionism.

Turning the cultural tide requires both formal and informal leadership. As a community, we can articulate common stressors, working toward organizational priorities that support authentic ways of being and that celebrate diversity. To sustain congruent and peaceful communities, where everyone can flourish as their best selves, requires a systemic change in the way we see each other. Rather than sizing each other up as we've learned to do, like-intentioned members can shift a group by mirroring unconditional positive regard.

PEACE IS NOT …

Establishing a sense of peace within homogenizing cultures differs greatly from the typical ways we learn to "keep the peace." According to *Peace and Power: A Handbook of Transformative Group Process*:

> It is important to recognize and move away from the old ways that create dis-ease and distrust. Peace is not:
>
> - Letting things slide for the sake of friendship
> - Doing whatever is required to keep on good terms
> - Criticizing people behind their backs
> - Being silent at a meeting only to rant and rave afterward
> - Letting things drift if they do not affect you personally
> - Playing it safe in order to avoid confrontation
> - Manipulating someone to avoid open conflict
> - Coercing someone to do what you want
> - Hearing distortions of truth without refuting them
> - Indulging another's behaviour when the behaviour is destructive
> - Withholding information to protect someone else. (Chinn, 2018)

In other words, denying ourselves in order to "keep the peace" only promotes discord and hostility within organizations. Flourishing organizations promote authentic expression, encouraging people to align their unique passions and abilities with their work roles. Another factor that promotes trust and therefore the confidence to put ourselves out there, aligning with our "real" selves as opposed to an "ideal" prescribed to us, is belief in a power greater than ourselves.

Spirituality and Living Our Calling

Even if we have different opinions on the elements that make a person "spiritual," we can all relate to the placebo effect. The placebo effect has a positive impact on our physical and mental health because it relates to our beliefs, and our beliefs have a powerful impact on health outcomes. Meditation enables us to capitalize on such placebo effects because it reorients our belief systems. Those who meditate with a spiritual focus (e.g., practitioners of Transcendental Meditation) aim to shift the mind away from physical concerns to spiritual enlightenment. As a result, they have a greater ability to reorient their belief systems and tend to experience more positive results from meditation than those who do not have a spiritual focus (Wachholtz et al., 2017).

In a study performed by Frecska et al. (2016), people who prayed could avoid the depleting effects of emotional labour and emotional suppression and had a greater ability to avoid temptation. They suggested that prayer was a social interaction with God and that social interactions promote cognitive function, improving our ability to change less favourable habits.

Prayer improves our concern for others, deepens our capacity to forgive, and promotes conflict resolution (Lambert et al., 2010). Feeling confident that we have the resources to manage our inner and outer world is a component of sense of coherence. Believing in a spiritual source greater than ourselves promotes two core components of sense of coherence: an ability to find meaning and an ability to comprehend life events. Finally, trusting that there is a benevolent spirit that has a plan beyond our control can help ground and secure us. From this more grounded place flows forgiveness, gratitude, comfort, acceptance, optimism, and hope.

Strengthening and Aligning Practices
Strengthening Practice

A. Getting to What Is Essential
Remember a time when you felt invigorated by a task. These moments provide clues about who you are, what you love, and what makes you unique, separate from the *doing* that comes from obligation. Each time we notice these moments, we add to the trail of breadcrumbs that are leading us home, back to the "signal" of who we are. Journalling about what types of activities energize us versus what types drain us can give us a lot of clarity.

Think of those times when you did something out of inspiration that had an impact on those around you. What qualities of self enabled that to emerge in the world? If it's too difficult to name these characteristics in yourself, move on—there are other techniques that can help provide you with clarity:

1. Consider what characteristics you most admire in others. What we most admire in others may mirror similar qualities within ourselves that have not yet fully emerged.

2. Ask those who had the chance to observe you before the age of 7 (i.e., before we become clouded by social conditioning) what unique characteristics stood out to them. What seemed to bring you joy? What environments and activities did you thrive in?

3. Find pictures of yourself as a child. See if you can capture the sense of joy and freedom that existed prior to incongruence. Often, we can even identify when the joy of living got clouded. Look closely—can you see a difference in the smiling eyes?

You are creating a trail of breadcrumbs made up of the moments in the past that struck you, where inspired *doing* in the world flowed from you *being* your "real" self.

Write down the past achievements you are most proud of (work or personal):

a. Do you notice any themes or patterns emerging from #1 and #2?
   What are your core values? See if you can notice your tendency to name what you "should" value. While there is nothing wrong with having "ideals," the point is to ensure that what you identified is congruent with your "real" self, not a list of values prescribed onto you by others/culture. Those that are real, that are essential to you, are the values and priorities you cannot put down; they are a part of your essence.

b. Dig deeper into your true self, connecting to desire and to love. What core values are true to you?
   Take a few moments to recognize where you have come from and where you are now, cultivating gratitude by looking back rather than looking forward. Take stock of all you are learning on the journey. Spend a few moments thinking about what you are most proud of in your life. Use these as clues to what is most essential about who you are, what you value, and the unique path you are destined for.

Goals that are congruent with your desires and values are far more likely to be achieved. Aim high! If fears arise, remember that courage is all about feeling the fear and acting anyway, when it is the right decision for you and others. Connect to your desire; do not settle for what seems easy. Connect to what excites you, to what you will fight for.

c. Write down one or two short-term goals (to be completed within the next 1 to 3 years).

d. Write down one or two long-term goals (to be completed beyond 3 years).

Aligning Practice

B. Roles That Fill Us and Roles That Empty Us
By reflecting on personal experiences, we get the opportunity to develop awareness and acceptance of unique belief systems, values, and resources and/or barriers that impact the ability to practise self-compassion and engage in thriving. Self-awareness is a component of mindfulness.

As for the roles we play, in what order would you say you 'actually' prioritize the roles in your life? Start by naming the roles you play on the surface of life, including the role of ensuring your basic human needs are met (Maslow, 1951). Your basic needs would include tending to your body (i.e food, exercise, warmth), and tending to your passions and esteem (i.e hobbies you enjoy, friendships, etc.).

Other types of roles might include looking after dependents, professional work, unpaid service work, life partner, etc.

Now that you have a list of roles. Put them in order of what take priority in your day. For example, in a typical day, without any conscious awareness, I'll often put professional work and caring for dependents ahead of my basic human needs.

Now that you've named how you actually prioritize these roles. Taking a step back, how might you shift these priorities to honor your basic human needs first, enabling the benefits of doing so to ripple out to the other roles in your life.

This activity intertwines with the "Working with our Incongruent Tendencies" exercise in Chapter 4. Much like we often subscribe to "ideal" characteristics, we do the same with the roles we play. Awareness of these roles is a component of mindfulness, which is a requirement of nonattachment and is necessary to determine whether these roles are continuing to serve us.

- When you describe who you are, what is your first response?
- Do you jump right to talking about what you do for work or do you describe what you love to do? Or perhaps you identify more with the familial and social roles you play (spouse, parent, partner)? How do you think others would describe you?

Most of us will identify with and promote the roles that are held in high social regard; in industrialized cultures, these are the roles that show the greatest contribution to society.

What roles are you playing? Are you able to decipher what roles you play based on a prescribed ideal versus a role that aligns with what is essential or "real" about you? List the roles that align with your "real" self (hint: those that align with our "real" selves are easy to get lost in, time flies, we tend to gain energy). Can you identify what part of the role is fulfilling you? What components feel fun or invigorating? Why are they providing meaning (compared with the roles that are not)? What core values do they align with?

Now list the roles that satisfy a prescribed "ideal." If you are struggling to decipher the difference, consider whether the roles you play align with what is essential (your desires, values, goals) and whether you find the role more energizing or more draining. Socially prescribed roles tend to take greater effort and often burn up our energy. Or perhaps you feel neutral about the role, but it burns up a great deal of time, making it difficult to play the role you are passionate about. The answers to these questions provide insight into our ability to live our calling and ultimately thrive.

Spending too much time in one role, especially a role that does not fulfill you, can be detrimental to your well-being. If efforts consistently outweigh rewards, you will eventually run out of energy stores, putting you at high risk for burnout.

What components of these roles feel incongruent with your values or essence? Deconstruct the role, getting to the qualities that feel effortful or that cause discomfort in your body.

If you had to pick one role or activity that takes up a great deal of your time and energy, or is out of line with your "real" values or essence, what would it be?

Drop in. Imagine your life without the role/activity you just identified. Imagine that every detail and worry was taken care of and that you were free of it. How would that feel?

Our courage comes from being so passionate about something that we are willing to act despite our fears. What are the obstacles in the way of removing this incongruent area of your life? What do you fear will happen if you remove the activity or role from your life?

If you cannot remove this role (i.e., parenting!), this is a moment to accept what cannot be changed and to look for ways to reorient yourself to the role (elaborated on in Chapter 7). By doing the significant thing to adjust a quality of the role we play, it can shift us from feeling like a victim of the role to a victor in the role.

- What inner and outer resources do you need to be able to remove the role? If it is not removable, then what resources do you need to be able to navigate the qualities that feel incongruent?
- What actions do you need to take in order to access the resources needed to remove the obstacle(s)?
- Will you take the action? If not, why? If so, when?

It is normal for this activity to cause "noise" within, stirring up all sorts of angst and insecurity. We live in a conditioned world, and for most of our lives we've learned to go with the flow. Even the thought of moving against the current of the status quo can activate the stress response. This is a great time to cultivate self-compassion. Perhaps do some loving-kindness practices, acknowledging your fear and comforting yourself like you would a dear friend.

C. Exploring Your Ikigai

The Japanese concept of ikigai (pronunciation: ick-ee-guy) has drawn a lot of attention in the West, in part because of a popular study that suggests it may correlate with longevity (Sone et al., 2008). Ikigai can be roughly translated as "life purpose," or "the reason you get up in the morning." It is important to acknowledge that I am not Japanese and cannot speak about this concept from a cultural perspective; it is therefore likely that much has been lost in translation.

Garcia and Miralles' (2017) popular interpretation of ikigai is a useful tool for finding balance between desire, purpose, and talent in our efforts to make a living. This model demonstrates the complexities of our essence and how our desires and values enable us to find meaning in what might otherwise feel like mundane daily routines.

In the West, we are prone to working to save money so that one day we can retire, at last free from obligational *doing*. However, as with the many centenarians devoted to ikigai, there is reason to believe that aligning all areas of our life with our passions and mission in the world is far more likely to improve our quality and quantity of life now as well as into our retirement years.

Finding your ikigai involves connecting to activities you love. Recognize and articulate the magic inside of you that the world needs right now. Identify what you are good at and how you can make a living with your skills, abilities, and passions. Use a practice that helps you drop into your felt sense so you can feel into innate (different from conditioned) values, skills, abilities, and passions. Tuning in is how we distinguish the "noise" of cultural obligations from the "signal" of who we are and what calls us.

Populate each of the circles (Figure 11.1). Start small. There is no need to dream up lofty goals. What is more important is keeping it simple and making it relevant to your

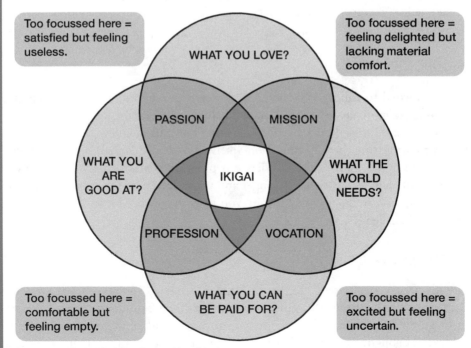

Fig. 11.1   A Useful Model for Finding Your Ikigai.

life here and now. Which areas are less clear? Can you relate to the symptoms of being too focused in certain areas?

As you continue to gain congruence, your answers will likely change. Keep coming back to ikigai (or another helpful tool) to challenge your previous assumptions.

D. Anchored by the "Means" of Calling, Propelled by the "Endpoint" of Vision

Connecting to our essence prompts and empowers us to live our calling. Our calling is our anchor, the lens through which we view the world. As such, calling focuses on the *means* to our end goals. Especially in the beginning, very few people will have a clear and succinct idea of what their calling is. Those of us who have subscribed to an "ideal" self in place of the "real" self will find it difficult to sort out what is a genuine call from within (signal) versus a prescribed call from external influences (noise). Forcing a calling might cause you to declare a calling that is out of sync with your "real" self. With this in mind, take your time, play with the idea, and hold your assumptions lightly. Calling work is deep and introspective, and as we gain congruence it becomes easier to separate the signal from the noise. Start broad and let the finer details fall into place over time. Be open to surprise and making changes. Your written calling should be short enough to memorize and easily call upon. This will act as your North Star, aligning your *doing* with your *being*.

Living your calling is a simple recipe: an inspired prompt leads you to take a significant action, and then you repeat the process.

VISION

A term related to calling is "vision." Our vision provides guidance and tangible milestones to motivate us, remind us, and help us celebrate the journey. Visions are descriptive and focused on achieving goals that move us to an *endpoint* rather than the *means* of getting there. We are more likely to achieve our goals if we own them, write them down, and regularly review our progress. Memorizing your vision can be more difficult, as it is typically longer and more detailed. However, keeping it in a place you visit frequently will inspire you to keep moving forward, especially in the face of challenges.

DEVELOPING A CALLING

Use the previous exercises ("Getting to What is Essential" and "Ikigai") as a treasure map, noting the patterns that emerge from what you are proudest of, what you are most grateful for, what values propel you forward, and what goals you aspire to achieve. Highlight key verbs that signify one or two core values that underscore your true self. These exercises will provide the structure necessary to formulate your calling statement, which you will begin developing by answering the following questions:

What value(s) are worth fighting for?

_____

_____

_____

Taking this one step further, consider the activities that feel meaningful and spark desire in you.

_____

_____

_____

What core values and principles drive your attraction to them?

_____

_____

_____

What areas can you assimilate without compromising who you are (i.e., maintaining congruence)?

_____

_____

_____

Your essence will emerge in a variety of ways in your life, reminding you who you are by creating angst in your body whenever you fall out of tune. Sometimes we must unwrap the cultural conditioning that shrouds it, but we all have this unique essence. A short calling statement can help tether you to your essence, empowering you to make decisions that are congruent with who you are. When congruent with your "real" self, a calling statement can empower your daily decisions and keep you motivated to reach your vision.

Articulating Your North Star: Creating a Calling Statement

1. Start with a verb (what you want to do).
2. Add an adjective (who you are aiming to engage).
3. State your desired outcome.

Combine the keywords into a short phrase as demonstrated in the framework below. Play with the words, feeling into what most resonates with your felt sense.

Sample Framework

My calling is to: (what you want to do?) (who are you wanting to do it for?) (your desired outcome?)

For example, my calling is: (To help) (people) (feel safe being authentic):

"My calling is to help people feel safe being authentic."

You aren't stuck with the framework; feel free to use what resonates and leave the rest. For instance, these statements are structured differently:

"To enable people to feel connected to others."
"To inspire others to be more than they thought they could be."
"To cultivate the self-worth in women."
"To help myself and others heal by practising self-compassion and freely providing unconditional positive regard to others."
"To promote congruence in myself and others by celebrating diversity."

Developing a Vision

A vision enables these causes to take form, providing guidance and forward movement. Knowing that the difficult work is an investment toward a worthy end provides the motivation to keep going. When vision aligns with calling, the likelihood of staying motivated to reach our goals is far greater. Clear visions enable people or organizations to make moment-to-moment decisions according to how they align with their calling and/or desired future state. When anchored in shared values (calling), visions empower and motivate employees to maintain the momentum required to reach the desired future state.

The core principles of making effective vision statements are as follows:

- Paint a mental picture of *your* ideal life >5 years from now.
- Reflect on your values, your essence, and your calling.
- Write the statement in the present tense.

Drop into your inner world, taking a few moments to connect to your heart, letting the outer world fall into the background. While this exercise requires us to be in thinking mode, try to come back to sensing mode as much as possible, reconnecting and ensuring that your written words are aligning with your essence.

Start by jotting down your calling:

My calling is _____.

Circle back to your core values. What is important to you? What can't you give up or put down? These are directly related to your essence and are often reflected in your calling statement. Now write some words that represent your ideal life. Try not to get too caught up in thinking by putting sentences together or trying to find the perfect word; just stick to single words, writing randomly and following your instincts. Are your words beginning to paint a mental picture of your ideal life? If not, what's missing?

You are now ready to interweave your calling, your essence, and the components of your ideal life into a vision statement, which is the mental picture that propels you forward. Play with the words, finding ones that resonate and motivate you. Using a vision framework is a great way to get you started; one is included here, but feel free to use whatever process works best for you! There are also examples provided, but remember this needs to be 100% true for you, so be careful not to let the examples sway you from what is "real" for you. Your vision statement will be especially powerful if it reflects *your* calling, *your* essence, and *your* ideal life. Do not get to stuck by trying to make it perfect. Your vision is a living statement that can be tweaked and adjusted as often as you like.

Sample Framework. In my daily life, I strive to be/honour/uphold **(your core value(s))** in all that I do. I am fulfilled by **(insert what you are passionate about, what motivates you)**. Each week, I work to progress toward **(what milestone/skill aligns with your calling)**. I am empowered and enriched when I connect to **(your superpower, your strengths)** by doing **(how you apply your strengths to your personal life and your work life)**. I am continuously working to refine/develop **(skill you are striving to improve)**, and I will strive to stay connected to who I am/my essence/my calling by **(activity/practice that enables you to connect to your inner world)**.

Here are some examples of calling statements (the means) followed by vision statements (the endpoint):

My Calling Statement. My calling is to cultivate relationships and work environments that help others feel safe being authentic.

My Vision Statement. In my day-to-day life, I strive to **be authentic** in all that I do. I am **fulfilled by meaningful and authentic connection with my self and others**. Each week I strive to **come to know, trust, and act from the essence** of who I am. I am empowered and enriched by connecting to **my calling, helping others feel safe being authentic**. I am continuously working to **develop my self-integrity**, and I strive to align with my calling by heartfully **connecting to my inner world and the desires** within it.

Another Example of a Calling Statement (contributed by Phillip Dames). My calling is to co-create spaces of unconditional positive regard for my community so that we can live free of obligation. Free to BE.

Phillip's Vision Statement. In my day-to-day life, I strive for the ability **to live free of obligational doing. Connecting to myself, my loved ones, nature, and music fulfills me**. Each week, I strive to **spend quality time in nature, and to gently lean beyond my comfort zones**. I am empowered and enriched when **I am in nature and by co-creating spaces of** unconditional positive regard. I am continually working to refine my ability to **expand my window of tolerance** and I **will stay connected to who I am through nature, music, and friendship**.

VISIONING WITH KIDS

Visioning can also be a valuable activity to do with children. It helps them dig into what is fun (taps into their desires), what their superpowers are (clues about their essence), and what motivates them (clues about their calling). Keep it light and make it fun—again, nothing is set in stone, and the statement can be adjusted as often as you or they like. Kids often have a much clearer idea of their essence (what they love, desire, and value) than adults do. Feel free to change the structure to make it more kid friendly.

9-Year-Old Piper's Vision Statement (she had parental assistance with wording). Each day, I try to be creative and unique in all that I do. I am excited by creating new things and then gifting them to others. Each week, I contribute to my household and earn an allowance so that I can buy art supplies and treats that I enjoy. I love making people feel noticed, and I stay connected to who I am by listening to music and doing arts and crafts.

8-Year-Old Beckett's Vision Statement (he also had parental assistance with wording). Each day, I try to be honest with other people and tidy with my things. Playing with others, building things, and going to new places excites me. Each week, I contribute to my household and earn my allowance, which helps me buy toys that I can build with. I show love to others through hugs and taking time with them. I honour who I am by speaking up about what is true for me and by doing what sounds fun for me.

A Meditation for the Road
By Dr. Crosbie Watler & Helen Watler

Let's begin by getting comfortable.
I invite you to close your eyes and make any adjustments you need to settle.
Pause.

Take a deep breath in …
And let it go …
Bring your awareness to your breath.
No need to change anything.
In and out.
Feel the rise and fall your breath creates in your body.
Pause.

Staying connected with your breath.
Relax your jaw and your cheeks, your face.
Brow relaxed.
Let your shoulders go.
Release tension from your arms. Feel your wrists and fingers relax.

Soften your stomach.
Feel your legs and feet get heavier,
Melting into the mat. Let the floor hold you.
Feel your body here ... warm ... relaxed ... soft.
Pause.

Notice any sensations in your body,
Any mental images ... emotions ... thoughts ...
Witness them without judgement, without resistance.
Bring your attention back to the flow of your breath.
In and out.
Feel the space in your body.
Notice the aliveness in your body.
Feel the spark of life within.
Connect with that spark, your inner pilot light.
Imagine your inner light ...
How does it look and feel?
What shape is it?
What colour is it?
How about a sound—what do you hear?
Is there a scent?
Connect with that inner light.
Breathing in, let it get stronger and brighter.
Feel it there within you.
Pause.

We are safe here.
We can trust this.
We have everything we need for this part of our journey.
The glow of our inner pilot light will show us the way.
We can return to it, again and again.
Pause.

Allow yourself to settle into a place of quiet awareness.
Stillness.
Being.
Presence.
The silent witness.
Your authentic self.
Nothing to do.
Nowhere to go.
Just ... be
Pause.

Here we are already whole.
No stories of success ... failure ... guilt or shame.

Simply "I am."
The pure spark of light.
Pause.

Here we are space without boundaries.
Awareness without thought.
Consciousness.
Connected within the web of life.
Pause.

With gratitude and quiet intention, we journey together.
To rediscover ourselves,
As if for the first time.
Remembering who we are.
Timeless ...
Thoughtless ...
Awareness ...
Feeling the connection with everything around us.

When you are in this place,
And I'm in this place,
We are one.

Namaste.

The Challenge: Navigation

By considering someone else's challenge, or working with another to consider ours, we cultivate nonattachment. We can often find comfort knowing we are not alone and that we can learn from and with each other. Coming from a more objective space, we can step back, reorienting from a position of strength with access to all our biological, intellectual, and spiritual capacities. With this benevolent orientation, we can face adversities with confidence, knowing we have the resources and support necessary to navigate life's challenges.

Let's circle back to the tree metaphor. We have now considered how our orientation influences our confidence in our abilities and our resources. As we come to believe that we are unconditionally positively regarded, we gain the courage to act authentically, closing the gap between our "real" self and our "ideal" self (congruence). Connecting more deeply with our "real" self expands our ability to connect outwardly, reminding us of how interconnected we are with each other, with the natural world, and with forces we feel but cannot fully comprehend. The more we tap into this expanded awareness, the more the day-to-day noise pales compared with the signal pulsing within us. The signal represents the values, desires, and passions that align us with our calling. From this orientation, the homogenizing forces endemic to Western culture can be seen for what they are—cultural preferences, not obligatory prescriptions. We can strategically navigate the weather, driven not by fear, but rather empowered with a renewed sense of confidence, enabling us to creatively resource with optimism, gratitude, and compassion.

 Attuning/Reflecting Opportunity

What are you noticing as you move through your days with a greater awareness of alignment and calling? What's working for you? What is coming up for clearing ("noise")? What areas are you wanting to strengthen?

Attuning for the Journey Ahead: Connecting Root Systems

We are *coming to know* how to live a calling by *aligning* our goals and actions with our desires and values. We have developed a calling statement that will anchor us to our essence and guide our steps as we move toward our desired future state (vision).

Now, we turn our focus to exploring how our roots intertwine with those of others. We *attune* and *align* collectively with like-intentioned others. Those we serve, those we lead, and those we work alongside. We *strengthen* our community of practice by establishing a shared vision, fortified by compassionate leadership strategies.

CHAPTER 12

Aligning in Community: Connecting Root Systems

Authentic relationships and supportive communities remind us who we are when we forget. (Demers, 2019)

So far, we have largely focused on establishing our personal roots (Figure 1.1), but managing the weather is equally important. The sequence is intentional. By feeling into the depth and capabilities of our roots, we can confidently and optimistically navigate challenging weather systems. As for the root systems of our neighbours, maintaining a collective perspective enables us to access resources within the larger community. By grounding individually and extending to resource collectively, we can remain calm in the eye of the storm. Focusing too much on individual capacities without feeling the support of a community is like expecting a fish to spend its entire life swimming upstream. It may happen for a time, but without collective momentum, the effort will become too burdensome, motivation will wane, and it (and we) will eventually succumb to the current. The better option is to maintain a healthy balance between self-reliance and mutuality. The inspiration of the whole is greater than the sum of the parts. It takes a like-intentioned community to turn the tide.

To feel connected, we need to be witnessed and to witness others in times of vulnerability. This is us, connecting in spirit, despite the physical borders that separate us. This is us sharing the sacred nature of our "real" selves. Doing so enables us to feel connected to others. This felt connection rewrites the story of separation that comes from *maya*—a Buddhist term for the visual *illusion* of separation. We establish trust and confidence in the process of manifesting our "real" selves in the world. When we share a part of ourselves that previously felt forbidden and are received with grace and compassion (unconditional positive regard), we learn to offer the same inwardly. Once we securely attach inwardly, tuning into the "signal" of who we are, we can then share this same confident and compassionate frequency with others. Although it starts with connection to just one person, it has a domino effect. Eventually, with more and more people attuning to unconditional positive regard, we reach the tipping point necessary to shift toxic cultures.

We have become the change we want to see in the world. This alone is our highest purpose.

Crosbie Watler MD, FRCPC

When informed by the individual and collective needs of the community, organizational structures can uphold healthy and empowered democracies. Those in formal positions of authority set the tone and standards necessary to sustain democracies that establish a shared community vision while also celebrating individual differences. This is required for individual members to lead according to their unique callings, in connection to a mosaic of like-intentioned others. To empower caregivers as leaders, we must shift the oppressive power structures. These power structures are evident in power-laden hierarchies and homogenizing cultural forces. We do this by turning from fear- and shame-based models toward communities of practice that empower every voice, honour transparency, and share leadership. To be clear, hierarchies have their place in improving efficiencies, establishing communication pathways, and limiting the stress that results from ambiguity. We can benefit from the order that hierarchical structures provide without behaving in ways that disempower those with less power. The distinguishing difference between helpful and unhelpful hierarchies is whether employees at the bottom of the hierarchy have an influential voice in the larger system. If the only way to feel heard is to move up the hierarchy, then the organization has a power-laden structure. Organizational momentum requires a shared leadership model, upheld by a far-reaching and practically relevant vision. The torchbearers of such a vision are the leaders, mentors, and educators who role model respectful communication and unconditional positive regard. From here, self- and other-compassionate leaders emerge, inspiring compassionate teams who are in turn inspired to provide compassionate care.

The Challenge: Orientation

By considering someone else's challenge, or working with another to consider ours, we cultivate nonattachment. We can often find comfort knowing we are not alone and that we can learn from and with each other. Working from this more objective space, we mitigate the stress response. We can then reorient from this position of strength, thus improving our ability to use all our biological, intellectual, and spiritual capacities. With this benevolent orientation, we can face adversities with confidence, knowing we have the resources and support necessary to navigate life's challenges.

Let's practise with Rachel and Todd. Rachel and Todd work as peer caregivers in a tertiary mental health institution. There is palpable tension between them stemming from a past misunderstanding that left Rachel believing that Todd complained to their manager about her.

When Rachel sees Todd, she gets activated, which sends her into fight mode. While she is careful to mind her words, she isn't shy about communicating her disapproval in subtle ways. She frequently sighs when Todd is talking and often criticizes his work, making her irritation clear.

Todd is intimidated by Rachel, who is a senior staff member and ringleader on the team. When Todd sees Rachel, he gets activated, which sends him into flight mode. He does his best to avoid her and the co-workers that seem to rally behind her hostile behaviours. But given their close work quarters, he finds himself constantly looking over his shoulder. To him, this feels like "bullying," but Rachel is so subtle that he doesn't feel he can call her behaviour out without making things worse for himself. Todd has kids to provide for. He needs this job. Rachel clearly has an axe to grind and has the **social capital** and seniority to do it.

Recently, Todd found a patient who was in his care lying on the floor. He rushed to attend to the patient, and Rachel and two other co-workers were right behind him. Rachel, standing with her two co-worker friends, pointed a finger at Todd and asked him why the bedrails weren't up. Todd felt wrongly accused, as the bedrails being up was not a requirement for this patient. However, he now sees that maybe it should have been. He is eager to escape the situation, as he feels attacked and guilty for missing this safety measure.

How do you think Todd should manage this challenge?

Consider a situation in your past or present where you could relate to Rachel (i.e., you felt betrayed to the point that you could not contain your hostility). What primary need is fuelling Rachel's resentment? How might she reorient herself in relationship to Todd?

Consider a relationship in your past or present where you can relate to Todd (i.e., you endured frequent bullying, but felt powerless to stop it). What primary need is fuelling Todd's felt sense of threat? How might he reorient himself in a way that helps him navigate this challenge?

Turning the Tide With Like-Intentioned Communities of Practice

A community of practice represents a like-intentioned group working under a shared vision. Refer back to Chapter 6, where we explored "signal" versus "noise," with "signal" representing the prompts of the spirt–body and "noise" representing external distractions and pressures and internal stress. When living in communities of *conditional* as opposed to *unconditional* positive regard, we will experience conflicts between our inner and outer worlds. We will surrender to the inner world, the outer world, or, depending on our navigation skills, carefully pendulate between the two.

Surrendering to the expectations of others leads us to ignore the prompts of the spirit–body so that we can say "yes" to others. As a result, we attain social ease. However, there is a cost: we become incongruent in that moment, fuelling shame and eroding self-trust. In this case, the noise from the outer world transitions into noise in the inner world (resentment). This leaves us feeling more secure in the outer world and less secure with ourselves. When the *be*ing self ("signal") is habitually quieted, deferring instead to the "noise," our subconscious *do*ing kicks in, requiring primal mechanisms to take the driver's seat. Enter fight, flight, freeze, and fawn.

Surrendering to the prompts of our inner world means that we show up with authenticity, expressing our "real" selves (including desires and values) with others. As a result, we say "yes" to the spirit–body despite the external noise. We then become congruent in that moment, which promotes self-compassion and self-trust. However, this scenario can lead to social dis-*ease* and can make us feel less secure with others, depending on our support systems. When we are feeling too vulnerable in the world, we can feel pushed beyond our window of tolerance for stress, resulting in fight, flight, freeze, or fawn.

Given that both choices can land us in an insecure way of being, leaving us prone to nervous system activation, how do we navigate this terrain? One thing is for certain: we cannot do it alone in this noisy world. Rather than pretending that we can swim upstream and not expect to get tired, eventually giving way to the cultural current, we can ground ourselves in a community of like-intentioned others. Together we turn the tide. This is group flow, which aligns with what polyvagal theory says about how human beings regulate one another (Flores & Porges, 2017). Those who know our "signal" can remind us of who we are when we forget. They fuel our sense of meaning and security in the world. From this connected place, we gain the courage to follow our calling ("signal") despite the "noise."

The *significant* thing represents the action we are called to take in any given moment that aligns with our "signal," despite noisy distractions and social pressures. Grounded in a secure community of practice characterized by unconditional positive regard, we take one significant action at a time. This is how we thrive. One thriving moment after another is how we learn to live a calling.

Connection to Others: Intertwining Roots

In utero, we are in constant physical connection with another being. At birth, we experience physical separation, a space between where we end and others begin. In death, when our spirit releases from the vessel hosting it, we again connect to all that is. Between birth and death, our physical separation and the stories that flow from it shape how we live, even though we remain energetically connected to all that is throughout our lives. While we are not alone, it can feel as though we are. As a result, out of fear of rejection, we often walk alone, afraid to show the parts of ourselves that might cause further separation. However, when we step into the light, exposing our spiritual nature, our core self, we plant the flag of who we are in the shared ground. When we show our "real" self to others, we share the pain born from separation, felt as shame in our physical form. It is in community that we release the shame that festers in isolation. When received with unconditional positive regard, the "real" self is witnessed, accepted, and loved. We remember our connection to all things, despite our physical boundaries, we, as human *be*ings, are in this together.

> ### A Holistic Approach to Mental Health
>
> **By Crosbie Watler, MD, FRCPC, a Canadian thought leader and psychiatrist**
>
> The newborn is fully immersed in awareness of authentic self—simply *I am*—no condition, no illusion of separation. In the same moment, nothing and everything. Perhaps we go back to that awareness of spirit, of *being* when we cast off our mortal cloak. Better not to wait. Self-awareness while still in human form is a formidable force. Seen and unseen allies will support you. You will never *prove this* to the doubters among you, so don't even try. There is a *noetic* quality—you deeply *feel* it to be true, and the constant flow of coincidence and divine serendipity confirms it.

Much of this text has focused on learning to tap into the richness of our inner worlds, expanding our awareness of our spiritual natures (essence) and our ability to respond to our felt senses. When grounded and resourced in this way, we forge deeper roots, improving our ability to manage stimuli before they evolve into stressors. We can self-soothe in times of stress. As a result, our *do*ing flows from an inspired *be*ing. In no time, with one *significant* action after another, we find that we are living our calling. However, our roots share the soil with others, intertwining and synchronizing, serving and being served. This intertwining is imperative, especially in times of scarcity. When working as a collective, we can pool our strengths and resources, enabling us to continue moving toward. We take only what we need and contribute what we can. This is connection in community. While we may get somewhere faster alone, we get much farther together.

> *This is how we have evolved to live—in community, with purpose and connection. In our modern world, we have lost our way. This is at the crux of our mental health and substance use crisi s. We need to look in the right place for solutions. Simply putting new funds into mental health care is a failed experiment. When we are supported to live the way, we were designed to live, everything heals.*
>
> Dr. Crosbie Watler, MD, FRCPC

Polyvagal theory (Flores & Porges, 2017; Porges, 2011), introduced in Chapter 1, underscores the role of connection and community in the healing process. When we connect with like-intentioned others who can mirror unconditional positive regard to one another, we calm and even rewire our nervous systems. When connected in this secure vessel, the "noise" within us settles, enabling us to attune to and express the "signal" of who we really are. We learn to see each other, separate from nervous system responses and cultural conditioning. In this seeing, we gain the courage necessary to manifest our authentic selves in the world.

In a review of 148 studies involving over 300 000 participants, Holt-Lunstad et al. (2010) found a 50% increase in likelihood of survival among those with strong social relationships. In other words, if half the members of a community died, those who survived were more likely to be the ones who had strong social relationships, while those who died were more likely to have weaker social ties. Supportive social relationships also improve our sense of coherence, which predicts a host of positive physical and mental health outcomes. In terms of the health of organizations, research conducted over several decades has shown us that those who feel more connected at work will have greater empathy for and trust in others, and they are also more likely to be cooperative (House et al., 1988). Those who feel connected, believing that others feel unconditional positive regard toward them, are more likely to contribute to a positive workplace than those who do not.

Social connection is not about how many friends we have—it is our sense of authentic and unconditional connection to at least one person. Those who prefer introversion may have only one person to whom they feel connected, while extroverts prefer many social connections. Some may find that they experience this connection with animals. That works too! We cannot feel connected at the level of the thinking mind. The ability to receive these benefits correlate with our experience of connection in the felt sense. The belief that we are connected, that we are resourced beyond our physical limitations, is a component of sense of coherence (our orientation to life). When we feel into the abundant resources of the collective, we gain security in the stability of our well-resourced root systems. From this orientation, we can confidently manage stimuli before they evolve into destabilizing stressors. As illustrated in Figure 1.1, deep and stable root systems are less likely to be threatened by the passing weather.

Quality is far more important than quantity here. A person who has one friend from whom they feel unconditional positive regard will reap more benefits than the person who has many conditional friendships. In the same way, workplace relationships characterized by unconditional positive regard that promote connectedness and a sense of belonging are exactly what is needed to transform the competitive ways of being that many of us have grown accustomed to.

In a study of novice caregiver resilience, Jessica, a new graduate caregiver and research participant, echoes this sentiment, demonstrating how feeling supported and safe at work reoriented her perspective and capacity to cope with workplace stress:

I was calling in sick often ... because I dreaded going into work. I got put on probation because of it. It was an unsupportive environment. I was super stressed out and burned out. There was no support there. There was no teamwork. There were no resources or senior nurses to ask questions. Now that I'm on floor [#], I feel safe, and it is so much better. No matter what happens, I can call for help, and someone will be there to help me. I don't call in sick now. I feel supported and excited to go to work now. (Dames, 2018a)

Relationships that promote connection while also encouraging authentic expression are essential in order for us to internalize (embody) unconditional positive regard from others. Once we have attuned to this felt sense, we can then pay it forward, gifting others with this more secure way of being. By cultivating a felt sense of connection with others, we are strengthening the two factors that determine how resilient we are. One, we gain congruence by showing up authentically in the world. Two, we improve our sense of coherence as we gain confidence in our inner collective resources, promoting a greater ability to navigate life's challenges without feeling chronically threatened by them.

Codependence Versus Interdependence

Relationships based on conditional acceptance, where loved ones must abide by social norms to gain approval, characterize codependence. Similar to what happens in homogenizing cultures, we continue to fuel codependence by subconsciously shaming each other into sameness. This way of being often results from observing and then internalizing the habits we picked up as children. We did not consciously choose to live this way; we were conditioned to do so. We allowed this conditioning to take over because we believed our survival depended on it. For those fighting to survive in an individualistic culture, anxiously attaching to or avoiding others is a natural outcome. Many of us have experience with codependence, beginning in childhood and then perpetuated via incongruence, habit, and familiarity in adulthood. Breaking codependent habits can be difficult, especially when we are unaware of them. As we journey toward congruence, we become uncomfortably aware of codependence. We cannot remain codependent and gain congruence. Codependency is a substantial roadblock to authentic expression. This newfound discomfort is normal and a sign that we are on the right path, leaning into the discomfort of birthing our authentic selves.

What are the common signs of codependence?

- Black and white thinking; feeling judged or judging other's actions as right or wrong based on rigid expectations (perfectionism)
- Avoidance of conflict; resistance to being accepted by others
- Avoiding expression of true opinions and desires because of fear of rejection, and
- Caving to a prescribed way of being to avoid rocking the boat.

When codependence runs rampant in work cultures that are characterized by the pressure to assimilate to a narrow way of being (through shaming), incongruence results. Once we become incongruent, the shame we feel inside becomes too much to bear, eventually leading to disembodiment. We lose our felt connection with ourselves and all that is. We cannot thrive in this disconnected state. From this fear-driven state, we will likely further contribute to the homogenizing forces that got us here.

On the other hand, interdependence is a balance of recognizing our dependence on others and honouring our independence as a unique individual. There is an innate tension between dependence and independence. It ebbs and flows as a normal part of any healthy relationship. Conflict is bound to arise within this tension. In fact, conflict is a healthy sign! It reminds us that we are both unique and the same. We learn to honour each other's unique needs and desires within a context characterized by connection. Through conflict, we work through the dependent–independent tensions, redefining where our boundaries end and others' boundaries begin. We learn to accept what we cannot change, and that we do not need to be the same to feel a sense of belonging in the world. From this secure place, we can agree to disagree without threatening our security in the larger human mosaic.

TESTING THE WATERS

In interdependent relationships, conflict is not as threatening because it does not require us to change who we are in order to be loved. We give and receive unconditional positive regard. If conditions arise, there is a safe space to discuss those, even test them out to reaffirm the safe nature of the relationship. This testing is necessary to internalize it, to believe in its unconditional nature. To reap the benefits of this secure way of *be*ing, we must believe it is unconditional. To believe it, we must experience it. Testing happens when we express ourselves authentically, ensuring that all parts of our "real" self are accepted as part of the bundle of characteristics that make us who we are. The bundle of who we are, as a whole, receives unconditional positive regard. To be clear, this does not mean that everyone will like all parts of us. No doubt we will irritate others (and others us). However, even our "unpopular" parts will be accepted as just that: parts of a much larger and positively regarded whole. Furthermore, when we are in states of threat, oftentimes it isn't the "real" self that is emerging; it is more likely our disembodied form, which is driven by the nervous system and largely disconnected from our "real" self. To mirror unconditional positive regard to ourselves in these challenging moments, we need to be able to detect the deeper "signal" beneath the surface "noise."

When we are interdependent, we can honour the differences and less favourable behaviours of others without feeling threatened by them. Communities of practice flourish only when such interdependent relationships are cultivated. We become unique *be*ings held together by creating a shared vision, underscoring priorities that promote authenticity through relationships of unconditional positive regard. It is this authentic connection between individuals that enables conflicts and challenges to be faced without the entire collective becoming destabilized. This is how we prevent ourselves as caregivers from feeling isolated and threatened when opinions and ways of being differ among us.

We will find common ground in our shared humanity. We all struggle with incongruence, working through the tension of feeling the need to compromise in order to feel safe in the world. In these common human experiences, we can take comfort that we are not alone. To illustrate this, consider a recent study where two novice caregivers and research participants, Candice and Jessica, felt empowered during the turbulent time when they were crossing the threshold into professional practice. They took comfort in knowing that they were not suffering alone, that what they were experiencing was quite normal among their peer group (Dames, 2018a): "Just being aware of it and seeing it in writing and doing the self-exploration has really helped me cope with it … it has really helped me grow" (Candice). "It is nice to know that I'm not the only one that who is dealing with this stuff" (Jessica).

Organizational Visioning

Living a calling moves us beyond our individual wants, cultivating our desire to contribute to a cause greater than ourselves. This calling anchors us, grounding our roots and providing the lens through which we view the world. It reminds us of who we are and what matters to us. It represents the "means" by which we live out our moments. We can have an individual calling and a collective calling. On the other hand, shared visions are more descriptive and focused on the "endpoint" rather than the means by which we get there. When organizations agree on a common vision, goals and actions take form, providing the guidance, inspiration, and momentum to work toward common goals. Effective visions provide a collective knowing that when the work gets difficult, the effort is a worthwhile investment. It provides the collective motivation to work through the tricky legs of the journey because the destination is worth it.

When anchored in clear collective visions, people and/or organizations are empowered and motivated make moment-to-moment decisions according to how they align with the person's and/or organization's calling and desired future state. Organizational visioning has three stages (NHS Improvement, 2018):

1. Formal leaders set the parameters for the vision.
2. A small group creates the main features of the vision, representing those with a stake in the future.
3. The vision is shared broadly and explained locally.

John Kotter's six key characteristics of visions further inform the development process. They are as follows:

1. Imaginable: It conveys a clear picture of the future.
2. Desirable: It appeals to the long-term interest of those involved.
3. Feasible: They are realistic and attainable.
4. Focused: They are clear enough to guide decision making.

5. **Flexible:** They allow individual initiative and alternative responses when conditions change.
6. **Communicable:** They are easy to communicate and can be explained quickly. (NHS Improvement, 2018)

Visioning Compassionate and Trauma-Informed Workplaces

Compassion is an antidote to the pervasive shaming that perpetuates social dominance and erodes workplace morale.

Social movements need a structure to support growth. Organizational leaders sustain that structure. Given the state of health care culture, pivoting to a more compassionate vision requires consistent maintenance, upheld and motivated by a shared leadership vision. Sustained change requires self-compassionate leaders to embody and extend compassion to others, underscoring the vision on a day-to-day basis. Michael West (2020), a key stakeholder in the NHS Improvement Process, outlined the characteristics of compassionate leadership:

- Attending: Paying attention to staff—"listening with fascination"
- Understanding: Finding a shared understanding of the situation they face
- Empathizing, and
- Helping: Taking intelligent action to help.

Research shows that the most powerful factor influencing culture is leadership. (NHS Improvement, 2017)

Compassionate work environments are sustained by congruent and compassionate leaders who are empowered by a supportive organizational structure and shared vision. Compassionate leaders model and promote relationships of unconditional positive regard, resulting in workplaces that celebrate authenticity and diversity. As discussed earlier, those who rank high in self-compassion are more likely to project the same unconditional positive regard outwardly. After England's National Health Service invested in a widespread effort to promote compassionate leadership, their program of research surrounding this effort showed significant improvements in caregiving culture and patient care outcomes. The research shows that when organizations embody compassion, supported and delivered by organizational leaders, they:

- Deliver high-quality care and value for money while supporting a healthy and engaged workforce
- Enable staff to show compassion, speak up, continuously improve, and create an environment where there is no bullying and where there is learning, quality, and the need for system leadership, and

- Contribute to cultural safety, improving diversity efforts and outcomes. (NHS Improvement, 2017, p. 3)

Workplaces can be viewed as communities of practice, as they are held together by common intentions to achieve common goals. In the same way, these intentions can expand to include other common priorities and values. For instance, in order to co-create a relational space that is trauma informed, the community needs to follow the principles of safety, trustworthiness, choice, collaboration, and empowerment (Vickers & Moyer, 2020). It is important to establish this safe space because when we show up more authentically with others, it can activate intense and often debilitating fears of rejection. If we lack security in our relational environment when these feelings arise, then we are likely to react, protecting ourselves from the potential danger. As a result, too much vulnerability too fast can cause us to emotionally shut down, or "freeze." Conversely, we will be far more likely to tolerate vulnerability when we move at the pace of trust. Inch by inch, as we come to believe that we are unconditionally positively regarded, we can put another "real" piece of ourselves on the collective table. This is the process of "testing" described earlier. Therefore, to co-create this type of community of practice, we must individually and collectively cultivate a belief in unconditional positive regard. Once this belief is internalized and then embodied (manifested in the physical world), we can shift into ways of being that (1) promote greater inner alignment and authentic expression (congruence) and (2) allow us to feel the agency and confidence necessary to successfully navigate life's challenges (sense of coherence).

Leadership: Role Modelling a New Way

Caregiving in today's high-stimulus and rapidly evolving health care environments requires leaders that are willing to role model a new way forward. Every health care provider is a leader capable of blooming where planted, but the soil they are planted in must be able to support their growth and development. When it does, these flourishing *be*ings will bear fruit, enabling them to share their abundance with the larger community.

We step into an informal leadership role the moment we cross the threshold into professional practice. Our capacity as leaders and change agents has a significant impact on our work culture. Despite the implicit expectations of caregivers to act as change agents, many report feeling unprepared for their role; this finding underscores the need for organizations to provide more support for leadership development (Sherman et al., 2011). The foundational components that will encourage employees to step out of their comfort zones, helping them to forge their paths as leaders, are cultivating trustworthiness, engaging in respectful communication, and normalizing conflict within a culture of unconditional positive regard.

Research shows that *trustworthiness* is associated with elevated levels of oxytocin, a hormone and neurotransmitter that improves empathy, prosocial behaviour, organizational commitment, and teamwork (Zak, 2018). High-trust organizations tend to have higher employee satisfaction rates, better morale, and better teamwork than low-trust organizations. The trustworthiness of leaders provides the relational blueprint that informs how the team will *be* together. Those who act in trustworthy ways—prioritizing transparency, openness, whole-heartedness, and relating from an empathetic place—set the tone for the workplace. As neuroscience has demonstrated, these qualities contribute significantly to the health of employees and the organization as a whole (Zak, 2018).

Role modelling direct and *respectful communication* provides an environment where employees feel safe authentically and assertively expressing themselves. Unfortunately, triangulated communication is the norm in many caregiving environments, eroding relational trust and safety. Triangulation occurs when we avoid addressing conflict with the person whom we feel threatened by. Instead, we report our disapproval of another to peers or to a manager, leaving the person with whom we are disagreeing (or disapproving of) out of the conversation while we build alliances behind their back. While building alliances with peers and management may feel safer—it enables us to avoid direct confrontation and therefore minimizes the risk of rejection—in the end, it fuels hostility and can do irreparable relational harm. When this scenario repeats itself over and over again in teams of caregivers, it makes for highly volatile and hostile relations. Furthermore, triangulated communication often inflames miscommunication and conflict, involving more people and adding offences to the initial injury. This conflict management strategy is a form of horizontal violence that runs rampant in many caregiving cultures.

NORMALIZING CONFLICT

Conflict is common in many caregiving environments because of the high-stimulus and fast-paced nature of the work. The pressure to perform is a source of stress for many, causing frequent nervous system activation. Because tasks are driven by client needs, which are continually changing, complex, and often unpredictable, decision making is frequent and often urgent (Sherman & Pross, 2010). On the one hand, differing opinions makes for a buffet of options, cultivating creative and flexible teams. On the other hand, if we view conflict as a threat, differing opinions will be an ongoing source of stress, leading to more tension and hostility. Our ability to resolve conflict hinges on our understanding of how it typically unfolds. It is also helpful to recognize the defensive tendencies (flight–flight–freeze–fawn) that we and our colleagues default to. When we recognize defensive patterns, we are more likely to interrupt and diffuse the stress response. For instance, consider the reactions that occur when a conflict-avoidant colleague has an emotional run-in with a co-worker who tends to go into fight when activated, or when two colleagues who both default to fighting stance engage in conflict.

CONFLICT THROUGH THE LENS OF UNMET NEEDS

The bulk of conflict and conflict resolution happens subconsciously. During a conflict, the person in a position of power, or the one who has traditionally taken the dominant role, will often direct the outcome. When these positions of power are directing the outcomes, both parties feel threatened. Nervous system tendencies will determine how members react, with varying combinations of fighting, fleeing, freezing, and fawning. If both people go into fight, the one driven by the most primal need will often dominate the conflict, as they are driven by a greater sense of threat (i.e., fighting for their survival). The one that has confidence that their primary needs are met will often (subconsciously) realize that backing down is not a choice for the other. It is a felt necessity that will likely endure despite reason. As a result, two people in fighting posture collide. When discomfort feels extreme, the one who can step back will do so. In another scenario, there may be a combination of fleeing and freezing, resulting in the conflict being avoided altogether. Or one may fight while the other flees or freezes, enabling the one fighting to feel a greater sense of resolution than the other. As a result, the one who fled or froze is more likely to hold the unresolved tension in their body, leading to resentment, which emerges as hostility in the workplace.

As you can see, conflict is often happening below the level of our conscious awareness. Furthermore, it is rarely about us. These are the moments when the capacity to embody *rational detachment* with others will prove to be an important skill. This form of nonattachment, first introduced in Chapter 3, is characterized by an ability to not take the behaviours of others personally. From this perspective, we recognize that the hostile behaviours of others are less about us and more about others' (or our own) unresolved hurts from the past being projected into the current situation. From this vantage point, we can keep things in perspective without getting stuck in our own assumptions and fears. Because it is not personal, it also doesn't threaten the nervous system. When grounded in this nonattached position, we can shift our focus from what is wrong to what can be done.

As we cultivate rational detachment, both parties can step back from the threat because they both understand that is not personal. When it feels personal, the "noise" of the moment will cloud our ability to see what is happening beneath the surface (our "signal"). When we keep things in perspective, it interrupts the nervous system, enabling us to move from reaction to actions that are more conscious and objective. This may require people to take some time away so that emotions stemming from fear can settle. If we cannot cultivate nonattachment on our own, reaching out to a friend or professional can help us attain the objectivity necessary to navigate the conflict more consciously. An example of a model that can help cultivate space and objective resources is WITS, described in the next section.

Navigating Conflict With WITS

The WITS program is a curriculum that focuses on promoting safe and healthy relationships in schools and communities. Studies show the positive impacts of helping children (and their families) to navigate conflict in a way that respects different ways of being. Doing so strengthens the social competence of the wider community (Leadbeater & Sukhawathanakul, 2011). WITS stands for walk away, ignore, talk it out, and seek help (https://witsprogram.ca). This simple acronym is easily memorized and provides a common language and clear shared intention. When our nervous systems are activated, diverting our attention to the acronym provides us with a greater ability to respond with conscious choice, as opposed to defaulting to our subconscious reaction. By stepping back, we become the observer rather than the victim of a looming threat.

The first two steps—walking away and ignoring—provide us with the space necessary to allow emotions to settle. These two steps help us to feel and then discharge the emotions we are feeling, which prevents them from accumulating as "noise" in the body. Creating space for emotions to come and go is healthier than resisting them. If we resist them, they are likely to get stuck in the body. In time, these emotions will likely emerge as a subconscious projection, and we have little to no influence over when that might happen. By contrast, if we allow the nervous system to settle, we can more effectively circle back to resolve the tension, enabling us to do the relational tending necessary for both parties to feel safe. Without this space between us and the conflict, we will remain in a defensive posture. If we cannot diffuse the threat response, we will remain attached to our side of the story. This attachment leads to a narrow perspective, preventing us from seeing the conflict from both sides and limiting our ability to acknowledge needs of the other. When this happens, when we cannot step back to talk things out, we can resource with the wider community. Seeking the help of more objective others helps us navigate the conflict in a way that is beneficial to both parties.

Recognizing Patterns Cultivates Choice

In reality, oversimplifying or compartmentalizing relational processes is not helpful. However, by recognizing and exploring trends, we can learn to recognize patterns early on before we become embroiled in stress states that we can't step back from. If we get to know the cues leading up to a stress state, we can interrupt the stress response, enabling us to step back before we get lost in a subjective spiral. From here, we are more able to maintain perspective, enabling us to better navigate common challenges. For this reason, it is important to understand how conflict typically unfolds.

Conflict typically occurs in distinct phases. It often begins with frustration, moves to conceptualization and then action, and ends at outcomes (Thomas, 1992). Knowing about the phases of conflict can help us cultivate nonattachment, as we realize that what we are going through is a normal part of being human. It does not define us, and like other common human challenges, we can learn to navigate it. When we can understand the phase of conflict we are in, it also helps us understand (and provide grace for) where other people are at. Rather than expecting them to be where we are, we can meet them where they are.

There are five distinct approaches to resolving conflict. Each approach relates to how assertive and cooperative we feel in a given scenario. Depending on preferences and habits, we can employ a mixture of approaches (Barsky, 2016; Thomas, 1992). The five approaches are as follows:

- Collaborating: Assertive, creative, and cooperative
- Competing: Aggressive, not cooperative
- Compromising: Negotiating assertively and cooperatively
- Accommodating: Passive but cooperative, and
- Avoiding: Passive, not cooperative.

This is a good time to expand your awareness by reflecting on how this information relates to your own tendencies during conflict. Use the attuning and strengthening practices below to explore your conflict style and assess how effective you are at resolving conflict.

Attuning and Strengthening Practices
Attuning Practice

A. Conflict Self-Assessment
Directions: Read each of the following statements. Assess yourself in terms of how often you tend to act similarly during conflict at work, at clinical placements, and at school. Place the number of the most appropriate response in the blank in front of each statement. Put "1" if the behaviour is never typical of how you act during a conflict, "2" if it is seldom typical, "3" if it is occasionally typical, "4" if it is frequently typical, or "5" if it is very typical of how you act during conflict.

_____ 1. Create new possibilities to address all important concerns.
_____ 2. Persuade others to see it and/or do it my way.
_____ 3. Work out some sort of give-and-take agreement.
_____ 4. Let other people have their way.
_____ 5. Wait and let the conflict take care of itself.
_____ 6. Find ways that everyone can win.
_____ 7. Use whatever power I have to get what I want.
_____ 8. Find an agreeable compromise among the people involved.

_____ 9. Give in so others get what they think is important.

_____ 10. Withdraw from the situation.

_____ 11. Cooperate assertively until everyone's needs are met.

_____ 12. Compete until I either win or lose.

_____ 13. Engage in "give a little and get a little" bargaining.

_____ 14. Let others' needs be met more than my own needs.

_____ 15. Avoid taking any action for as long as I can.

_____ 16. Partner with others to find the most inclusive solution.

_____ 17. Put my foot down assertively for a quick solution.

_____ 18. Negotiate for what all parties value and can live without.

_____ 19. Agree to what others want to create harmony.

_____ 20. Keep as far away from others involved as possible.

_____ 21. Stick with it to get everyone's highest priorities.

_____ 23. Argue and debate over the best way.

_____ 23. Create some middle position everyone agrees to.

_____ 24. Put my priorities below those of other people.

_____ 25. Hope the issue does not come up.

_____ 26. Collaborate with others to achieve our goals together.

_____ 27. Compete with others for scarce resources.

_____ 28. Emphasize compromise and trade-offs.

_____ 29. Cool things down by letting others do it their way.

_____ 30. Change the subject to avoid the fighting.

Conflict Self-Assessment Scoring Tool: Look at the numbers you placed in the blanks on the conflict assessment. Write the number you placed in each blank on the appropriate line below. Add up your total for each column and enter that total on the appropriate line. The greater your total is for each approach, the more often you tend to use that approach when conflict occurs at work. The lower the score is, the less often you tend to use that approach when conflict occurs at work.

Collaborating	Competing	Compromising	Accommodating	Avoiding
1. _____	2. _____	3. _____	4. _____	5. _____
6. _____	7. _____	8. _____	9. _____	10. _____
11. _____	12. _____	13. _____	14. _____	15. _____
16. _____	17. _____	18. _____	19. _____	20. _____
21. _____	22. _____	23. _____	24. _____	25. _____
26. _____	27. _____	28. _____	29. _____	30. _____
Total _____	Total _____	Total _____	Total _____	Total _____

Adapted from Hurst, J. B. (1993). *Conflict self-assessment.* University of Toledo; Dames, S. (2019). Understanding and resolving conflict. In P. Yoder-Wise, J. Waddell, & N. Walton (Eds.), *Yoder-Wise's leading and managing in Canadian nursing* (2nd ed., pp. 433-451). Elsevier.

Strengthening Practice

This second strengthening practice is designed to assess and reflect on the quality of decisions and relationships that inform the outcome of conflict resolution efforts.

B. A Framework to Assess Conflict Resolution
1. Quality of decisions
    a. How creative are planning efforts?
    b. How practical and realistic are the goals?
    c. Were intended goals achieved?
    d. What surprising results were achieved?
2. Quality of relationships
    a. How have efforts helped cultivate understanding?
    b. How have efforts impacted people's willingness to work together?
    c. How have mutual respect, unconditional positive regard, and cooperation been generated?

Adapted from Hurst, J., & Kinney, M. (1989). *Empowering self and others*. University of Toledo.

In a culture of unconditional positive regard, collaboration and compromise are the preferred conflict resolution methods because they both promote assertive and authentic expression. If we share a common vision, empowered and underscored by unconditional regard for all team members, differing opinions are an opportunity for creativity and growth rather than a cultural threat. When we lead with this orientation, we minimize the fear that tends to lead to competitive or avoidant behaviours. As a result, people are more likely to address conflict before it festers into personal offences.

Caregiving culture will be changed through systemic efforts that address old ways of being and use new tools and techniques to support a new shared vision. This will provide the momentum necessary to create lasting change. To illustrate the value investing in a shared vision, Ceravolo et al. (2012) carried out a study involving a health system in the United States that was well known for the lateral violence occurring among caregivers. The authors spent 3 years providing workshops to strengthen communication methods in the workplace, delivering the curriculum to over 4 000 nurses and over 1 000 nursing students. As a result, they had a 14% decrease in reports of lateral violence and a significant decrease in vacancy and turnover rates.

Forging new cultural habits where we as caregivers are addressing conflict in a respectful and productive fashion requires a shared vision and shared tools to reach that vision. For example, if the shared vision involves compassionate relationships, then co-workers will collectively and intentionally practise active listening and open dialogues that promote differing perspectives. As these tools actualize in the workplace, employees stay motivated to continue investing in the effort. In additional to shared tools, role modelling is equally important. Organizational leaders who model these behaviours have a significant impact on workplace culture; this is the crux of leadership.

Effective Mentors: It's Not About Perfection

Mentorship as a concept has been defined in a variety of ways. For our purposes, mentorship means a relationship between two people, where one person invests their resources (time, knowledge, energy) to help another grow and develop to be their best, most authentic self. Mentorship is actualized through coaching, role modelling, and collaboration (Henry-Noel et al., 2019).

On the felt sense level, effective mentors—those that inspire and support their mentee with unconditional positive regard—focus on progress, not perfection. They promote a feeling of safety. Mentors that are congruent will mirror unconditional positive regard, providing the empathy and safety required to encourage authentic (and thus vulnerable) ways of being. These mentorship qualities align with Rogers' (1959) work, where relationships of unconditional positive regard improve congruence between the "real" self and "ideal" self. This congruence then prevents feelings of shame, which is the typical feeling that emerges when we believe we have failed to meet the conditions set for us by others. Candice, Mary, and Sarah, three new graduate caregivers and research participants (Dames, 2018a), shared their reflections on their mentorship experiences:

Having an authority figure [as a mentor] who really sees who I am, accepts me, and encourages me, [really] encouraged my growth. (Candice)

If it weren't for [my work mentor], I wouldn't be where I am today. (Mary)

I found that just having a mentor or someone you can go to is helpful, even just to vent about … even just to ask questions that you might not be comfortable asking. (Sarah)

Mentors that offer unconditional positive regard, despite a mentee's obvious shortcomings, provide an emotionally safe space to make mistakes, ask questions, and resolve areas of dissonance that might otherwise go unaddressed. Besides encouraging authenticity, a mentor with social capital (a high degree of respect in the workplace) promotes a greater ability to take on the more vulnerable advocate roles that are required to challenge unhelpful social conditions (Dames, 2018b). Mentors that support authenticity promote self-efficacy and goal achievement (Zimmerman et al., 1992). Retention rates positively correlate with the assignment of a formal mentor for new caregivers, with benefits compounding the longer mentors are available (Salt et al., 2008; Scott et al., 2008). Furthermore, support systems that provide a nurturing space to be vulnerable enhance feelings of security and belonging (Brown, 2010; Rogers, 1959). Another factor that enables thriving is familiarity, acceptance, and feelings of belonging to the team, which requires relational and environmental consistency.

Educators as Cultural Seed Tenders

Teaching ... emerges from one's inwardness, for better or worse. As I teach, I project the condition of my soul onto my students, my subject, and our way of being together. The entanglements I experience in the classroom are often no more or less than the convolutions of my inner life. Viewed from this angle, teaching holds a mirror to the soul. If I am willing to look in that mirror and not run from what I see, I have a chance to gain self-knowledge—and knowing myself is as crucial to good teaching as knowing my students and my subject. (Palmer, 2007)

By empowering individual voices and affirming collective values, educators promote a greater ability for trainees to bloom wherever their careers plant them. In this context, educators include undergraduate faculty, workplace supervisors, and the experienced providers that mentor novices in their field of practice. These educators have an enormous influence on the conditions and conditioning that inform the growth of novice caregivers.

Educators are the seed tenders within health care culture. They can use their power either to sustain or to challenge the status quo.

We need a shift in our collective thinking in order to successfully change culture. Currently, particularly in the West, there is more pressure to assimilate than to show up authentically. To change our culture, we need an interruption that addresses and deconstructs the perfectionistic and rigid social conditions we find ourselves in. Perfectionism is often compounded in postsecondary settings, especially among those who lacked a felt sense of unconditional positive regard in their upbringings (causing greater incongruence). Research suggests that the stressors leading to burnout may begin during undergraduate education. Those who are experiencing feelings of burnout before entering the profession are at higher risk of leaving their position after only 10 to 15 months (Rudman & Gustavsson, 2012). The socialization of caregivers informs their ability to be congruent, to align their "real" values with professional "ideals." When the practice of being who one should be rather than who one really is becomes a well-established way of life, then these caregivers "can no longer rely on their emotions to provide them with an accurate sense of their real attitudes, values, and feelings about other people or events. They have learned how to con themselves, and no longer know who they really are" (Bergquist, 1993, pp. 72–73). Feeling ambiguous about ourselves, how we feel, and the values that drive us prevents us from resolving emotional tension. Conversely, in cultures that promote and celebrate diverse ways of being, thinking, and doing, it is likely that we as caregivers will express our personality traits and personal values in our professional roles.

O'Callaghan (2013) has described a hidden curriculum in health care culture that promotes emotional incongruence. When students incubate in an environment of intimidation and shame during their training, emotional incongruence is likely. They are then prone to using the same incongruent behaviours within the workplace and toward their clients. The implicit curriculum shapes student identity and informs what kind of person they will be as a professional caregiver. The implicit components that make up the hidden curriculum include program culture, customs, rituals, and how people relate to one another.

The highest form of love is the love that allows for intimacy without the annihilation of difference. (Palmer, 2007)

Palmer (1998), an important author in the field of education, described the need to develop the hearts of educators. By doing so, we can reach new members early on in their habit development, which is imperative for cultivating and sustaining flourishing cultures. A more heart-centred culture promotes congruence of the heart, mind, and emotions of teachers and learners. This focus on habits of the heart provides a pathway toward a healthy democracy. From this framework, the path forward is clearer, as it is led by a common vision to co-create a nourishing work culture. A shared vision among health care educators that is informed by the collective value of nourishing and tending to the newest members will promote deep roots (congruence and sense of coherence) so that caregivers can thrive in today's high-stimulus work environments:

We must understand that we are all in this together.
We must develop an appreciation of the value of otherness.
We must cultivate the ability to hold tension in life-giving ways.
We must generate a sense of personal voice and agency.
We must strengthen our capacity to create community. (Palmer, 1998, pp. 44–45)

Leading with heart and authenticity means enabling individuals to freely live their callings, which contributes to fulfillment of the collective vision. Authentic leaders and educators who mirror unconditional positive regard in their relationships create the safe and secure environment necessary to draw like-intentioned others toward their shared vision. This visioning process enables members to articulate shared values such as diversity and authenticity. These shared values act as the glue that holds healthy democracies together and buffers cultures from homogeniz-ing tendencies. Healthy democracies are sustained by members who can live with the tensions that emerge in organizations that encourage diversity, which implies that members have the capacity to manage their emotions and have an awareness and acceptance of the emotions of others (Taylor & Cranton, 2012). This recipro-cal respect of our own and others' emotions as they are (minimizing the surface act-ing) takes a degree of individual and collective cultural congruence. These cultural habits provide the rich soil for individuals to bloom where planted.

Because educators are in a position of authority, their actions and behaviours have powerful ripple effects. Therefore, they have an opportunity to model and perpetuate empathy and congruence, promoting environments where relationships of unconditional positive regard can flourish. Role modelling enables a mirror-ing effect (mirror transference), inspiring others to tune into the same frequency. Through a process of attunement, role modelling emotional congruence promotes reciprocal behaviours, which in turn promotes authentic displays of emotion and perpetuates nurturing and respectful behaviours between co-workers and clients.

For example, when we teach students about what it means to care for self, we must go beyond talk; it must be implicitly built into our ways of being as care-givers. In a recent qualitative study with novice caregivers (Dames, 2018a), study participant Mary found that the sheer amount of work in the program did not jive with self-care: "It didn't feel like you could succeed in the program and make time for self-care." Sarah, another study participant, found that she learned self-care through role modelling:

> My [clinical mentor] would say, "Are they sick? Can it wait? Yes, it can wait, go on your break!" I always thought more practice would be better in that way because you get to apply what you're learning, including self-care. The application is what really nails it in. (Dames, 2018a)

Role modelling is the most powerful form of teaching. It promotes learned behaviours that promote congruent or incongruent caregivers and caregiving work cultures. However, if educators do not feel congruent or are not working toward congruence themselves, then they cannot mentor students and novice providers to do the same.

Aligning and Strengthening Practices
Aligning Practice

A. Workplace Alignment
- Can you recall any components of the vision within the organizations you've worked for? What implicit ("real") values are reflected in your workplace culture?
- Are these values congruent with your calling and the values that sustain it?

- Are there workplace factors that encourage authentic ways of being, where you feel you can be vulnerable, creative, and playful (*being* vs. *doing*) at work?
- What components of your work life cause you to feel emotionally unsafe/unable to be your authentic self? If you can pinpoint specific times when feelings of threat arise, take note of them. What thought patterns do these uncomfortable feelings represent?

Feelings of threat are often less about what is actually happening in the moment and more about a previous unresolved event. When we did not feel safe enough to feel a difficult emotion in the past, it can lead to an assumption of threat in the thinking mind and a stuck energy in the body. This assumption and felt energy in the body emerges when a current-day event leads us to believe that we may be walking into the same challenge (with a similar lack of resources). But in reality, the current-day event may not be an actual threat. These unresolved events and resulting stuck energies are *somaticized* (psychological tensions expressed in the body) as trauma, which will continue to spring up until the energy can be discharged. Awareness of emotional energy, whether ours or others', helps us recognize when transference is happening. Transference happens when you feel the emotion of another person, or they feel an emotion of yours. How we address emotional energy arising within us is often different from navigating emotional energy that is flowing to us. Both emerge in our internal alert system, where our emotional messages cue us to pay attention, but how we resolve them can be quite different. For instance, if someone is experiencing an intense emotion and we are finding ourselves getting activated as a result, we can settle our bodies by creating a physical or at least energetic space, reminding ourselves of where they end and we begin. However, if the source of energy is arising within us, whether because of an actual or past threat, feeling and tending to the energy is necessary to discharge it.

- What events at work tend to activate strong emotions in you (whether those emotions originate in you or in another person)?
- How might emotional transference be a factor?
- How might these activations be related to your past experience of events that possibly remain unresolved?

Strengthening Practice

B. Circling Back to Move Forward
"Living a calling" is a way of *being* in which we stay connected to the present moment, aligned with our authentic self while creating and moving toward a larger vision. Although the means of getting there is important, having an endpoint in mind is necessary to maintain forward momentum. This is where visioning comes in. Before you begin, remember that the goal of practice is progress, not perfection. If you get stuck in discontentment, cultivate an attitude of gratitude by reflecting on how far you've come. Remember that practising creates habits; it is a process. In time, habits happen, but they take repetition. Eventually, habits become an intuitive response, enabling us to move from effort to ease. Investing in their development is well worth the effort if it moves us closer to our vision.

At first, reorienting can take great effort: effort to stay focused, effort to connect to our inner voice, effort to lean in to the gentle whispers that bubble up from inside. At first, we lack the trust necessary to invest in feeling the discomfort when it arises. To manage this discomfort, we can work with the nervous system, settling the felt sense of threat at the root of our discomfort. When we are calm and embodied once more, we keep moving. When the body says stop, we listen. By doing so, we gain trust in the process at the level of the body. While the thinking mind may want to forge ahead to the end, we must prioritize the felt sense, choosing to move at the pace of trust in the body.

Ultimately, we must feel safe enough to be willing to be vulnerable, to live with the questions the process creates, and to move at a pace that enables us to stay embodied. If we do not, then the thinking mind will splinter from the vessel of our spirit, and our healing will be delayed.

The Challenge: Navigation

By considering someone else's challenge, or working with another to consider ours, we cultivate nonattachment. We can often find comfort knowing we are not alone and that we can learn from and with each other. Coming from a more objective space, we can step back and reorient ourselves from a position of strength with access to all of our biological, intellectual, and spiritual capacities. With this benevolent orientation, we can face adversities with confidence, knowing we have the resources and support necessary to navigate life's challenges.

Let's return to Todd and Rachel's challenge to explore the source of their conflict and come up with a potential solution. In this situation, Todd's needs are to satisfy the basic physiological needs of his family and to feel a sense of approval (prescribed esteem) from the authority figure that enables him to meet the needs of his family. While he may want to assertively address the situation, which will address his secondary need, his primary need as the main provider for his family will continue to take precedence. He likely fears that using his voice to protect himself may threaten the security of those he feels responsible for. As a result, it is reasonable to assume that he will remain stuck until the primary threat dissipates.

In Rachel's view, when Todd went above her to their manager, it threatened her sense of safety in their relationship. She felt hurt that he didn't come to her first. Now, she doesn't feel safe around him, worrying that if she makes a mistake, he could do it again. Rather than addressing Todd directly, so that the emotional energy could be felt, communicated, and released, she avoided the situation and that energy became stuck in her body. As a result, the emotional energy transitioned to resentment, which is expressed on the surface as hostility.

As we can see, both Rachel and Todd feel threatened, which is causing them to react by fighting and fleeing, respectively. Neither party is inherently good or bad, right or wrong. When both parties are fused—for instance, when Rachel was accusing Todd of negligence—the WITS framework can help them navigate the challenge. If patient safety were not a consideration, then *walking away* may have worked for one or both parties. However, given the urgency of the situation, Todd could then *ignore* Rachel's comments, enabling him to attend to the patient and to his nervous system at the same time. The first two responses create a space, interrupting the routinized response. Once their nervous systems settle, they can *talk it out* with greater objectivity. Because their situation is more than just tension between two parties, they would be wise to seek help from an objective and congruent other. Doing so would enable a safe space for them to feel into, express, and eventually discharge the hostile energy moving between them.

LOOKING BACK TO MOVE FORWARD

Reflect on your progress on this journey, which started long before you picked up this book. Before you do, drop in and clear any outer distractions by moving into a low-stimulus space. Use some of the stress mitigation tools you've learned to tend to and clear any inner angst. Feel into your heart space. From this more spacious place, you will be more able to feel into your inherent worth, separate from conditions of worth.

- How have your personal and professional intentions (means of getting there) and goals (desired endpoint) changed?
- How about your awareness and felt sense of the mind–body–spirit connection?

Progress takes many forms, such as increased mindfulness, nonattachment, and awareness as well as new ways of relating to yourself. If you find yourself measuring your worth against constructed "ideals," come back to the grounding and clearing practices you've been using.

Reflect back on what congruence means to you, observing the thoughts and emotions that arise from looking for security in prescribed "ideals." Speak to these emotions as dear friends, letting them come and just as easily letting them go.

Consider when you felt the most connected to desire, when you felt the most alive. What quality of those moments called you in?

What practices felt rewarding? What helps to shift you from *do*ing to *be*ing? Which practices will you hold close as you journey on?

These moments reflect thriving. Notice what you notice. Like a trail of breadcrumbs, these clues are leading you back to the body and to the spiritual inspirations you feel there. Each breadcrumb is like a treasure on the path, providing the courage and desire to continue on, despite the challenges along the way. By continuing to do our significant things—those things that call us, regulate us, and empower us—we tap into the abundant treasure box of the inner self. This is you, thriving.

Anchor to your inner world (the felt sense of the body); lift your eyes to your North Star (calling); carve an intentional path that propels you toward a worthy cause (vision). This is you, thriving.

The Invitation by Oriah "Mountain Dreamer" House

It doesn't interest me what you do for a living.
I want to know what you ache for
and if you dare to dream of meeting your heart's longing.

It doesn't interest me how old you are.
I want to know if you will risk looking like a fool
for love
for your dream
for the adventure of being alive.

It doesn't interest me what planets are squaring your moon …
I want to know if you have touched the centre of your own sorrow
if you have been opened by life's betrayals
or have become shriveled and closed
from fear of further pain.

I want to know if you can sit with pain
mine or your own
without moving to hide it
or fade it
or fix it.

I want to know if you can be with joy
mine or your own
if you can dance with wildness
and let the ecstasy fill you to the tips of your fingers and toes
without cautioning us
to be careful
to be realistic
to remember the limitations of being human.

It doesn't interest me if the story you are telling me
is true.
I want to know if you can

disappoint another
to be true to yourself.
If you can bear the accusation of betrayal
and not betray your own soul.
If you can be faithless
and therefore trustworthy.

I want to know if you can see Beauty
even when it is not pretty
every day.
And if you can source your own life
from its presence.

I want to know if you can live with failure
yours and mine
and still stand at the edge of the lake
and shout to the silver of the full moon,
"Yes."

It doesn't interest me
to know where you live or how much money you have.
I want to know if you can get up
after the night of grief and despair
weary and bruised to the bone
and do what needs to be done
to feed the children.

It doesn't interest me who you know
or how you came to be here.
I want to know if you will stand
in the centre of the fire
with me
and not shrink back.

It doesn't interest me where or what or with whom
you have studied.
I want to know what sustains you
from the inside
when all else falls away.

I want to know if you can be alone
with yourself

and if you truly like the company you keep
in the empty moments.
Source: Oriah "Mountain Dreamer" House. From The Invitation. © 1999.
HarperONE. All rights reserved. Presented with permission of the author.
www.oriah.org.

Putting It All Together

This book has presented several tools designed to nurture our root systems, encouraging them to grow deep so that we can feel secure when external stressors, or "weather" systems, blow in. These feelings of safety enable us to cultivate meaning, desire, and confidence. We are developing strong root systems, learning how to thrive and navigate challenges so they do not activate our nervous systems. We are shifting our attention away from the churning mind, to the felt sense—to *knowingness*. We are becoming harmonious within the mind–body–spirit ecosystem. We are moving from *dis*-ease. We are nurturing congruence with self-compassion—I will never be perfect at *do*ing, yet I am already whole. We are navigating the "weather" with grounding and clearing practices. We are supporting our sense of coherence through mindfulness. We are tilling the soils of our childhoods, reparenting as we go. We are reorienting to trauma from a place of resilience and self-awareness. The unresolved "weather" of our past is dissipating. We are reframing the stories that have kept us small. We are no longer helpless—we are becoming anchored, held. We are learning to live our calling. We are learning to trust our connected roots systems, leading within communities that are connected and empowered. We are becoming a tribe with shared vision and intention, in an energetic field of unconditional positive regard.

Final Words

None of us can do this alone. The journey requires a felt sense of unconditional positive regard, and we cannot generate this frequency on our own. We receive it from those who received it before us. My greatest hope is that you can attune to this grounding and empowering frequency, and that you will mirror it for others so that they can do the same. This is how we heal as individuals, as caregivers, as organizations, as communities, as cultures—we do it together.

Individually and collectively, we are *be*ing called in. Called into the life we were born to live. Come to know your inner world. What it feels. What it desires. What it fears. Whom it feels safe with. How it is soothed. How it wants to be loved. What calls it out of the shadows each day.

Resource broadly! Find the rituals that bring you back to *be*ing, those that anchor you securely to your essence. From this embodied place, may your *do*ing be inspired with meaning and empowered by connection to all that is. When you do, you will find all the courage you need to accept the invitation, to do the *significant* thing that propels you into your calling. To this end, may you forge deeper roots.

Resourcing With Deep Roots

Sense of Coherence (Orientation to World)	Congruence (Orientation to Self)
Increasing nonattachment/objectivity through mindfulness	Cultivating healthy relationships, a sense of belonging, and connection to community, land, and culture
Feeling confident navigating challenges before they become overwhelming	Deepening unconditional positive regard inwardly (self-compassion) and outwardly
Allowing gratitude and optimism to reorient our perspective	Using tools and practices to ground, regulate, release, soothe, introspect
Balancing order and chaos; cultivating acceptance and inspiration	Cultivating our sense of wholeness, life purpose, values, beauty, spirituality
Creatively fulfilling our life's calling in response to the needs of the world	Working with our body and physiology; regulating the stress response
Drawing on internal (e.g., intuition) and external (e.g., visual) senses to make meaning	Asking, "Who am I?"
	Becoming our authentic self, pursuing our calling

Sense of coherence centres on our orientation to life: our sense of meaning, comprehension, predictability, confidence, and self-efficacy. Growing confidence and awareness of our resources through mindfulness promotes sense of coherence.

Congruence centres on our orientation to self. It is the aligning of our "real" (actual) self and "ideal" (potential) self. Deepening relationships of unconditional positive regard and self-compassion promote congruence.

When combined, congruence and sense of coherence enable us to thrive. *Thriving roots* are deeply rooted in personal authenticity and in connection with the world. From this grounded place, we can mindfully live with purpose, joy, courage, and compassion.

How Practices Promote Sense of Coherence and Congruence Development

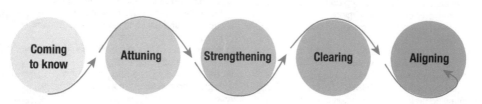

The objectives of this book are realized through a process by which we **come to know** the heart of our identities by:

- **Attuning** to personal and collective resources. This includes dropping into our bodies and inner worlds, attuning to our authentic selves (e.g., values, calling, spirituality) and inner and outer sense capacities (e.g., intuition, insight, physical senses). As we attune, we can distinguish the imprints of social conditioning and habitual, survival/stress behaviours. This also includes attuning to healthy relationship support: the wisdom, compassion, witnessing, and mirroring of unconditional positive regard.
- **Strengthening** our relationship with self and others and our confidence in our resourcing capacities. We do this by cultivating mindfulness; understanding "the weather" of our workplace environments and trauma, stress, and the process of recovery. We engage in practices to help us stay embodied, to regulate our nervous systems, and to connect inwardly and outwardly.
- **Clearing** by working with unresolved events (trauma) from the past, and letting go of the coping strategies that no longer serve us through self-compassion, insight, shadow work, and the release of shame.
- **Aligning** our personal and professional identities with our "real" selves and living a meaningful calling that aligns with our values, talents, and desires.

Objectives Within the Journey

Objective	Theory/Concept	Examples of Practices
Strengthen your sense of coherence and congruence	• Coming to know **congruence and sense of coherence; pendulating** between inner and outer awareness (orientation to self and world)	• Basic mindfulness • Mindful walking (pendulating) • Reorientation through gratitude and strategic optimism
Strengthen self-compassion and have a greater understanding of the meaning and value of relationships of unconditional positive regard with others	• Defining self-compassion and unconditional positive regard • The **weather** of health care/social culture and context • **Real** and **ideal selves** aligning (including social programming, racism, "shadow"/disowned parts) • **Moral injury** • **Shame**	• Loving-kindness exercises • Forgiveness • Clearing exercises • Authentic expression
Learn to attune to your inner world in order to strengthen and align with your inner resources	• **Spirituality** as **authenticity**, values, meaning-making, wholeness, interconnectedness • **Loving-kindness**	• Notice what you notice • Immersing in felt sense • Mindfulness • Loving-kindness exercises
Come to know and strengthen stress management tools and strategies to better handle current stressors and facilitate the healing of past adversities	• **Stress** regarding perception and meaning-making of stimulus; physiological process • **Trauma** • Working with fight–flight–freeze–fawn • **Vicarious trauma** and **projection** • Working with **emotions** • **Cultivating choice;** improving your ability to *act* vs. *react* in moments of stress	• Reflect on your resources • Breathing exercises • RAIN • Emotional freedom technique (EFT) • Listening to music • Connecting to nature • Group work: practising debriefing, establishing safety (group norms), emotional expression, awareness of self and others
Attune and align with a calling statement, providing you with guidance on your journey	• **Calling** as "North Star"; creative and authentic response to the needs of the world • **Enjoy (living in joy)**	• Exploring desires, preferences, and tendencies • Working with holistic frameworks to identify one's vision and calling • Being witnessed as you embody and voice your authentic self

Glossary

Acupuncture: Acupuncture involves the insertion of fine needles into various parts of the body. The needles are then stimulated using the hands or electrical impulses.

Agency: The degree to which a person feels empowered to act congruently, according to their genuine values, beliefs, and preferences.

Aromatherapy: Aromatherapy involves the smelling of extracts made from natural sources to calm the limbic system, promoting relaxation and reducing stress.

Attachment: Attachment reflects how securely rooted we are in our "real" selves (congruence) and how confident we are navigating life's challenges (sense of coherence).

Attachment tendencies: Adult relational attachment tendencies range from an addictive/anxious orientation to an avoidant orientation, depending on one's view of self and others. When our adult relational style is anxiously attached, we long to have a less secure part of the self filled by another. When our relational style is avoidant attachment, vulnerability from or with others doesn't feel safe, which causes us to emotionally flee or freeze when another person seeks greater intimacy. Secure attachment occurs when two people heartfully connect from a place of wholeness, not needing something from, nor avoiding vulnerability with, the other person.

Authentic: Relating to congruence, we are most authentic when our "*doing*" in the world comes from an inspired state of "*being*." In this state, we lack self-consciousness. How we manifest in the external world is a natural expression of the values, desires, and emotions that emerge from our inner world.

Binaural beats: An auditory tool that uses two different beat/tone frequencies in each ear. As a result, it can alter brainwaves, enabling people to enter specific brain wave states. Binaural beats can be used to improve cognitive flexibility and focus, reduce anxiety, and promote the ability to enter relaxed/meditative states.

Brain chunking: Brain chunking represents our subconscious tendency to organize stimuli or information into patterns that represent a meaningful whole. Reactions and tendencies emerge from the brain organizing, or chunking, data into belief systems. Brain chunking enables us to act quickly from these belief systems and assumptions, often before conscious thought can occur.

Burnout: Burnout results from workplace stress that has not been successfully managed. It consists of three components: (1) emotional exhaustion, (2) depersonalization (detachment from the "real" self), and (3) reduced professional efficiency and diminished sense of accomplishment (Maslach & Jackson, 1986; World Health Organization, 2019).

Child-centred upbringing: A child-centred upbringing happens when the care of a child centres on their unique qualities and developmental needs, promoting the child's confidence and autonomy in the process. Unconditional positive regard enables the child to self-actualize according to their natural preferences and talents, as opposed to those prescribed by parents or the culture at large. This is not to be confused with permissive parenting. Because boundaries and clear expectations that promote respect and responsibility are required for children to flourish, they are essential components of a child-centred upbringing.

Cognitive behavioural therapy (CBT): A therapeutic approach that brings awareness to the relationship between thoughts (conscious, automatic, underlying core beliefs) and behaviours. This technique aims to change behaviour through self-monitoring, scheduling, and exposure–response prevention.

Community of practice: A community of practice describes a group of people who share an intention for something they do together and learn how to integrate into their daily lives, learning to do it better as they interact regularly (Wenger-Trayner & Wenger-Trayner, 2015). In the context of this book, a community of practice describes a group of people with a shared intention to cultivate a space of unconditional positive regard, aiming to minimize stress and other barriers to thriving and to maximize one's ability to flourish individually and in community. As a group, they facilitate the ability to operate from this place in their day-to-day lives through relationships and practices that expand awareness and promote self-regulation/stress mitigation, heartful connectedness, and an ability to live one's calling.

Complex post-traumatic stress disorder (PTSD): Complex PTSD differs from PTSD in that the former stems from feeling unable to escape ongoing traumatic events such as chronic abuse and negligence (National Health Service, 2018). Symptoms are similar to those of PTSD but can also include feelings of shame or guilt, difficulty controlling emotions, dissociation, isolation, relationship difficulties, risky behaviour, self-harm, and suicidal thoughts.

Congruence (Rogers, 1959): Congruence represents our orientation to self. It is the aligning of our "real" (actual) self and "ideal" (potential) self. Deepening self-compassion is key to the development of congruence.

Dialectical behavioural therapy (DBT): A modified version of CBT that combines emotional regulation, reality testing, mindfulness, acceptance, and stress tolerance.

Dissociation: When we feel threatened or stressed, the nervous system subconsciously mounts a defensive response (fight–flight–freeze–fawn). Dissociation is a form of "freeze" response. It occurs when we react by detaching from our felt sense, including our emotions. When we are dissociated, our ability to creatively think and resource is limited.

Dissociation versus nonattachment: Dissociation is a subconscious reaction to fear. Nonattachment occurs when we step back from emotions to work with them objectively. Dissociation occurs subconsciously and leads to impulsive and involuntary reactions. Nonattachment is conscious, enabling mindful action, which cultivates the ability to choose. Mindful action enables emotions to come and go, without our feeling attached to or threatened by them.

Distress: Distress occurs when our experience of stress extends beyond the threatening event or exceeds our capacity to cope.

Embodiment: To embody healing, we must express or manifest the healing in a tangible way, at the level of the felt sense. For example, this may occur through emotional expression or a change in one's way of being and behaviours.

Emotional intelligence: Emotional intelligence describes our degree of awareness of and ability to control our emotions. When we are emotionally intelligent, we are more apt to express our emotions and navigate others' emotions with discernment and compassion.

Emotional freedom technique (EFT): A technique that involves tapping various energy points on the body while repeating a mantra that correlates with a desired emotional state. During the process, one addresses a current stressor or brings up a stressful memory from the past (at the root of the stressor) with compassionate awareness while tapping on acupressure points.

Emotional labour (Hochschild, 2012): Emotional labour is the practice of emoting states of being that are incongruent with our genuine feelings.

Emotional transference: The subconscious redirection of feelings from one person to another. It also occurs when present-day stimuli remind us of an unhealed wound from the past, causing us to project the felt threat of unmet needs from the past onto the present moment.

Empathy: The ability to put oneself in another's shoes, especially in times of suffering. We cultivate empathy by imagining what another person is feeling or by imagining that we can feel what another person is feeling, taking on the feeling as if it were our own.

Essence: Our intrinsic nature. The part of us that remains constant from birth to death. Our "real" self, separate from our behaviours and cultural conditioning.

Eye movement desensitization and reprocessing (EMDR): EMDR involves a variety of techniques that direct a person's eyes back and forth while they reimagine an activating event.

Fight–flight–freeze–fawn: The fight–flight–freeze–fawn responses are known as stress responses. These physiological responses evolved millions of years ago to enable humans to sense and respond to threats or danger. They are controlled by the brain's autonomic nervous system and are part of the limbic system.

Forest bathing: Forest bathing, the English translation for the Japanese practice of "shinrin-yoku" (森林浴), involves spending contemplative time immersed in nature, at a leisurely pace, paying special attention to the sensory experience.

Also called "forest therapy," forest bathing is effective for reducing anxiety, depression, and anger while increasing vigour and boosting the immune system, with benefits lasting even after the immersion experience is over.

Freeze: A primitive stress response that occurs when the parasympathetic nervous system remains activated, causing a form of cognitive immobility.

Homogenization: The process of making things uniform. Homogenization and perfectionism are cyclical and mutually reinforcing. Extreme forms of perfectionism incubate in homogenizing cultures where we learn to view the world through a black and white lens with little tolerance for shades of grey. Similarly, cultural homogenization is fuelled by perfectionistic individuals who have learned to prescribe their unrealistically high expectations ("ideals") onto others.

Horizontal violence: Hostile and often harmful behaviour toward a co-worker.

Incongruence: Incongruence, which emerged from a concept developed by Carl Rogers (1959), describes the shame that results when there is a discrepancy between one's real self and one's ideal self. The greater the discrepancy, the greater the shame one feels.

Liminality: Liminality represents the threshold between what is known and the mystery of what is yet to come. It is in this space that most of our significant embodied transformations emerge. Staying embodied in this space is essential in order to shift from one way of being to another. To do so, we must navigate, not shut down, the felt chaos that arises in the "in between."

Meditation: Sustained mindfulness, or mindfully tending to our *being* state for sustained periods of time. While the term mindfulness suggests that meditation is a form of thinking, it is in fact the opposite. *Awareness* is a more accurate term for this state of consciousness than *mindfulness*, as it is not limited to the thinking mind. We can observe the thinking mind, the same way we can observe our emotions, sense perceptions, and intuition, energetically sensing and noticing things both internally and externally.

Mindfulness: The process of stepping back from passing thoughts and emotions to cultivate nonattachment. From this place, we can investigate stimuli objectively, which prevents them from feeling stressful or threatening.

Mirroring transference (Kohut, 1984): Mirroring transference occurs when we fulfill a function for a person that they cannot yet perform themselves. By doing this, the other person can attune to the felt sense and, as result, direct this same felt sense inwardly to themselves and outwardly to others.

Moral injury: Moral injury occurs when a person acts in a way that is incongruent with their personal values and beliefs. When unresolved, moral injury fuels shame.

Negativity bias: A negativity bias means that negative events have a greater emotional impact on us than positive ones, with the effect of negative events lingering longer than that of positive ones. People with a negativity bias are more likely to pick up on fear and sadness than on pleasant emotions.

Neuroception: Our subconscious ability to sense potential threats. The inner radar that aims to protect us and keep us safe (Flores & Porges, 2017).

Neurofeedback: The use of devices such as electroencephalogram (EEG) headbands to provide instant feedback on the electrical activity of the brain. The theory behind using neurofeedback, similar to biofeedback, is that by connecting our brain states to specific activities and feeling states, we are more likely to enter our desired states quickly and confidently.

Noise: In this book, "noise" refers to that which distracts us from the "signal" of our *be*ing. This can be in our environment, whether tangible stimuli or energetic transference from others. This can also be experienced within as the angst created by a threatened nervous system.

Nonattachment: The ability to step back from emotions in order to work with them objectively. From this space, we can observe stimuli without attaching or identifying with them, then ground and tap into the inner resources necessary to navigate challenges.

Optimism: The inclination to view intentions, events, behaviours, and outcomes in a positive frame. Common optimistic metaphors include the ability to see the "silver lining" or to view things through "rose-coloured glasses." To optimistically reframe one's orientation to a difficult scenario requires looking for the positive aspects within the situation so that it can be viewed from a more positive vantage point.

Perfectionism: The endless pursuit of flawlessness, whereby anything short of perfect is not good enough. This mindset often promotes an unrealistic and critical view of oneself and others.

Polyvagal theory (Porges, 2009): Polyvagal theory describes how the autonomic nervous system interacts with the face–heart connection, facilitating a social engagement system, which then enables social interactions to regulate visceral states.

Post-traumatic stress disorder (PTSD): A condition whereby one re-experiences the threat of a past event in the here and now, causing nervous system activation and emotional avoidance. As a result, individuals tend to be hypervigilant and easily threatened. Diagnosis criteria include symptoms that reflect re-experiencing, avoidance, reactivity, and cognitive and mood impacts (National Institute of Mental Health, 2019b).

Priming: A technique that aims to replicate feelings of secure attachment either subliminally or explicitly. Developing and promoting secure attachment cues through priming has been shown to reduce avoidant and anxious tendencies.

Projection: Emotional projections are a subconscious and defensive coping mechanism that occurs as a result of unresolved adversities (past wounds). When someone feels emotions that are too difficult to own and deal with, they are prone to subconsciously blaming others for these undesirable feelings.

Rational detachment: A form of nonattachment characterized by the ability to not take the behaviours of others personally. We can recognize that behaviours in others are generally projections of their past experiences. From this vantage point, we can keep things in perspective without getting stuck in our own assumptions and fears. Because other people's behaviours aren't personal, they also don't need to threaten our nervous systems. When we are grounded in this nonattached position, we can shift our focus from what is wrong to what can be done.

Reflexology: A noninvasive technique whereby practitioners apply pressure to points on the feet and hands that correlate to internal organs and other parts of the body.

Reparenting: The process of directing unconditional positive regard inwardly, from a well-resourced and relatively nonattached place, in order to work *with* the wounded self rather than *as* the wounded self.

Reiki: A form of therapy that shows promise as a strategy to promote relaxation and reduce stress. Practitioners gently lay their hands some distance above or directly on the body and use various hand movements to work with the body's energy.

Resilience: Resilience means embodying a way of being that views challenges optimistically, as opportunities to attune, strengthen, clear, and align. Resilience promotes an ability to adapt in the face of adversity, emerging from a benevolent orientation and a felt confidence that we have the resources and support system necessary to navigate challenges as they arise.

Self-compassion (Neff, 2016): Self-compassion is compassion turned inward. It describes how we treat ourselves when we are suffering or experiencing moments of perceived inadequacy. It consists of three components: (1) self-kindness over judgement, (2) common humanity over isolation, and (3) mindfulness versus overidentification.

Self-efficacy: Self-efficacy is the confidence and belief in our ability to achieve our goals.

Self-integrity: A quality that develops when one acts congruently, which means living according to one's authentic values, beliefs, and preferences. Self-integrity stems from self-compassion. Conversely, perfectionism stems from fear. Integrity happens when our *do*ing flows from our *be*ing rather than the reverse. In this way, when we act congruently, we have self-integrity.

Sense of coherence (Antonovsky, 1979): Sense of coherence represents our orientation to life: our sense of meaning, comprehension, predictability, confidence, and self-efficacy. Mindfulness practice is key to developing our sense of coherence.

Shame: The painful feelings that occur when we become conscious of behaviours that are incongruent with our core beliefs and values.

Signal: In this book, "signal" is that which arises from our unconditioned essence. This can come forward as a *significant* action that we are called to do or as an emotion we are called to tend to. It is the inner prompt born from desire and compassion.

Significant action/thing: The inspired *do*ing that is called from our *be*ing state. This thing is often the *significant* thing—that thing that will empower us, unstick us, move us from being a victim to a victor. How do we know what the significant thing is? As we become more accustomed to how the "signal" of desire and inner knowing resonates in the body, it becomes more obvious. Every moment is different. The significant thing in one moment may be different from that in the next. However, if we do not do the significant thing, it often calls to us until we do.

Social capital: The ability of individuals to influence those around them. Those that have more social capital set the etiquette and display rules in the groups or social units they are a part of.

Somaticized: The process of psychological tensions being expressed in the felt sense of the body.

Stigma: A complex construct that can come from a variety of sources, including oneself. It occurs when certain circumstances or qualities of people are labelled with a mark of disgrace. While it starts as a social phenomenon, it can quickly become self-ascribed.

Stimuli: The events, the interactions that move and change around us, and the resulting thoughts and feelings about the events that then arise within us. Stimuli in and of themselves don't cause stress; it is the interpretation of the stimuli—the related thoughts and feelings—that provoke the stress response.

Stress: Stress can be defined in two ways: as the stressor (external source of "bad weather") or as the experience of distress. In this book, we distinguish the *source* of stress from the *experience* of stress. A combination of extrinsic and intrinsic factors activates the perception of threat. Extrinsic factors are things that happen outside our inner workings (the "weather"), and intrinsic factors come from within (congruence and sense of coherence, or the "roots"). We have little control over extrinsic factors, but those with well-developed intrinsic factors are less likely to feel intimidated and threatened by unpredictable and often challenging "weather" patterns. When extrinsic factors do feel threatening, those with strong roots will have more confidence to resolve the threat before it becomes a chronic stressor.

Trauma: An unmet need or unhealed wound from the past. If we cannot integrate past adversities by allowing related emotions to be expressed and for meaning-making to occur, the emotion becomes trapped. As a result, when an event subconsciously reminds us of this unresolved past adversity, we unconsciously project the trapped emotional energy onto the present moment. The experience of trauma presents an opportunity to recognize an unhealed wound from the past so that when we feel ready (i.e., adequately resourced), we can tend to the unmet need.

Two-Eyed Seeing: The ability "to see from one eye with the strengths of Indigenous ways of knowing, and to see from the other eye with the strengths of Western ways of knowing, and to use both of these eyes together" (Bartlett et al., 2012, p. 335).

Unconditional positive regard: The act of accepting ourselves and one another for who we are. Positive regard is not withdrawn if another person makes a mistake or if they show up in an irritating way. It's not about liking each other or accepting all behaviours. It's about respecting one another as human beings with free will and operating under the assumption that we are all doing the best we can with the tools we have. In environments of unconditional positive regard, we feel that we are accepted as we are, quirks and wounds alike; we have the ability to see our and others' inherent human worth, separate from behaviours and achievements; and we have the ability to assertively and kindly set boundaries that honour our needs and desires, which also prevents hostility or resentment. In this space, people feel freer to try things out, despite the vulnerability felt and the risk of missteps.

Vicarious trauma: Vicarious trauma occurs when the traumatic experience of another person negatively impacts a care provider's identity and beliefs. When unresolved, the experience of vicarious trauma can lead to cynicism and despair (McCann & Pearlman, 1990; Pearlman & Saakvitne, 1995).

Victim–perpetrator cycle: The victim–perpetrator cycle describes what happens when someone (the perpetrator) who feels oppressed, and hence experiences a loss of their sense of personal power, subconsciously attempts to take back their power by exerting dominance over another (the victim). The victim–perpetrator cycle describes the vacillation between these two roles.

References

Adamson, J., & Clark, H. A. (1999). *Scenes of shame: Psychoanalysis, shame, and writing*. State University of New York Press.

Ahmad, R., Naqvi, A. A., Al-Bukhaytan, H. M., et al. (2019). Evaluation of aromatherapy with lavender oil on academic stress: A randomized placebo controlled clinical trial. *Contemporary Clinical Trials Communications, 14*,100346. https://doi.org/10.1016/j.conctc.2019.100346.

Ainsworth, M. D. (1964). Patterns of attachment behavior shown by the infant in interaction with his mother. *Merrill–Palmer Quarterly of Behavior and Development, 10*(1), 51–58.

Alcoholics Anonymous. (2001). *Alcoholics anonymous* (4th ed.). A.A. World Services.

Aldao, A., Nolen-Hoeksema, S., & Schweizer, S. (2010). Emotion regulation strategies across psychopathology: A meta-analysis. *Clinical Psychology Review, 30*, 217–237. https://doi.org/10.1016/j.cpr.2009.11.004.

Allan, B. A., Duffy, R. D., & Douglass, R. (2015). Meaning in life and work: A developmental perspective. *The Journal of Positive Psychology, 10*(4), 323–331. https://doi.org/10.1080/17439760.2014.950180.

Amato, P. R., & Kane, J. B. (2011). Life-course pathways and the psychosocial adjustment of young adult women. *Journal of Marriage and Family, 73*(1), 279–295. https://doi.org/10.1111/j.1741-3737.2010.00804.x.

American Association of Colleges of Nurses. (2020). *Fact sheet: Nursing shortage*. https://www.aacnnursing.org/Portals/42/News/Factsheets/Nursing-Shortage-Factsheet.pdf.

American Psychiatric Association. (1980). *Diagnostic and statistical manual of mental disorders* (3rd ed.). Author.

Anand, H. (2014). Effect of meditation ("OM" chanting) on alpha EEG and galvanic skin response: Measurement of an altered state of consciousness. *Indian Journal of Positive Psychology, 5*(3), 255.

Andersen, S., & Berg, J. E. (2001). The use of a sense of coherence test to predict drop-out and mortality after residential treatment of substance abuse. *Addiction Research & Theory, 9*(3), 239–251. https://doi.org/10.3109/16066350109141752.

Antonovsky, A. (1979). *Health, stress and coping*. Jossey-Bass.

Antonovsky, A. (1987). *Unraveling the mystery of health: How people manage stress and stay well*. Jossey-Bass.

Aspy, D. J., & Proeve, M. (2017). Mindfulness and loving-kindness meditation. *Psychological Reports, 120*(1), 102–117. https://doi.org/10.1177/0033294116685867.

Avey, J. B., Luthans, F., Smith, R. M., et al. (2010). Impact of positive psychological capital on employee's well-being over time. *Journal of Occupational Health Psychology, 15*(1), 17–28. https://doi.org/10.1037/a0016998.

Bakker, A., Killmer, C., Siegrist, J., et al. (2000). Effort–reward imbalance and burnout among nurses. *Journal of Advanced Nursing, 31*(4), 884–891. https://doi.org/10.1046/j.1365-2648.2000.01361.x.

Baldwin, C., Linnea, A., & Wheatley, M. J. (2010). *The circle way: A leader in every chair*. Berrett-Koehler Publishers.

Bandura, A. (1997). *Self-efficacy: The exercise of control*. Freeman.

Barnett, L. A. (2007). The nature of playfulness in young adults. *Personality and Individual Differences, 43*, 949–958. https://doi.org/10.1016/j.paid.2007.02.018.

Barsky, A. (2016). *Conflict resolution for the helping profession: Negotiation, mediation, advocacy, facilitation, and restorative justice* (3rd ed.). Oxford University Press.

Bartels, J. B. (2014). The pause. *Critical Care Nurse, 34*(1), 74–75. https://doi.org/10.4037/ccn2014962.

Bartlett, C., Marshall, M., & Marshall, A. (2012). Two-Eyed Seeing and other lessons learned within a co-learning journey of bringing together indigenous and mainstream knowledges and ways of knowing. *Journal of Environmental Studies and Sciences, 2*, 331–340.

Bartlett, M. Y., & DeSteno, D. (2006). Gratitude and prosocial behavior. *Psychology Science, 17*(4), 319–325. https://doi.org/10.1111/j.1467-9280.2006.01705.x.

Basso, J. C., & Suzuki, W. A. (2017). The effects of acute exercise on mood, cognition, neurophysiology, and neurochemical pathways: A review. *Brain Plasticity, 2*(2), 127–152. https://doi.org/10.3233/BPL-160040.

Baum, A., Cohen, L., & Hall, M. (1993). Control and intrusive memories as possible determinants of chronic stress. *Psychosomatic Medicine, 55*(3), 274–286. https://doi.org/10.1097/00006842-199305000-00005.

Baumeister, R. F., & Leary, M. R. (1995). The need to belong: Desire for interpersonal attachments as a fundamental human motivation. *Psychological Bulletin, 117*(3), 497–529. https://doi.org/10.1037/0033-2909.117.3.497.

B.C. Ministry of Health. (2014). *Setting priorities for the B.C. Health System.* https://www.health.gov.bc.ca/library/publications/year/2014/Setting-priorities-BC-Health-Feb14.pdf.

Beck, A. T. (1970). Cognitive therapy: Nature and relation to behavior therapy. *Behavior Therapy, 1*(2), 184–200.

Beecroft, P. C., Dorey, F., & Wenten, M. (2008). Turnover intention in new graduate nurses: A multivariate analyses. *Journal of Advanced Nursing, 61*(1), 41–52. https://doi.org/10.1111/j.1365-2648.2007.04570.x.

Beecroft, P. C., Kunzman, L., & Krozek, C. (2001). RN internship: Outcomes of a one-year pilot program. *Journal of Nursing Administration, 31*(12), 575–576. https://doi.org/10.1097/00005110-200112000-00008.

Belgers, M., Leenaars, M., Homberg, J. R., et al. (2016). Ibogaine and addiction in the animal model, a systematic review and meta-analysis. *Translational Psychiatry, 6*(5), e826. https://doi.org/10.1038/tp.2016.71.

Benard, B. (2004). *Resiliency: What we have learned.* WestEd.

Benner, P., Sutphen, M., Leonard, V., et al. (2010). *Educating nurses: A call for radical transformation.* Jossey-Bass.

Berceli, D., Salmon, M., Bonifas, R., et al. (2014). Effects of self-induced unclassified therapeutic tremors on quality of life among non-professional caregivers: A pilot study. *Global Advances in Health and Medicine, 3*(5), 45–48. https://doi.org/10.7453/gahmj.2014.032.

Bergh, H., Baigi, A., Fridlund, B., et al. (2006). Life events, social support and sense of coherence among frequent attenders in primary health care. *Public Health, 120*(3), 229–236. https://doi.org/10.1016/j.puhe.2005.08.020.

Bergquist, W. (1993). *The postmodern organization: Mastering the art of invisible change.* Jossey-Bass.

Berkovich-Ohana, A., Glicksohn, J., & Goldstein, A. (2012). Mindfulness-induced changes in gamma band activity—Implications for the default mode network, self-reference and attention. *Clinical Neurophysiology, 123*(4), 700–710. https://doi.org/10.1016/j.clinph.2011.07.048.

Besen, E., Matz-Costa, C., Brown, M., et al. (2013). Job characteristics, core self-evaluations, and job satisfaction: What's age got to do with it? *The International Journal of Aging and Human Development, 76*(4), 269–295. https://doi.org/10.2190/AG.76.4.a.

Beyer, K. M. M., Kaltenbach, A., Szabo, A., et al. (2014). Exposure to neighbourhood green space and mental health: Evidence from the survey of the health of Wisconsin. *International Journal of Environmental Research and Public Health, 11*, 3453–3472. https://doi.org/10.3390/ijerph110303453.

Bianchi, R., Schonfeld, I. S., & Laurent, E. (2015). Is burnout separable from depression in cluster analysis? A longitudinal study. *Social Psychiatry and Psychiatric Epidemiology, 50*(6), 1005–1011. https://doi.org/10.1007/s00127-014-0996-8.

Binswanger, H. (1991). Volition as cognitive self-regulation. *Organizational Behavior and Human Decision Processes, 50*, 154–178. https://doi.org/10.1016/0749-5978(91)90019-P.

Bisson, J. I., Ehlers, A., Matthews, R., et al. (2007). Psychological treatments for chronic post-traumatic stress disorder: Systematic review and meta-analysis. *The British Journal of Psychiatry, 190*(2), 97–104. https://doi.org/10.1192/bjp.bp.106.021402.

Blatchford, C. (2019). *Rolling with the waves.* Lorian Press.

Blatz, W. E. (1967). *Human security: Some reflections.* University of Toronto Press.

Bluth, K., Campo, R. A., Futch, W. S., & Gaylord, S. A. (2017). Age and gender differences in the associations of self-compassion and emotional well-being in a large adolescent sample. *Journal of Youth and Adolescence, 46*(4), 840–853. https://doi.org/10.1007/s10964-016-0567-2.

Bly, R. (1989). *A little book on the human shadow.* Harper & Row.

BMG Research. (2013). *NHS Wales staff survey 2013—National overview.* Author.

Boamah, S. A., & Laschinger, H. (2016). The influence of areas of worklife fit and worklife interference on burnout and turnover intentions among new graduate nurses. *Journal of Nursing Management, 24*(2), E164–E174. https://doi.org/10.1111/jonm.12318.

Bodenheimer, T., & Sinsky, C. (2014). From triple to quadruple aim: Care of the patient requires care of the provider. *Annals of Family Medicine, 12*(6), 573–576. https://doi.org/10.1370/afm.1713.

Bond, M. E. (2009). Exposing shame and its effect on clinical nursing education. *The Journal of Nursing Education, 48*(3), 132–140. https://doi.org/10.3928/01484834-20090301-02.

Bowden, D., Goddard, L., & Gruzelier, J. (2010). A randomised controlled single-blind trial of the effects of reiki and positive imagery on well-being and salivary cortisol. *Brain Research Bulletin, 81*(1), 66–72. https://doi.org/10.1016/j.brainresbull.2009.10.002.

Bowlby, J. (2012). *A secure base.* Taylor & Francis.

Brach, T. (2013). *The RAIN of self-compassion.* https://www.tarabrach.com/selfcompassion1/.

Brach, T. (2016, February 6). *How to meditate FAQ: A definitive guide for a gratifying practice!* https://www.tarabrach.com/faq-for-meditation-2/.

Brady, M. J., Peterman, A. H., Fitchett, G., et al. (1999). A case for including spirituality in qual-ity of life measurement in oncology. *Psycho-Oncology*, *8*(5), 417–428. https://doi.org/10.1002/(SICI)1099-1611(199909/10)8:5%3C417::AID-PON398%3E3.0.CO;2-4.

Breslau, N., Chilcoat, H. D., Kessler, R. C., et al. (1999). Previous exposure to trauma and PTSD effects of subse-quent trauma: Results from the Detroit area survey of trauma. *American Journal of Psychiatry*, *156*(6), 902–907. https://doi.org/10.1176/ajp.156.6.902.

Bretherton, I., & Munholland, K. A. (1999). Internal working models in attachment relationships: A construct revisited. In J. Cassidy & P. R. Shaver (Eds.), *Handbook of attachment: Theory, research, and clinical applications* (pp. 89–111). The Guilford Press.

British Columbia Nurses' Union. (2019). *BCNU applauds government decision to include nurses in mental injury presumption legislation*. https://www.bcnu.org/news-and-events/news/2019/bcnu-applauds-government-deci-sion-to-include-nurses-in-mental-injury-presumption-legislation.

Brotheridge, C. M., & Grandey, A. A. (2002). Emotional labor and burnout: Comparing two perspectives of 'people work'. *Journal of Vocational Behavior*, *60*(1), 17–39. https://doi.org/10.1006/jvbe.2001.1815.

Brown, B. (2006). Shame resilience theory: A grounded theory study on women and shame. *Families in Society*, *87*(1), 43–52. https://doi.org/10.1606/1044-3894.3483.

Brown, B. (2010). *The gifts of imperfection: Let go of who you think you're supposed to be and embrace who you are*. Hazelden Publishing.

Bruskas, D., & Tessin, D. H. (2013). Adverse childhood experiences and psychosocial well-being of women who were in foster care as children. *The Permanente Journal*, *17*(3), e131–e141. https://doi.org/10.7812/TPP/12-121.

Bryant, R. A., & Foord, R. (2016). Activating attachments reduces memories of traumatic images. *PLoS One*, *11*(9), e0162550. https://doi.org/10.1371/journal.pone.0162550.

Bryant, R. A., & Hutanamon, T. (2018). Activating attachments enhances heart rate variability. *PLoS One*, *13*(2), e0151747. https://doi.org/10.1371/journal.pone.0151747.

Buffone, A. E. K., Poulin, M., DeLury, S., et al. (2017). Don't walk in her shoes! Different forms of perspective tak-ing affect stress physiology. *Journal of Experimental Social Psychology*, *72*, 161–168. https://doi.org/10.1016/j.jesp.2017.04.001.

Campbell, D. G., Felker, B. L., Liu, C. F., et al. (2007). Prevalence of depression–PTSD comorbidity: Implica-tions for clinical practice guidelines and primary care-based interventions. *Journal of General Internal Medicine*, *22*(6), 711–718. https://doi.org/10.1007/s11606-006-0101-4.

Canadian Institute for Health Information. (2015). *Registered nurses: Backgrounder*. https://www.cihi.ca/en/nurs-es_2014_background_en.pdf.

Canadian Institute for Health Information. (2018). *Nursing in Canada, 2018: A lens on supply and workforce*. https://www.cihi.ca/sites/default/files/document/regulated-nurses-2018-report-en-web.pdf.

Canadian Mental Health Association. (2020). *Fast facts about mental health and mental illness*. https://cmha.ca/fast-facts-about-mental-illness.

Cardador, M. T., Dane, E., & Pratt, M. G. (2011). Linking calling orientations to organizational attachment via organizational instrumentality. *Journal of Vocational Behavior*, *79*(2), 367–378. https://doi.org/10.1016/j.jvb.2011.03.009.

Carnelley, K. B., Bejinaru, M., Otway, L., et al. (2018). Effects of repeated attachment security priming in outpa-tients with primary depressive disorders. *Journal of Affective Disorders*, *234*, 201–206. https://doi.org/10.1016/j.jad.2018.02.040.

Carter-Scott, C. (1998). *If life is a game, these are the rules*. Dell Publishing Group.

Carvalho, F., Weires, K., Ebling, M., et al. (2013). Effects of acupuncture on the symptoms of anxiety and de-pression caused by premenstrual dysphoric disorder. *Acupuncture in Medicine*, *31*(4), 358–363. https://doi.org/10.1136/acupmed-2013-010394.

Castle, S., Wilkins, S., Heck, E., et al. (1995). Depression in caregivers of demented patients is associated with altered immunity: Impaired proliferative capacity, increased CD8, and a decline in lymphocytes with surface signal transduction molecules (CD38+) and a cytotoxicity marker (CD56+, CD8+). *Clinical and Experimental Immunology*, *101*(3), 487–493. https://doi.org/10.1111/j.1365-2249.1995.tb03139.x.

Cavanagh, J. F., Eisenberg, I., Guitart-Masip, M., et al. (2013). Frontal theta overrides Pavlovian learning biases. *Journal of Neuroscience*, *33*(19), 8541–8548. https://doi.org/10.1523/Jneurosci.5754-12.2013.

Cebolla, A., Campos, D., Galiana, L., et al. (2017). Exploring relations among mindfulness facets and various meditation practices: Do they work in different ways? *Consciousness and Cognition*, *49*, 172–180. https://doi.org/10.1016/j.concog.2017.01.012.

Center for Addiction and Mental Health. (2017). *Moral injury.* https://www.camh.ca/en/camh-news-and-stories/moral-injury.

Center for Addiction and Mental Health. (2019). *The crisis is real.* https://www.camh.ca/en/driving-change/the-crisis-is-real.

Centers for Disease Control and Prevention. (2014). About the study. https://web.archive.org/web/20151221202610/http://www.cdc.gov/violenceprevention/acestudy/about.html.

Ceravolo, D. J., Schwartz, D. G., Foltz-Ramos, K. M., et al. (2012). Strengthening communication to overcome lateral violence. *Journal of Nursing Management, 20*(5), 599–606. https://doi.org/10.1111/j.1365-2834.2012.01402.x.

Chachula, K. M., Myrick, F., & Yonge, O. (2015). Letting go: How newly graduated registered nurses in Western Canada decide to exit the nursing profession. *Nurse Education Today, 35*(7), 912–918. https://doi.org/10.1016/j.nedt.2015.02.024.

Chaieb, L., Wilpert, E. C., Hoppe, C., et al. (2017). The impact of monaural beat stimulation on anxiety and cognition. *Frontiers in Human Neuroscience, 11*, 251. https://doi.org/10.3389/fnhum.2017.00251.

Chandler, G. E. (2012). Succeeding in the first year of practice: Heed the wisdom of novice nurses. *Journal for Nurses in Staff Development, 28*(3), 103–107. https://doi.org/10.1097/NND.0b013e31825514ee.

Chang, Y. (2012). The relationship between maladaptive perfectionism with burnout: Testing mediating effect of emotion-focused coping. *Personality and Individual Differences, 53*(5), 635–639. https://doi.org/10.1016/j.paid.2012.05.002.

Chao, S., & Chen, P. (2013). The reliability and validity of the Chinese version of the nonattachment scale: Reliability, validity, and its relationship with mental health. *Bulletin of Educational Psychology, 45*(1), 121–139.

Chekroud, S. R., Gueorguieva, R., Zheutlin, A. B., et al. (2018). Association between physical exercise and mental health in 1.2 million individuals in the USA between 2011 and 2015: A cross-sectional study. *Lancet Psychiatry, 5*(9), 739–746. https://doi.org/10.1016/S2215-0366(18)30227-x.

Chen, P., Chou, C., Yang, L., et al. (2017). Effects of aromatherapy massage on pregnant women's stress and immune function: A longitudinal, prospective, randomized controlled trial. *The Journal of Alternative and Complementary Medicine, 23*(10), 778–786. https://doi.org/10.1089/acm.2016.0426.

Chikovani, G., Babuadze, L., Iashvili, N., et al. (2015). Empathy costs: Negative emotional bias in high empathisers. *Psychiatry Research, 229*(1), 340–346. https://doi.org/10.1016/j.psychres.2015.07.001.

Chinn, P. L. (2018). Peace. In *Peace and power: A handbook of transformative group process* (pp. 3–5). https://peaceandpowerblog.files.wordpress.com/2017/11/2018-handbook.pdf.

Chiu, M., Lebenbaum, M., Cheng, J., et al. (2017). The direct healthcare costs associated with psychological distress and major depression: A population-based cohort study in Ontario, Canada. *PLoS One, 12*(9), e0184268. https://doi.org/10.1371/journal.pone.0184268.

Cho, J., Laschinger, H. K. S., & Wong, C. (2006). Workplace empowerment, work engagement and organizational commitment of new graduate nurses. *Canadian Journal Nursing Leadership, 19*(3), 43–60. https://doi.org/10.12927/cjnl.2006.18368.

Chopra, D. (2004). *The seven spiritual laws of success.* Amber-Allen Publishing/New World.

Chozen Bays, J. (2009). *Mindful eating: A guide to rediscovering a healthy and joyful relationship with food.* Shambhala.

Church, D., Hawk, C., Brooks, A. J., et al. (2013). Psychological trauma symptom improvement in veterans using emotional freedom techniques: A randomized controlled trial. *The Journal of Nervous and Mental Disease, 201*(2), 153–160. https://doi.org/10.1097/NMD.0b013e31827f6351.

Cilliers, F., & Coetzee, F. C. (2003). The theoretical–empirical fit between three psychological wellness constructs: Sense of coherence, learned resourcefulness and self-actualization. *South African Journal of Labor Relations, 27*(1), 4–24. https://www.researchgate.net/publication/280482583_The_theoreticalempirical_fit_between_three_psychological_wellness_constructs_sense_of_coherence_learned_resourcefulness_and_self-actualisation.

Clark, L. A., & Watson, D. (1999). Temperament: A new paradigm for trait psychology. In L. A. Pervin & O. P. John (Eds.), *Handbook of personality: Theory and research* (2nd ed., pp. 399–423). The Guilford Press.

Clark, P. K., Leddy, K., Drain, M., et al. (2007). State nursing shortages and patient satisfaction: More RNs—Better patient experiences. *Journal of Nursing Care Quality, 22*(2), 128–129. https://doi.org/10.1097/01.NCQ.0000263101.29181.aa.

Clond, M. (2016). Emotional freedom techniques for anxiety: A systematic review with meta-analysis. *The Journal of Nervous and Mental Disease, 204*(5), 388–395. https://doi.org/10.1097/NMD.0000000000000483.

Colier, N. (2018). *Choosing love over fear: Responding from love not reacting from fear.* http://nancycolier.com/choosing-love-fear-responding-love-not-reacting-fear/

Cooke, M., Holzhauser, K., Jones, M., et al. (2007). The effect of aromatherapy massage with music on the stress and anxiety levels of emergency nurses: Comparison between summer and winter. *Journal of Clinical Nursing, 16*(9), 1695–1703. https://doi.org/10.1111/j.1365-2702.2007.01709.x.

Corey, S. M., Epel, E., Schembri, M., et al. (2014). Effect of restorative yoga vs. stretching on diurnal cortisol dynamics and psychosocial outcomes in individuals with the metabolic syndrome: The PRYSMS randomized controlled trial. *Psychoneuroendocrinology, 49*, 260–271. https://doi.org/10.1016/j.psyneuen.2014.07.012.

Corey, T. P., Shoup-Knox, M. L., Gordis, E. B., et al. (2012). Changes in physiology before, during, and after yawning. *Frontiers in Evolutionary Neuroscience, 3*, 7. https://doi.org/10.3389/fnevo.2011.00007.

Corroon, J., James, M., Mischley, L. K., et al. (2017). Cannabis as a substitute for prescription drugs—A cross-sectional study. *Journal of Pain Research, 10*, 989–998. https://doi.org/10.2147/JPR.S134330.

Costa, D. K., & Moss, M. (2018). The cost of caring: Emotion, burnout, and psychological distress in critical care clinicians. *Annals of the American Thoracic Society, 15*(7), 787–790. https://doi.org/10.1513/AnnalsATS.201804-269PS.

Cowin, L. S., & Hengstberger-Sims, C. (2006). New graduate nurse self-concept and retention: A longitudinal survey. *International Journal of Nursing Studies, 43*(1), 59–70. https://doi.org/10.1016/j.ijnurstu.2005.03.004.

Cruceanu, V. D., & Rotarescu, V. S. (2013). Alpha brainwave entrainment as cognitive performance activator. *Cognition, Brain, Behavior, 17*(3), 249–261. https://www.researchgate.net/publication/289030858_Alpha_brainwave_entrainment_as_a_cognitive_performance_activator.

Curran, T., & Hill, A. P. (2019). Perfectionism is increasing over time: A meta-analysis of birth cohort differences from 1989 to 2016. *Psychological Bulletin, 145*(4), 410–429. https://doi.org/10.1037/bul0000138.

Currie, E. J., & Carr Hill, R. A. (2012). What are the reasons for high turnover in nursing? A discussion of presumed causal factors and remedies. *International Journal of Nursing Studies, 49*(9), 1180–1189. https://doi.org/10.1016/j.ijnurstu.2012.01.001.

Curtis, R., Zeh, D., Miller, M., et al. (2004). Examining the validity of a computerized chakra measuring instrument: A pilot. *Subtle Energies & Energy Medicine, 15*(3), 209–223. http://journals.sfu.ca/seemj/index.php/seemj/article/viewFile/387/349.

Dahl, C. J., Lutz, A., & Davidson, R. J. (2015). Reconstructing and deconstructing the self: Cognitive mechanisms in meditation practice. *Trends in Cognitive Sciences, 19*(9), 515–523. https://doi.org/10.1016/j.tics.2015.07.001.

Dames, S. (2018a). *A study of the interplay between new graduate life experience, context, and the experience of stress in the workplace: Exploring factors towards self-actualizing as a novice nurse.* University of Calgary. [Unpublished doctoral thesis].

Dames, S. (2018b). THRIVEable work environments: A study of interplaying factors that enable novice nurses to thrive. *The Journal of Nursing Management, 26*(6), 567–574. https://doi.org/10.1111/jonm.12712.

Dames, S. (2019). Understanding and resolving conflict. In P. Yoder-Wise, J. Waddell, & N. Walton (Eds.), *Yoder-Wise's leading and managing in Canadian nursing* (2nd ed., Chap. 24). Elsevier Inc.

Dames, S. (2020, July 15). Suffering to bliss: Transforming trauma to grit. *Roots to Thrive.* https://rootstothrive.com/2020/07/15/suffering-to-bliss-transforming-trauma-to-grit/.

Dames, S., & Hunter, K. (2020, August 30). Turning to the trees. *Roots to Thrive.* https://rootstothrive.com/2020/08/30/turning-to-the-trees/.

Dames, S., & Javorski, S. (2018). Sense of coherence, a worthy factor toward nursing student and new graduate satisfaction with nursing, goal setting affinities, and coping tendencies. *Quality Advancement in Nursing Education, 4*(1). https://doi.org/10.17483/2368-6669.1108.

Deary, I., Watson, R., & Hogston, R. (2003). A longitudinal cohort study of burnout and attrition in nursing students. *Journal of Advanced Nursing, 43*(1), 71–81. https://doi.org/10.1046/j.1365-2648.2003.02674.x.

Delli Pizzi, S., Padulo, C., Brancucci, A., et al. (2016). GABA content within the ventromedial prefrontal cortex is related to trait anxiety. *Social Cognitive and Affective Neuroscience, 11*(5), 758–766. https://doi.org/10.1093/scan/nsv155.

Demers, L., & Roper, M. (2018). *A pause for grounding and connection.* Vancouver Island Health Authority. [Unpublished manuscript].

Dev, V., Fernando, A. T., Lim, A. G., et al. (2018). Does self-compassion mitigate the relationship between burnout and barriers to compassion? A cross-sectional quantitative study of 799 nurses. *International Journal of Nursing Studies, 81*, 81–88. https://doi.org/10.1016/j.ijnurstu.2018.02.003.

Dickerson, S. S., Gruenewald, T. L., & Kemeny, M. E. (2009). Psychobiological responses to social self-threat: Functional or detrimental? *Self and Identity, 8*(2), 270–285. https://doi.org/10.1080/15298860802505186.

Dickerson, S. S., Kemeny, M. E., Aziz, N., et al. (2004). Immunological effects of induced shame and guilt. *Psychosomatic Medicine, 66*(1), 124–131. https://doi.org/10.1097/01.PSY.0000097338.75454.29.

Dispenza, J. (2012). *Breaking the habit of being yourself: How to lose your mind and create a new one.* Hay House Publishing.

Dixon-Woods, M., Baker, R., Charles, K., et al. (2013). Culture and behavior in the English National Health Service: Overview of lessons from a large multimethod study. *British Medical Journal Quality and Safety, 23*, 106–115. https://doi.org/10.1136/bmjqs-2013-001947.

Drake, D., Ocampo, E., Donaldson, J., et al. (2017). The effect of aromatherapy on anxiety experienced by hospital nurses. *MedSurg Nursing, 26*(3), 201.

Drapkin, J., McClintock, C., Lau, E., et al. (2016). Spiritual development through the chakra progression. *Open Theology, 2*(1), 605–620. https://doi.org/10.1515/opth-2016-0048.

Dückers, M. L., Alisic, E., & Brewin, C. R. (2016). A vulnerability paradox in the cross-national prevalence of post-traumatic stress disorder. *The British Journal of Psychiatry, 209*(4), 300–305. https://doi.org/10.1192/bjp.bp.115.176628.

Duffy, R. D., Allan, B. A., Autin, K. L., et al. (2013). Calling and life satisfaction: It's not about having it, it's about living it. *Journal of Counseling Psychology, 60*(1), 42. https://doi.org/10.1037/a0030635.

Dunn, C., Haubenreiser, M., Johnson, M., et al. (2018). Mindfulness approaches and weight loss, weight maintenance, and weight regain. *Current Obesity Reports, 7*(1), 37–49. https://doi.org/10.1007/s13679-018-0299-6.

Dyrbye, L. N., Shanafelt, T. D., Johnson, P. O., et al. (2019). A cross-sectional study exploring the relationship between burnout, absenteeism, and job performance among American nurses. *BMC Nursing, 18*(1), 57. https://doi.org/10.1186/s12912-019-0382-7.

Dzurec, L. C., Kennison, M., & Gillen, P. (2017). The incongruity of workplace bullying victimization and inclusive excellence. *Nursing Outlook, 65*(5), 588–596. https://doi.org/10.1016/j.outlook.2017.01.012.

Eda, N., Ito, H., Shimizu, K., et al. (2018). Yoga stretching for improving salivary immune function and mental stress in middle-aged and older adults. *Journal of Women & Aging, 30*(3), 227–241. https://doi.org/10.1080/08952841.2017.1295689.

Electris, A. C. (2013). *Vicarious trauma: A relationship between emotional empathy and emotional overidentification in mid-career trauma clinicians* (Publication No. 3536157) [Doctoral dissertation, Long Island University]. ProQuest Dissertations & Theses Global.

Ellis, A. (1962). *Reason and emotion in psychotherapy.* Lyle Stuart.

Ellis, A. (2002). The role of irrational beliefs in perfectionism. In G. L. Flett & P. L. Hewitt (Eds.), *Perfectionism: Theory, research, and treatment* (pp. 217–229). American Psychological Association. https://doi.org/10.1037/10458-000.

Embong, N. H., Soh, Y. C., Ming, L. C., et al. (2015). Revisiting reflexology: Concept, evidence, current practice, and practitioner training. *Journal of Traditional and Complementary Medicine, 5*(4), 197–206. https://doi.org/10.1016/j.jtcme.2015.08.008.

Emet, J. (2012). Calming the mind: A meditation exercise. In *Buddha's book of sleep* (pp. 98–104). https://www.gaiam.com/blogs/discover/calming-the-mind-a-meditation-exercise.

Emmons, R. A., & Stern, R. (2013). Gratitude as a psychotherapeutic intervention. *Journal of Clinical Psychology, 69*(8), 846–855. https://doi.org/10.1002/jclp.22020.

Encyclopaedia Britannica. (2020, May 6). Spiritualism. In *Britannica.com encyclopedia.* https://www.britannica.com/topic/spiritualism-philosophy.

Erickson, R., & Grove, W. (2007). Why emotions matter: Age, agitation, and burnout among registered nurses. *Online Journal of Issues in Nursing, 13*(1). https://doi.org/10.3912/OJIN.Vol13No01PPT01.

Eriksson, M., & Lindström, B. (2005). Validity of Antonovsky's sense of coherence scale: A systematic review. *Journal of Epidemiology and Community Health, 59*(6), 460–466. https://doi.org/10.1136/jech.2003.018085.

Eriksson, M., & Lindström, B. (2006). Antonovsky's sense of coherence scale and the relation with health: A systematic review. *Journal of Epidemiology and Community Health, 60*(5), 376–381. https://doi.org/10.1136/jech.2005.041616.

Eriksson, M., & Lindström, B. (2007). Antonovsky's sense of coherence scale and its relation to quality of life: A systematic review. *Journal of Epidemiology and Community Health, 61*(11), 938–944. https://doi.org/10.1136/jech.2006.056028.

Erim, Y., Tagay, S., Beckmann, M., et al. (2010). Depression and protective factors of mental health in people with hepatitis C: A questionnaire survey. *International Journal of Nursing, 47*(3), 342–349. https://doi.org/10.1016/j.ijnurstu.2009.08.002.

Erol, R. Y., & Orth, U. (2011). Self-esteem development from age 14 to 30 years: A longitudinal study. *Journal of Personality and Social Psychology, 101*(3), 607–619. https://doi.org/10.1037/a0024299.

Eshkevari, L., Permaul, E., & Mulroney, S. E. (2013). Acupuncture blocks cold stress-induced increases in the hypothalamus–pituitary–adrenal axis in the rat. *Journal of Endocrinology, 217*(1), 95–104. https://doi.org/10.1530/JOE-12-0404.

Feigenbaum, K. D., & Smith, R. A. (2019). Historical narratives: Abraham Maslow and Blackfoot interpretations. *The Humanistic Psychologist, 48*(3), 232–243. https://doi.org/10.1037/hum0000145.

Feldt, T., Kokko, K., Kinnunen, U., et al. (2005). The role of family background, school success, and career orientation in the development of sense of coherence. *European Psychologist, 10*(4), 298–308. https://doi.org/10.1027/1016-9040.10.4.298.

Fergusson, D. M., & Horwood, L. J. (2003). Resilience to childhood adversity: Results of a 21-year study. In S. S. Luthar (Ed.), *Resilience and vulnerability: Adaptation in the context of childhood adversities* (pp. 130–155). Cambridge University Press.

Finegood, E., Rarick, J., & Blair, C. (2017). Exploring longitudinal associations between neighborhood disadvantage and cortisol levels in early childhood. *Development and Psychopathology, 29*(5), 1649–1662. https://doi.org/10.1017/S0954579417001304.

Fischer, R., Colzato, L. S., Hommel, B., et al. (2016). High-frequency binaural beats increase cognitive flexibility: Evidence from dual-task crosstalk. *Frontiers in Psychology, 7,* 1287. https://doi.org/10.3389/fpsyg.2016.01287.

Fitts, P. M., & Posner, M. I. (1967). *Human performance.* Brooks/Cole Publishing.

Flett, G. L., Madorsky, D., Hewitt, P. L., et al. (2002). Perfectionism cognitions, rumination, and psychological distress. *Journal of Rational-Emotive and Cognitive-Behavior Therapy, 20*(1), 33–47. https://doi.org/10.1023/A:1015128904007.

Flores, P. J., & Porges, S. W. (2017). Group psychotherapy as a neural exercise: Bridging polyvagal theory and attachment theory. *International Journal of Group Psychotherapy, 26,* 1–21. https://doi.org/10.1080/00207284.2016.1263544.

Flory, J. D., & Yehuda, R. (2015). Comorbidity between post-traumatic stress disorder and major depressive disorder: Alternative explanations and treatment considerations. *Dialogues in Clinical Neuroscience, 17*(2), 141. https://doi.org/10.31887/dcns.2015.17.2/jflory.

Fossion, P., Leys, C., Kempenaers, C., et al. (2014). Psychological and socio-demographic data contributing to the resilience of Holocaust survivors. *The Journal of Psychology: Interdisciplinary and Applied, 148*(6), 641–657. https://doi.org/10.1080/00223980.2013.819793.

Fournier, J. C., DeRubeis, R. J., Hollon, S. D., et al. (2010). Antidepressant drug effects and depression severity: A patient-level meta-analysis. *The Journal of the American Medical Association, 303*(1), 47–53. https://doi.org/10.1001/jama.2009.1943.

Frecska, E., Bokor, P., & Winkelman, M. (2016). The therapeutic potentials of ayahuasca: Possible effects against various diseases of civilization. *Frontiers in Pharmacology, 7,* 35. https://doi.org/10.3389/fphar.2016.00035.

Freud, A. (1937). *The ego and the mechanisms of defence.* Hogarth Press and Institute of Psycho-Analysis.

Freud, S. (1926). *Inhibitions, symptoms, and anxiety. The Psychoanalytic Quarterly, 5*(1), 1–28. https://doi.org/10.1080/21674086.1936.11925270.

Friese, M., Schweizer, L., Arnoux, A., et al. (2014). Personal prayer counteracts self-control depletion. *Consciousness and Cognition, 29,* 90–95. https://doi.org/10.1016/j.concog.2014.08.016.

Frost, R. O., Marten, P., Lahart, C., et al. (1990). The dimensions of perfectionism. *Cognitive Therapy and Research, 14,* 449–468. https://doi.org/10.1007/BF01172967.

Fujimaru, C., Okamura, H., Kawasaki, M., et al. (2012). Self-perceived work-related stress and its relation to salivary IgA, cortisol and 3-methoxy-4-hydroxyphenyl glycol levels among neonatal intensive care nurses. *Stress and Health, 28*(2), 171–174. https://doi.org/10.1002/smi.1414.

Gallace, A., Torta, D. M. E., Moseley, G. L., et al. (2011). The analgesic effect of crossing the arms. *Pain, 152*(6), 1418–1423. https://doi.org/10.1016/j.pain.2011.02.029.

Garcia, H., & Miralles, F. (2017). *Ikigai: The Japanese secret to a long and happy life.* Penguin Books.

Gardner, B., Lally, P., & Wardle, J. (2012). Making health habitual: The psychology of "habit formation" and general practice. *The British Journal of General Practice, 62*(605), 664–666. https://doi.org/10.3399/bjgp12X659466.

Garrosa, E., Moreno-Jiménez, B., Rodríguez-Muñoz, A., et al. (2011). Role stress and personal resources in nursing: A cross-sectional study of burnout and engagement. *International Journal of Nursing Studies, 48*(4), 479–489. https://doi.org/10.1016/j.ijnurstu.2010.08.004.

Gates, D. M., Gillespie, G. L., & Succop, P. (2011). Violence against nurses and its impact on stress and productivity. *Nursing Economics, 29*(2), 59–67.

Geuens, N., Braspenning, M., Van Bogaert, P., et al. (2015). Individual vulnerability to burnout in nurses: The role of type D personality within different nursing specialty areas. *Burnout Research, 2*(2–3), 80–86. https://doi.org/10.1016/j.burn.2015.05.003.

Gillespie, B. M., Chaboyer, W., & Wallis, M. (2007). Development of a theoretically derived model of resilience through concept analysis. *Contemporary Nurse, 25*(1–2), 124–135. https://doi.org/10.5172/conu.2007.25.1-2.124.

Goetz, J. L., Keltner, D., & Simon-Thomas, E. (2010). Compassion: An evolutionary analysis and empirical review. *Psychological Bulletin, 136*(3), 351–374. https://doi.org/10.1037/a0018807.

Goleman, D. (1996). *Emotional intelligence: Why it can matter more than IQ.* Bantam Books.

Gollan, J. K., Hoxha, D., Hunnicutt-Ferguson, K., et al. (2016). Twice the negativity bias and half the positivity offset: Evaluative responses to emotional information in depression. *Journal of Behavior Therapy and Experimental Psychiatry, 52,* 166170. https://doi.org/10.1016/j.jbtep.2015.09.005.

Gong, Y., Han, T., Yin, X., et al. (2014). Prevalence of depressive symptoms and work-related risk factors among nurses in public hospitals in southern China: A cross-sectional study. *Scientific Reports*, *4*, 7109. https://doi.org/10.1038/srep07109.

Gould, D., Tuffey, S., Udry, E., et al. (1996). Burnout in competitive junior tennis players: I. A quantitative psychological assessment. *Sport Psychologist*, *10*, 322–340.

Gouveia, M. J., Carona, C., Canavarro, M. C., et al. (2016). Self-compassion and dispositional mindfulness are associated with parenting styles and parenting stress: The mediating role of mindful parenting. *Mindfulness*, *7*(3), 700–712. https://doi.org/10.1007/s12671-016-0507-y.

Grady, D. (2020). *Where is the medicine?* [Conference presentation]. Psychedelic Psychotherapy Forum, Vancouver Island Conference Centre, Nanaimo, BC, Canada.

Gray, B. (2009). The emotional labor of nursing—Defining and managing emotions in nursing work. *Nurse Education Today*, *29*(2), 168–175. https://doi.org/10.1016/j.nedt.2008.08.003.

Green, B. (2013). Post-traumatic stress disorder: New directions in pharmacotherapy. *Advances in Psychiatric Treatment*, *19*(3), 181–190. https://doi.org/10.1192/apt.bp.111.010041.

Green, B. L., Goodman, L. A., Krupnick, J. L., et al. (2000). Outcomes of single versus multiple trauma exposure in a screening sample. *Journal of Traumatic Stress*, *13*(2), 271–286. https://doi.org/10.1023/A:1007758711939.

Grevenstein, D., Aguilar-Raab, C., & Bluemke, M. (2018). Mindful and resilient? Incremental validity of sense of coherence over mindfulness and Big Five personality factors for quality of life outcomes. *Journal of Happiness Studies*, *19*(7), 1883–1902. https://doi.org/10.1007/s10902-017-9901-y.

Griffin, M. (2004). Teaching cognitive rehearsal as a shield for lateral violence: An intervention for newly licensed nurses. *Journal of Continuing Education in Nursing*, *35*(6), 257. https://doi.org/10.3928/0022-0124-20041101-07.

Griffiths, R. R., Johnson, M. W., Carducci, M. A., et al. (2016). Psilocybin produces substantial and sustained decreases in depression and anxiety in patients with life-threatening cancer: A randomized double-blind trial. *Journal of Psychopharmacology*, *30*(12), 1181–1197. https://doi.org/10.1177/0269881116675513.

Gruzelier, J. (2014). EEG-neurofeedback for optimising performance. I: A review of cognitive and affective outcome in healthy participants. *Neuroscience and Biobehavioral Reviews*, *44*, 124–141. https://doi.org/10.1016/j.neubiorev.2013.09.015.

Gunnell, K. E., Mosewich, A. D., McEwen, C. E., et al. (2017). Don't be so hard on yourself! Changes in self-compassion during the first year of university are associated with changes in well-being. *Personality and Individual Differences*, *107*(2017), 43–48. https://doi.org/10.1016/j.paid.2016.11.032.

Hakanen, J. J., & Bakker, A. B. (2016). Born and bred to burn out: A life-course view and reflections on job burnout. *Journal of Occupational Health Psychology*, *22*(3), 354–364. https://doi.org/10.1037/ocp0000053.

Hall, L. (2019). *Chakra healing guided meditation*. https://www.the-guided-meditation-site.com/.

Hammarlund, R. A., Crapanzano, K. A., Luce, L., et al. (2018). Review of the effects of self-stigma and perceived social stigma on the treatment-seeking decisions of individuals with drug- and alcohol-use disorders. *Substance Abuse and Rehabilitation*, *9*, 115–136. https://doi.org/10.2147/sar.s183256.

Harari, D., Swider, B. W., Steed, L. B., et al. (2018). Is perfect good? A meta-analysis of perfectionism in the workplace. *The Journal of Applied Psychology*, *103*(10), 1121–1144. https://doi.org/10.1037/apl0000324.

Harmon-Jones, E., & Peterson, C. K. (2009). Supine body position reduces neural response to anger evocation. *Psychological Science*, *20*(10), 1209–1210. https://doi.org/10.1111/j.1467-9280.2009.02416.x.

Harne, B. P., & Hiwale, A. S. (2018). EEG spectral analysis on OM mantra meditation: A pilot study. *Applied Psychophysiology and Biofeedback*, *43*(2), 123–129. https://doi.org/10.1007/s10484-018-9391-7.

Hassmén, P., Koivula, N., & Uutela, A. (2000). Physical exercise and psychological well-being: A population study in Finland. *Preventive Medicine*, *30*(1), 17–25. https://doi.org/10.1006/pmed.1999.0597.

Heavy Head, R. (2018, March 28). *Naamitapiikoan Blackfoot influences on Abraham Maslow* [Video]. https://www.youtube.com/watch?v=WTO34FLv5a8.

Helali, A. (2016). *The effects of daily self-reiki practice on nurses' level of burnout*. (Publication No. 10259455) [Doctoral dissertation, University of Phoenix]. ProQuest Dissertations & Theses Global.

Helliwell, J., Layard, R., & Sachs, J. (2017). *World happiness report 2017*. Sustainable Development Solutions Network.

Henry-Noel, N., Bishop, M., Gwede, C. K., et al. (2019). Mentorship in medicine and other health professions. *Journal of Cancer Education*, *34*, 629–637.https://doi.org/10.1007/s13187-018-1360-6

Hess, U., Kafetsios, K., Mauersberger, H., et al. (2016). Signal and noise in the perception of facial emotion expressions: From labs to life. *Personality and Social Psychology Bulletin*, *42*(8), 1092–1110. https://doi.org/10.1177/0146167216651851.

Hewitt, P. L., & Flett, G. L. (1993). Dimensions of perfectionism, daily stress, and depression: A test of the specific vulnerability hypothesis. *Journal of Abnormal Psychology*, *102*, 58–65. https://doi.org/10.1037/0021-843X.102.1.58.

Heyman, M., Dill, J., & Douglas, R. (2018). *Ruderman white paper on mental health and suicide of first responders*. Ruderman Family Foundation. https://dir.nv.gov/uploadedFiles/dirnvgov/content/WCS/TrainingDocs/First%20Responder%20White%20Paper_Final%20(2).pdf.

Higgins, E. T., Klein, R., & Strauman, T. (1985). Self-concept discrepancy theory: A psychological model for distinguishing among different aspects of depression and anxiety. *Social Cognition, 3*, 51–76. https://doi.org/10.1521/soco.1985.3.1.51.

Hochschild, A. R. (2012). *The managed heart: Commercialization of human feeling*. University of California Press.

Hoge, C. W., Grossman, S. H., Auchterlonie, J. L., et al. (2014). PTSD treatment for soldiers after combat deployment: Low utilization of mental health care and reasons for dropout. *Psychiatric Services, 65*(8), 997–1004. https://doi.org/10.1176/appi.ps.201300307.

Holt-Lunstad, J., Smith, T. B., & Layton, J. B. (2010). Social relationships and mortality risk: A meta-analytic review. *PLoS Med, 7*(7), e1000316. https://doi.org/10.1371/journal.pmed.1000316.

Hölzel, B. K., Carmody, J., Vangel, M., et al. (2011). Mindfulness practice leads to increases in regional brain gray matter density. *Psychiatry Research, 191*(1), 36–43. https://doi.org/10.1016/j.pscychresns.2010.08.006.

Homan, K. J., & Sirois, F. M. (2017). Self-compassion and physical health: Exploring the roles of perceived stress and health-promoting behaviors. *Health Psychology Open, 4*(2). https://doi.org/10.1177/2055102917729542.

Hoskins, M., Pearce, J., Bethell, A., et al. (2015). Pharmacotherapy for post-traumatic stress disorder: Systematic review and meta-analysis. *The British Journal of Psychiatry, 206*(2), 93–100. https://doi.org/10.1192/bjp.bp.114.148551.

House, J. S., Landis, K. R., & Umberson, D. (1988). Social relationships and health. *Science, 241*(4865), 540–545. https://doi.org/10.1126/science.3399889.

Houston, J. (1992). *Godseed: The journey of Christ*. Quest Books.

Hurst, J. B. (1993). *Conflict self-assessment*. University of Toledo.

Hurst, J., & Kinney, M. (1989). *Empowering self and others*. University of Toledo.

Hurst, Y., & Fukuda, H. (2018). Effects of changes in eating speed on obesity in patients with diabetes: A secondary analysis of longitudinal health check-up data. *BMJ Open, 8*, e019589. https://doi.org/10.1136/bmjopen-2017-019589.

Hutcherson, C. A., Seppala, E. M., & Gross, J. J. (2008). Loving-kindness meditation increases social connectedness. *Emotion, 8*(5), 720–724. https://doi.org/10.1037/a0013237.

Hwang, S., Kim, G., Yang, J., et al. (2016). The moderating effects of age on the relationships of self-compassion, self-esteem, and mental health: Self-compassion and age. *Japanese Psychological Research, 58*(2), 194–205. https://doi.org/10.1111/jpr.12109.

Iranmanesh, S., Tirgari, B., & Bardsiri, H. S. (2013). Post-traumatic stress disorder among paramedic and hospital emergency personnel in south-east Iran. *World Journal of Emergency Medicine, 4*(1), 26–31. https://doi.org/10.5847/wjem.j.issn.1920-8642.2013.01.005.

Jackson, D., Clare, J., & Mannix, J. (2002). Who would want to be a nurse? Violence in the workplace—A factor in recruitment and retention. *Journal of Nursing Management, 10*(1), 13–20. https://doi.org/10.1046/j.0966-0429.2001.00262.x.

Jacobs, D., & Kyzer, S. (2010). Upstate AHEC lateral violence among nurses project. *South Carolina Nurse, 17*(1), 1–3. https://cdn.ymaws.com/www.scnurses.org/resource/resmgr/imported/JacobsLateralViolenceProjectSCNurse0Articlfinal.pdf.

Jahromi, F. G., Naziri, G., & Barzegar, M. (2012). The relationship between socially prescribed perfectionism and depression: The mediating role of maladaptive cognitive schemas. *Social and Behavioral Sciences, 32*, 141–147. https://doi.org/10.1016/j.sbspro.2012.01.023.

Jakobsen, J. C., Gluud, C., & Kirsch, I. (2020). Should antidepressants be used for major depressive disorder? *BMJ Evidence-Based Medicine, 25*(4), 130. https://doi.org/10.1136/bmjebm-2019-111238.

Jesse, M. T., Abouljoud, M. S., Hogan, K., et al. (2015). Burnout in transplant nurses. *Progress in Transplantation, 25*(3), 196–202. https://doi.org/10.7182/pit2015213.

Jirakittayakorn, N., & Wongsawat, Y. (2017). Brain responses to a 6-Hz binaural beat: Effects on general theta rhythm and frontal midline theta activity. *Frontiers in Neuroscience, 11*, 365. https://doi.org/10.3389/fnins.2017.00365.

Johnston, L., Miles, L., & Macrae, C. N. (2010). Why are you smiling at me? Social functions of enjoyment and non-enjoyment smiles. *The British Journal of Social Psychology, 49*(1), 107–127. https://doi.org/10.1348/014466609X412476.

Judge, T. A., & Bono, J. E. (2001). Relationship of core self-evaluations traits—self-esteem, generalized self-efficacy, locus of control, and emotional stability—with job satisfaction and job performance: A meta-analysis. *Journal of Applied Psychology, 86*(1), 80–92. http://citeseerx.ist.psu.edu/viewdoc/download?doi=10.1.1.705.776&rep=rep1&type=pdf.

Jung, C. G. (1954). *The collected works of C.G. Jung. Volume 17: The development of personality.* Princeton University Press.

Jung, C. G. (1970). *The collected works of C.G. Jung. Volume 17: Mysterium coniunctionis.* Princeton University Press.

Katie, B., & Mitchell, S. (2003). *Loving what is: Four questions that can change your life.* Harmony Books.

Katzman, M. A., Bleau, P., Blier, P., et al. (2014). Canadian clinical practice guidelines for the management of anxiety, posttraumatic stress and obsessive-compulsive disorders. *BMC Psychiatry, 14,* S1.

Keane, T. M., Caddell, J. M., & Taylor, K. L. (1988). Mississippi Scale for combat-related posttraumatic stress: Three studies in reliability and validity. *Journal of Consulting and Clinical Psychology, 56,* 85–90. https://doi. org/10.1037//0022-006x.56.1.85.

Kearney, D. J., Malte, C. A., McManus, C., et al. (2013). Loving-kindness meditation for posttraumatic stress disorder: A pilot study. *Journal of Traumatic Stress, 26*(4), 426–434. https://doi.org/10.1002/jts.21832.

Kelly, J. (2018). Forgiveness: A key resiliency builder. *Clinical Orthopaedics and Related Research, 476*(2), 203–204. https://doi.org/10.1007/s11999.0000000000000024.

Kelly, A. C., Vimalakanthan, K., & Miller, K. E. (2014). Self-compassion moderates the relationship between body mass index and both eating disorder pathology and body image flexibility. *Body Image, 11*(4), 446–453. https://doi.org/10.1016/j.bodyim.2014.07.005.

Kemp, A. (2019). *The Quantum K2 experience.* https://quantumk.co.uk/quantum-k2/.

Khalid, A., Kim, B. S., Seo, B. A., et al. (2016). Gamma oscillation in functional brain networks is involved in the spontaneous remission of depressive behavior induced by chronic restraint stress in mice. *BMC Neuroscience, 17*(1), 4. https://doi.org/10.1186/s12868-016-0239-x.

Khan, A., Faucett, J., Lichtenberg, P., et al. (2012). A systematic review of comparative efficacy of treatments and controls for depression. *PLoS One, 7*(7), e41778. https://doi.org/10.1371/journal.pone.0041778.

Khan, A. M., Dar, S., Ahmed, R., et al. (2018). Cognitive behavioral therapy versus eye movement desensitiza- tion and reprocessing in patients with post-traumatic stress disorder: Systematic review and meta-analysis of randomized clinical trials. *Cureus, 10*(9), e3250. https://doi.org/10.7759/cureus.3250.

Kiecolt-Glaser, J. K., McGuire, L., Robles, T. F., et al. (2002). Psychoneuroimmunology: Psychological influences on immune function and health. *Journal of Consulting and Clinical Psychology, 70*(3), 537–547. https://doi. org/10.1037//0022-006X.70.3.537.

Killingsworth, M. A., & Gilbert, D. T. (2010). A wandering mind is an unhappy mind. *Science, 330*(6006), 932. https://doi.org/10.1126/science.1192439

Kious, B. M., Sabic, H., Sung, Y., et al. (2017). An open-label pilot study of combined augmentation with creatine monohydrate and 5-hydroxytryptophan for selective serotonin reuptake inhibitor- or serotonin–norepineph- rine reuptake inhibitor-resistant depression in adult women. *Journal of Clinical Psychopharmacology, 37*(5), 578–583. https://doi.org/10.1097/JCP.0000000000000754.

Kohut, H. (1984). *How does analysis cure?* University of Chicago Press.

Kornfield, J. (2008). *The art of forgiveness, lovingkindness, and peace.* Bantam Dell.

Kovner, C. T., Brewer, C. S., Greene, W., et al. (2009). Understanding new nurses' intent to stay at their jobs. *Nursing Economics, 27*(2), 81–98.

Kovner, C. T., Fairchild, S., Poornima, H., et al. (2007). Newly licensed RNs' characteristics, work attitudes, and intentions to work. *The American Journal of Nursing, 107*(9), 58–70. http://www.rwjf.org/content/dam/farm/ articles/journal_articles/2007/rwjf13494.

Kozlowska, K., Walker, P., McLean, L., & Carrive, P. (2015). Fear and the defense cascade: Clinical im- plications and management. *Harvard Review of Psychiatry, 23*(4), 263–287. https://doi.org/10.1097/ HRP.0000000000000065.

Kral, T. R. A., Schuyler, B. S., Mumford, J. A., et al. (2018). Impact of short- and long-term mindfulness meditation training on amygdala reactivity to emotional stimuli. *NeuroImage, 181,* 301–313. https://doi. org/10.1016/j.neuroimage.2018.07.013.

Kyu, H. H., Bachman, V. F., Alexander, L. T., et al. (2016). Physical activity and risk of breast cancer, colon cancer, diabetes, ischemic heart disease, and ischemic stroke events: Systematic review and dose–response meta-analysis for the Global Burden of Disease Study. *British Medical Journal, 354.* https://doi.org/10.1136/bmj.i3857.

Lacey, B. C., & Lacey, J. I. (1974). Studies of heart rate and other bodily processes in sensorimotor behavior. In P. A. Obrist, A. H. Black, J. Brener, & L. V. DiCara (Eds.), *Cardiovascular psychophysiology* (pp. 538–564). Aldine.

Lai, J., Ma, S., Wang, Y., et al. (2020). Factors associated with mental health outcomes among health care work- ers exposed to coronavirus disease 2019. *JAMA Network Open, 3*(3), e203976. https://doi.org/10.1001/ jamanetworkopen.2020.3976.

Lally, P., van Jaarsveld, C. H. M., Potts, H. H. W., et al. (2010). How are habits formed: Modelling habit formation in the real world? *European Journal of Social Psychology, 40,* 998–1009. https://doi.org/10.1002/ ejsp.674.

Lambert, N. M., Fincham, F. D., Stillman, T. F., et al. (2010). Motivating change in relationships: Can prayer increase forgiveness. *Psychological Science, 21*(1), 126–132. https://doi.org/10.1177/0956797609355634.

Lamott, A. (1999). *Traveling mercies: Some thoughts on faith.* Pantheon.

Lampariello, L. R., Cortelazzo, A., Guerranti, R., et al. (2012). The magic velvet bean of *Mucuna pruriens. Journal of Traditional and Complementary Medicine, 2*(4), 331–339. https://doi.org/10.1016/s2225-4110(16)30119-5.

Lane, P. (2019). Indigenous wisdom for compassionate living and unified action [Online course]. https://theshiftnetwork.com/course/13371.

Laneri, D., Schuster, V., Dietsche, B., et al. (2016). Effects of long-term mindfulness meditation on brain's white matter mictrostructure and the aging. *Frontiers in Aging Neuroscience, 7,* 254. https://doi.org/10.3389/fnagi.2015.00254.

Laposa, J. M., Alden, L. E., & Fullerton, L. M. (2003). Work stress and posttraumatic stress disorder in ED nurses/personnel (CE). *Journal of Emergency Nursing, 29*(1), 23–28. https://doi.org/10.1067/men.2003.7.

Larm, P., Åslund, C., Starrin, B., et al. (2016). How are social capital and sense of coherence associated with hazardous alcohol use? Findings from a large population-based Swedish sample of adults. *Scandinavian Journal of Public Health, 44*(5), 525. https://doi.org/10.1177/1403494816645221.

Laschinger, H. K., Grau, A. L., Finegan, J., et al. (2010). New graduate nurses' experiences of bullying and burnout in hospital settings. *Journal of Advanced Nursing, 66*(12), 2732–2742. https://doi.org/10.1111/j.1365-2648.2010.05420.x.

Laschinger, H. K. S., Borgogni, L., Consiglio, C., et al. (2015). The effects of authentic leadership, six areas of work life, and occupational coping self-efficacy on new graduate nurses' burnout and mental health: A cross-sectional study. *International Journal of Nursing Studies, 52*(6), 1080–1089. https://doi.org/10.1016/j.ijnurstu.2015.03.002.

Laschinger, H. K. S., Grau, A. L., Finegan, J., et al. (2012). Predictors of new graduate nurses' workplace wellbeing: Testing the job demands–Resources model. *Health Care Management Review, 37*(2), 175–186. https://doi.org/10.1097/HMR.0b013e31822aa456.

Lea, J., & Cruickshank, M. T. (2017). The role of rural nurse managers in supporting new graduate nurses in rural practice. *Journal of Nursing Management, 25*(3), 176–183. https://doi.org/10.1111/jonm.12453.

Leadbeater, B., & Sukhawathanakul, P. (2011). Multicomponent programs for reducing peer victimization in early elementary school: A longitudinal evaluation of the WITS primary program. *Journal of Community Psychology, 39*(5), 606–620. https://doi.org/10.1002/jcop.20447.

Lee, L., James, P., Zevon, E., et al. (2019). Optimism is associated with exceptional longevity in 2 epidemiologic cohorts of men and women. *Proceedings of the National Academy of Sciences of the United States of America, 116*(37), 18357–18362. https://doi.org/10.1073/pnas.1900712116.

Lee, Y.-J., Kim, H-G., Cheon, E-J., et al. (2019). The analysis of electroencephalography changes before and after a single neurofeedback alpha/theta training session in university students. *Applied Psychophysiology and Biofeedback, 44*(3), 173–184. https://doi.org/10.1007/s10484-019-09432-4.

Leininger, M. (1994). The tribes of nursing in the USA culture of nursing. *Journal of Transcultural Nursing, 6*(1), 18–22. https://doi.org/10.1177/104365969400600104.

Leiter, M. P., Jackson, N. J., & Shaughnessy, K. (2009). Contrasting burnout, turnover intention, control, value congruence and knowledge sharing between Baby Boomers and Generation X. *Journal of Nursing Management, 17*(1), 100–109. https://doi.org/10.1111/j.1365-2834.2008.00884.x.

Leiter, M. P., Price, S. L., & Laschinger, H. K. S. (2010). Generational differences in distress, attitudes and incivility among nurses: Generational differences among nurses. *Journal of Nursing Management, 18*(8), 970–980. https://doi.org/10.1111/j.1365-2834.2010.01168.x.

Letvak, S., Ruhm, C. J., & McCoy, T. (2012). Depression in hospital-employed nurses. *Clinical Nurse Specialist, 26*(3), 177–182. https://doi.org/10.1097/nur.0b013e3182503ef0.

Leung, M., Chan, C. C. H., Yin, J., et al. (2013). Increased gray matter volume in the right angular and posterior parahippocampal gyri in loving-kindness meditators. *Social Cognitive and Affective Neuroscience, 8*(1), 34–39. https://doi.org/10.1093/scan/nss076.

Levine, P. A. (2010). *In an unspoken voice: How the body releases trauma and restores goodness.* North Atlantic Books.

Lewig, K. A., & Dollard, M. F. (2003). Emotional dissonance, emotional exhaustion and job satisfaction in call center workers. *European Journal of Work and Organizational Psychology, 12*(4), 366–392. https://doi.org/10.1080/13594320344000200.

Li, C-Y., Chen, S-C., Li, C-Y., et al. (2011). Randomised controlled trial of the effectiveness of using foot reflexology to improve quality of sleep amongst Taiwanese postpartum women. *Midwifery, 27*(2), 181–186. https://doi.org/10.1016/j.midw.2009.04.005.

Li, Q. (2010). Effect of forest bathing trips on human immune function. *Environmental Health and Preventive Medicine, 15*(1), 9–17. https://doi.org/10.1007/s12199-008-0068-3.

Li, X., Ma, R., Pang, L., et al. (2017). Delta coherence in resting-state EEG predicts the reduction in cigarette craving after hypnotic aversion suggestions. *Scientific Reports, 7*(1), 2430. https://doi.org/10.1038/s41598-017-01373-4.

Li, Y., & Jones, C. B. (2012). A literature review of nursing turnover costs. *Journal of Nursing Management, 21,* 405–418. https://doi.org/10.1111/j.1365-2834.2012.01411.x.

Lighthall, N., Gorlick, M., & Schoeke, A. (2013). Stress modulates reinforcement learning in younger and older adults. *Psychology and Aging, 28*(1), 35–46. https://doi.org/10.1037/a0029823.

Lin, W., Hu, J., & Gong, Y. (2015). Is it helpful for individuals with minor depression to keep smiling? An event-related potentials analysis. *Social Behavior and Personality, 43*(3), 383–396. https://doi.org/10.2224/sbp.2015.43.3.383.

Lindmark, U., Stenström, U., Wärnberg-Gerdin, E., et al. (2010). The distribution of "sense of coherence" among Swedish adults: A quantitative cross-sectional population study. *Scandinavian Journal of Public Health, 38*(1), 1. https://doi.org/10.1177/1403494809351654.

Lindmark, Y., Hakebearg, M., & Hugoson, A. (2001). Sense of coherence and its relationship with oral health-related behavior and knowledge of and attitudes towards oral health. *Community Dentistry and oral Epidemiology, 39,* 542–553. https://doi.org/10.1111/j.1600-0528.2011.00627.x.

Linehan, M. M., Dimeff, L., Koerner, K., et al. (2016). *Research on DBT: Summary of non-RCT studies.* https://behavioraltech.org/downloads/Research-on-DBT_Summary-of-Data-to-Date.pdf.

Liu, Y.-Z., Wang, Y.-X., & Jiang, C.-L. (2017). Inflammation: The common pathway of stress-related diseases. *Frontiers in Human Neuroscience, 11,* 316. https://doi.org/10.3389/fnhum.2017.00316.

Lively, K. J. (2000). Reciprocal emotion management: Working together to maintain stratification in private law firms. *Work and Occupations, 27*(1), 32–63. http://isites.harvard.edu/fs/docs/icb.topic155590.files/Lively_ReciprocalEmotionManagement.pdf.

Lo, R. (2002). A longitudinal study of perceived level of stress, coping and self-esteem of undergraduate nursing students: An Australian case study. *Journal of Advanced Nursing, 39*(2), 119–126. https://doi.org/10.1046/j.1365-2648.2000.02251.x.

Locke, E. A. (1996). Motivation through conscious goal setting. *Applied and Preventive Psychology, 5*(2), 117–124. https://doi.org/10.1016/S0962-1849(96)80005-9.

Locke, E., & Latham, G. P. (2002). Building a practically useful theory of goal setting and task motivation: A 35-year odyssey. *American Psychologist, 57*(9), 705–717. https://doi.org/10.1037/0003-066X.57.9.705.

Loeb, S. J., Penrod, J., Falkenstern, S., et al. (2003). Supporting older adults living with multiple chronic conditions. *Western Journal of Nursing Research, 25*(1), 8–29. https://doi.org/10.1177/0193945902238830.

Lund, I., Yu, L-C., Uvnas-Moberg, K., et al. (2002). Repeated massage-like stimulation induces long-term effects on nociception: Contribution of oxytocinergic mechanisms. *European Journal of Neuroscience, 16,* 330–338. https://doi.org/10.1046/j.1460-9568.2002.02087.x.

Luthans, K. W., & Jensen, S. M. (2005). The linkage between psychological capital and commitment to organization mission: A study of nurses. *Journal of Nursing Administration, 35*(6), 304–310. https://doi.org/10.1097/00005110-200506000-00007.

Lutz, A., Brefczynski-Lewis, J., Johnstone, T., et al. (2008). Regulation of the neural circuitry of emotion by compassion meditation: Effects of meditative expertise. *PLoS One, 3*(3). https://doi.org/10.1371/journal.pone.0001897.

Lutz, A., Greischar, L. L., Rawlings, N. B., et al. (2004). Long-term meditators self-induce high-amplitude gamma synchrony during mental practice. *Proceedings of the National Academy of Sciences of the United States of America, 101*(46), 16369–16373. https://doi.org/10.1073/pnas.0407401101.

Ly, C., Greb, A. C., Cameron, L. P., et al. (2018). Psychedelics promote structural and functional neural plasticity. *Cell Reports, 23*(11), 3170–3182. https://doi.org/10.1016/j.celrep.2018.05.022.

Ma, X., Yue, Z.-Q., Gong, Z.-Q., et al. (2017). The effect of diaphragmatic breathing on attention, negative affect and stress in healthy adults. *Frontiers in Psychology, 8,* 874. https://doi.org/10.3389/fpsyg.2017.00874.

MacDonald, D. A., & Friedman, H. L. (2020). Growing up and waking up: A conversation with Ken Wilber about leaving transpersonal to form integral psychology. *Journal of Humanistic Psychology.* https://doi.org/10.1177/0022167820902287.

Magnuson, C. D., & Barnett, L. A. (2013). The playful advantage: How playfulness enhances coping with stress. *Leisure Sciences, 35*(2), 129–144. https://doi.org/10.1080/01490400.2013.761905.

Mahli, J. (2013). *Horizontal violence in the nursing profession* [Unpublished master's thesis]. The University of British Columbia. https://doi.org/10.14288/1.0073751.

Mahipalan, M., & Sheena, S. (2018). Workplace spirituality and subjective happiness among high school teachers: Gratitude as A moderator. *Explore, 15*(2), 107–114. https://doi.org/10.1016/j.explore.2018.07.002.

Manczak, E. M., DeLongis, A., & Chen, E. (2016). Does empathy have a cost? Diverging psychological and physiological effects within families. *Health Psychology, 35*(3), 211–218. https://doi.org/10.1037/hea0000281.

Manitoba Nurses' Union. (2015). *Helping Manitoba's wounded healers: Post-traumatic stress disorder in the nursing profession.* https://manitobanurses.ca/system/files/MNU-%20PTSD%20Report%20-%20Web%20Version. pdf.

Marshall, D. (2019). *High performance habits: Future self—Becoming a new story leader.* http://www.highperfor mancehabits.com.au/meditation/Future%20Self%20Meditation.pdf.

Maslach, C., & Jackson, S. E. (1986). *Maslach burnout inventory manual* (2nd ed.). Consulting Psychologists Press.

Maslach, C., Jackson, S. E., Leiter, M. P., et al. (1996). *Maslach burnout inventory* (3rd ed.). Consulting Psychologists Press.

Maslow, A. H. (1943). A theory of human motivation. *Psychological Review, 50*(4), 370–396. https://doi. org/10.1037/h0054346.

Maslow, A. H. (1954). *A preface to motivation theory.* Harper & Row.

Maslow, A. H. (1968). *Toward a psychology of being.* D. Van Nostrand Company.

Maslow, A. H. (1971). *The farther reaches of human nature.* Viking.

Matthews, B. (2006). *Engaging education: Developing emotional literacy, equity and co-education.* Open University Press.

McCabe, I. (2015). *Carl Jung and Alcoholics Anonymous: The twelve steps as a spiritual journey of individuation.* Karnac Books.

McCann, L. I., & Pearlman, L. A. (1990). Vicarious traumatization: A framework for understanding the psychological effects of working with victims. *Journal of Traumatic Stress, 3*(1), 131–149. https://doi.org/10.1002/ jts.2490030110.

McCraty, R. (2015). *Science of the heart: Exploring the role of the heart in human performance.* (Vol. 2). HeartMath Institute. https://www.heartmath.org/research/science-of-the-heart/.

McCraty, R. (2017). New frontiers in heart rate variability and social coherence research: Techniques, technologies, and implications for improving group dynamics and outcomes. *Frontier in Public Health, 5,* 267. https:// doi.org/10.3389/fpubh.2017.00267.

McCraty, R., Atkinson, M., Tomasino, D., et al. (2009). The coherent heart: Heart–brain interactions, psychophysiological coherence, and the emergence of system-wide order. *Integral Review, 5*(2). https://www.integral- review.org/issues/vol_5_no_2_mccraty_et_al_the_coherent_heart.pdf.

McCraty, R., & Childre, D. (2010). Coherence: Bridging personal, social and global health. *Alternative Therapies in Health and Medicine, 16*(4), 10–24. https://www.heartmath.org/assets/uploads/2015/01/coherence-bridg- ing-personal-social-global-health.pdf.

McKenna, L., & Newton, J. M. (2007). After the graduate year: A phenomenological exploration of how new nurses develop their knowledge and skill over the first 18 months following graduation. *Australian Journal of Advanced Nursing, 25*(4), 9–15. http://www.ajan.com.au/Vol25/Vol_25-4_McKenna.pdf.

McKinley, S. (2020, April 16). Canadian healthcare workers on COVID-19 front line say they need mental health support, poll indicates. *Toronto Star.* https://www.thestar.com/news/canada/2020/04/16/canadian-health- workers-on-covid-19-front-line-say-they-need-mental-health-support-poll-indicates.html.

McManus, D. E. (2017). Reiki is better than placebo and has broad potential as a complementary health therapy. *Journal of Evidence-Based Complementary and Alternative Medicine, 22*(4), 1051–1057. https://doi. org/10.1177/2156587217728644.

Meesters, A., den Bosch-Meevissen, Y. M. C. I., Weijzen, C. A. H., et al. (2017). The effect of mindfulness- based stress reduction on wound healing: A preliminary study. *Journal of Behavioral Medicine.* https://doi. org/10.1007/s10865-017-9901-8.

Melander, H., Ahlqvist-Rastad, J., Meijer, G., et al. (2003). Evidence b(i)ased medicine—selective reporting from studies sponsored by pharmaceutical industry: Review of studies in new drug applications. *British Medical Journal, 326*(7400), 1171–1173. https://doi.org/10.1136/bmj.326.7400.1171.

Melrose, S. (2011). Perfectionism and depression: Vulnerabilities nurses need to understand. *Nursing Research and Practice, 2011,* 858497. https://doi.org/10.1155/2011/858497.

Mental Health Commission of Canada. (2018). *Caring for healthcare workers; the National Standard for Psychological Health and Safety in Healthcare.* https://healthstandards.org/leading-practice/caring-healthcare-workers- national-standard-psychological-health-safety-healthcare/.

Merakou, K., Xefteri, E., & Barbouni, A. (2016). Sense of coherence in religious Christian orthodox women in Greece. *Community Mental Health Journal, 53,* 353–357. https://doi.org/10.1007/s10597-016-0051-1.

Mesmer-Magnus, J. R., DeChurch, L. A., & Wax, A. (2012). Moving emotional labor beyond surface and deep acting: A discordance–congruence perspective. *Organizational Psychology Review, 2*(1), 6–53. https://doi. org/10.1177/2041386611417746.

Miller, T. Q., Smith, T. W., Turner, C. W., et al. (1996). Meta-analytic review of research on hostility and physical health. *Psychology Bulletin, 119*(2), 322–348. https://doi.org/10.1037/0033-2909.119.2.322.

Mitchell, M. (2010). Ingratitude and the death of freedom. In Adam Bellow (Ed.), *New threats to freedom* (pp. 181–188). Templeton Press.

Mitchell, A., Ahmed, A., & Szabo, C. (2014). Workplace violence among nurses, why are we still discussing this? Literature review. *Journal of Nursing Education and Practice, 4*(4), 147–150. https://doi.org/10.5430/jnep.v4n4p147.

Miyata, S., Kumagaya, R., Kakizaki, T., et al. (2019). Loss of glutamate decarboxylase 67 in somatostatin-expressing neurons leads to anxiety-like behavior and alteration in the Akt/GSK3β signaling pathway. *Frontiers in Behavioral Neuroscience, 13*, 131. https://doi.org/10.3389/fnbeh.2019.00131.

Modi, S., Rana, P., Kaur, P., et al. (2014). Glutamate level in anterior cingulate predicts anxiety in healthy humans: A magnetic resonance spectroscopy study. *Psychiatry Research: Neuroimaging, 224*(1), 34–41. https://doi.org/10.1016/j.pscychresns.2014.03.001.

Montero-Marin, J., Zubjaga, F., Cereceda, M., et al. (2016). Burnout subtypes and absence of self-compassion in primary healthcare professionals: A cross-sectional study. *PLoS One, 11*(6), e0157499. https://doi.org/10.1371/journal.pone.0157499.

Morina, N., Schnyder, U., Schick, M., et al. (2016). Attachment style and interpersonal trauma in refugees. *Australian & New Zealand Journal of Psychiatry, 50*(12), 1161–1168. https://doi.org/10.1177/0004867416631432.

Mortier, A. V., Vlerick, P., & Clays, E. (2016). Authentic leadership and thriving among nurses: The mediating role of empathy. *Journal of Nursing Management, 24*(3), 357–365. https://doi.org/10.1111/jonm.12329.

Munn, S. L. (2013). Unveiling the work–life system: The influence of work–life balance on meaningful work. *Advances in Developing Human Resources, 15*(4), 401–417. https://doi.org/10.1177/1523422313498567.

Myrin, B., & Lagerström, M. (2006). Health behavior and sense of coherence among pupils aged 14–15. *Scandinavian Journal of Caring Sciences, 20*(3), 339–346. https://doi.org/10.1111/j.1471-6712.2006.00413.x.

Nahlén, C., & Saboonchi, F. (2009). Coping, sense of coherence, and the dimensions of affect in patients with chronic heart failure. *European Journal of Cardiovascular Nursing, 9*(2), 118–125. https://doi.org/10.1016/j.ejcnurse.2009.11.006.

Najavits, L. (2015). The problem of dropout from "gold standard" PTSD therapies. *F1000Prime Reports, 7*(43). https://doi.org/10.12703/P7-43.

National Health Service. (2018). *Complex PTSD—Post-traumatic stress disorder.* https://www.nhs.uk/conditions/post-traumatic-stress-disorder-ptsd/complex/.

National Institute of Mental Health. (2019a). *Generalized anxiety disorder: When Worry Gets Out of Control.* https://www.nimh.nih.gov/health/publications/generalized-anxiety-disorder-gad/index.shtml.

National Institute of Mental Health. (2019b). *Post-traumatic stress disorder.* https://www.nimh.nih.gov/health/topics/post-traumatic-stress-disorder-ptsd/index.shtml.

National Institute of Mental Health. (2020). *Post-traumatic stress disorder.* https://www.nimh.nih.gov/health/publications/post-traumatic-stress-disorder-ptsd

Navarro-Gil, M., Escolano Marco, C., Montero-Marín, J., et al. (2018). Efficacy of neurofeedback on the increase of mindfulness-related capacities in healthy individuals: A controlled trial. *Mindfulness, 9*(1), 303–311. https://doi.org/10.1007/s12671-017-0775-1.

Neath, I., & Surprenant, A. M. (2003). *Human memory: An introduction to research, data, and theory* (2nd ed.). Wadsworth.

Neff, K. D. (2016). The Self-Compassion Scale is a valid and theoretically coherent measure of self-compassion. *Mindfulness, 7*, 264–274. https://doi.org/10.1007/s12671-015-0479-3.

Neff, K.D. (2018). *Definition of self-compassion.* http://self-compassion.org/the-three-elements-of-self-compassion-2/.

Neff, K.D. (2019). *Exercise 2: Self-compassion break.* https://self-compassion.org/exercise-2-self-compassion-break/

Neff, K. D., & Germer, C. (2018). *The mindful self-compassion workbook: A proven way to accept yourself, build inner strength, and thrive.* The Guildford Press.

Nett, R. J., Witte, T. K., Holzbauer, S. M., et al. (2015). Risk factors for suicide, attitudes toward mental illness, and practice-related stressors among US veterinarians. *Journal of the American Veterinary Medical Association, 247*(8), 945–955. https://doi.org/10.2460/javma.247.8.945.

Neuman, B. (1995). *The Neuman systems model* (3rd ed.). Appleton & Lange.

Newson, J. J., & Thiagarajan, T. C. (2019). EEG frequency bands in psychiatric disorders: A review of resting state studies. *Frontiers in Human Neuroscience, 12*, 521. https://doi.org/10.3389/fnhum.2018.00521.

Nguyen Van, H., Dinh Le, M., Nguyen Van, T., et al. (2018). A systematic review of effort–reward imbalance among health workers. *The International Journal of Health Planning and Management, 33*(3), e674–e695. https://doi.org/10.1002/hpm.2541.

NHS Improvement. (2017). *Culture and leadership program, phase I: Discover.* https://www.england.nhs.uk/culture/culture-leadership-programme/discovery-phase/.

NHS Improvement. (2018). *Culture and leadership program, phase II: Design.* https://www.england.nhs.uk/culture/culture-leadership-programme/design-phase/.

Niemiec, R. M. (2014). *Mindfulness and character strengths: A practical guide to flourishing.* Hogrefe.

Nowrouzi, B., Giddens, E., Gohar, B., et al. (2016). The quality of work life of registered nurses in Canada and the United States: A comprehensive literature review. *International Journal of Occupational and Environmental Health, 22*(4), 341–358. https://doi.org/10.1080/10773525.2016.1241920.

Nursing Solutions Inc. (2018). *2018 National healthcare retention & RN staffing report.* https://pdf4pro.com/view/2018-national-health-care-retention-amp-rn-staffing-1292b3.html.

O'Brien-Pallas, L., Murphy, G. T., Shamian, J., et al. (2010). Impact and determinants of nurse turnover: A Pan-Canadian study. *Journal of Nursing Management, 18*(8), 1073–1086. https://doi.org/10.1111/j.1365-2834.2010.01167.x.

O'Brien-Pallas, L., Tomblin Murphy, G., & Shamian, J. (2008). *Understanding the costs and outcomes of nurses' turnover in Canadian hospitals.* University of Toronto: Nursing Health Services Research Unit.

O'Callaghan, A. (2013). Emotional congruence in learning and health encounters in medicine: Addressing an aspect of the hidden curriculum. *Advances in Health Sciences Education, 18*(2), 305–317. https://doi.org/10.1007/s10459-012-9353-4.

Odland, L.-V., Sneltvedt, T., & Sorlie, V. (2014). Responsible but unprepared: Experiences of newly educated nurses in hospital care. *Nurse Education in Practice, 14*(5), 538–543. https://doi.org/10.1016/j.nepr.2014.05.005.

O'Leary, O. F., Dinan, T. G., & Cryan, J. F. (2015). Faster, better, stronger: Towards new antidepressant therapeutic strategies. *European Journal of Pharmacology, 753*, 32–50. https://doi.org/10.1016/j.ejphar.2014.07.046.

Olson, M. A., Kemper, K. J., & Mahan, J. D. (2015). What factors promote resilience and protect against burnout in first year pediatric and medicine-pediatric residents? *Journal of Evidence-Based and Complementary Alternative Medicine, 20*(3), 192–198. https://doi.org/10.1177/2156587214568894.

O'Malley, D., Dowd, D., Brungardt, H., & Cox, K. (2015). Changing the game for population health. *Health Progress, 96*(2), 31. https://doi.org/10.1016/j.nepr.2014.05.005.

Oriah "Mountain Dreamer." (1999). *The invitation* (1st ed.). HarperOne. http://www.oriahmountaindreamer.com.

Palhano-Fontes, F., Barreto, D., Onias, H., et al. (2019). Rapid antidepressant effects of the psychedelic ayahuasca in treatment-resistant depression: A randomized placebo-controlled trial. *Psychological Medicine, 49*(4), 655–663. https://doi.org/10.1017/S0033291718001356.

Pallant, J. F., & Lae, L. (2002). Sense of coherence, well-being, coping and personality factors: Further evaluation of the sense of coherence scale. *Personality and Individual Differences, 33*(1), 39–48. https://doi.org/10.1016/S0191-8869(01)00134-9.

Palmer, P. J. (1998). *The courage to teach: Exploring the inner landscape of a teacher's life* (1st ed.). Jossey-Bass.

Palmer, P. J. (2000). *Let your life speak: Listening for the voice of vocation.* Jossey-Bass.

Palmer, P. J. (2004). *A hidden wholeness: The journey toward an undivided life.* Jossey-Bass.

Palmer, P. J. (2007). *The courage to teach: Exploring the inner landscape of a teacher's life* (10th ed.). Wiley.

Palmer, P. J., Zajonc, A., & Scribner, M. (2010). *The heart of higher education: A call to renewal* (1st ed.). Jossey-Bass.

Paris, J. (2015). *The intelligent clinician's guide to the DSM-5.* Oxford University Press.

Park, A. T., Leonard, J. A., Saxler, P., et al. (2018). Amygdala–medial prefrontal connectivity relates to stress and mental health in early childhood. *Social Cognitive and Affective Neuroscience, 13*(4), 430–439. https://doi.org/10.1093/scan/nsy017.

Park, B. J., Tsunetsugu, Y., Kasetani, T., et al. (2007). Physiological effects of Shinrin-yoku (taking in the atmosphere of the forest)—Using salivary cortisol and cerebral activity as indicators. *Journal of Physiological Anthropology, 26*, 123–128. https://doi.org/10.2114/jpa2.26.123.

Parker, V., Giles, M., Lantry, G., et al. (2014). New graduate nurses' experiences in their first year of practice. *Nurse Education Today, 34*(1), 150–156. https://doi.org/10.1016/j.nedt.2012.07.003.

Pearlman, L. A., & Mac Ian, P. S. (1995). Vicarious traumatization: An empirical study of the effects of trauma work on trauma therapists. *Professional Psychology: Research and Practice, 26*(6), 558–565. https://doi.org/10.1037/0735-7028.26.6.558.

Pearlman, L. A., & Saakvitne, K. W. (1995). *Trauma and the therapist: Countertransference and vicarious traumatization in psychotherapy with incest survivors.* W.W. Norton & Company.

Pemberton, E., & Turpin, P. G. (2008). The effect of essential oils on work-related stress in intensive care unit nurses. *Holistic Nursing Practice, 22*(2), 97–102. https://doi.org/10.1097/01.HNP.0000312658.13890.28.

Perciavalle, V., Blandini, M., Fecarotta, P., et al. (2017). The role of deep breathing on stress. *Neurological Sciences, 38*(3), 451–458. https://doi.org/10.1007/s10072-016-2790-8.

Perret, J. L., Best, C. O., Coe, J. B., et al. (2020). Prevalence of mental health outcomes among Canadian veterinarians. *Journal of the American Veterinary Medical Association, 256*(3), 365–375. https://doi.org/10.2460/javma.256.3.365.

Perry, B. D., Pollard, R. A., Blakley, T. L., et al. (1995). Childhood trauma, the neurobiology of adaptation, and "use-dependent" development of the brain: How "states" become "traits." *Infant Mental Health Journal, 16*(4), 271–291. https://doi.org/10.1002/1097-0355(199524)16:4%3C271::AID-IMHJ2280160404%3E3.0.CO;2-B.

Perry, G. S., Presley-Cantrell, L. R., & Dhingra, S. (2012). Guest editorial: Addressing mental health promotion in chronic disease prevention and health promotion. *Public Health Reviews, 34*(2), 1–7. http://www.publichealthreviews.eu/upload/pdf_files/12/00_Perry.pdf.

Petersson, S., Perseius, K., & Johnsson, P. (2014). Perfectionism and sense of coherence among patients with eating disorders. *Nordic Journal of Psychiatry, 68*(6), 409–415. https://doi.org/10.3109/08039488.2013.851738.

Porath, C. L., & Pearson, C. M. (2012). Emotional and behavioral responses to workplace incivility and the impact of hierarchical status. *Journal of Applied Social Psychology, 42*, 326–357. https://doi.org/10.1111/j.1559-1816.2012.01020.x.

Porath, C., Spreitzer, G., Gibson, C., et al. (2012). Thriving at work: Toward its measurement, construct validation, and theoretical refinement. *Journal of Organizational Behavior, 33*(2), 250–275. https://doi.org/10.1002/job.756.

Porges, S. W. (2009). The polyvagal theory: New insights into adaptive reactions of the autonomic nervous system. *Cleveland Clinic Journal of Medicine, 76*(Suppl 2), S86–S90. https://doi.org/10.3949/ccjm.76.s2.17.

Porges, S. W. (2011). *The polyvagal theory: Neurophysiological foundations of emotions, attachment, communication, and self-regulation.* W.W. Norton & Company.

Pratt, L. A., Brody, D. J., & Gu, Q. (2017). *Antidepressant use among persons aged 12 and over: United States, 2011–2014.* National Center for Health Statistics. NCHS Data Brief No. 283.

Providence Health. (2019, April 26). *B.C. extends presumptive PTSD coverage to dispatchers, nurses, healthcare aids.* http://www.providencehealthcare.org/news/20190426/bc-extends-presumptive-ptsd-coverage-dispatchers-nurses-health-care-aids.

Proyer, R. T. (2013). The well-being of playful adults: Adult playfulness, subjective well-being, physical well-being, and the pursuit of enjoyable activities. *European Journal of Humour Research, 1*, 84–98. https://doi.org/10.7592/EJHR2013.1.1.proyer.

Proyer, R. T., Gander, F., Bertenshaw, E. J., et al. (2018). The positive relationships of playfulness with indicators of health, activity, and physical fitness. *Frontiers in Psychology, 9*, 1440. https://doi.org/10.3389/fpsyg.2018.01440.

PTSD United. (2020). *PTSD statistics.* https://ptsdunited.org/ptsd-statistics-2/.

Public Health Agency of Canada. (2020). *Federal Framework on Posttraumatic Stress Disorder.* https://www.canada.ca/en/public-health/services/publications/healthy-living/federal-framework-post-traumatic-stress-disorder.html.

Rabb, K. (2014). Mindfulness, self-compassion and empathy, among health care professionals: A review of the literature. *Journal of Health Care Chaplaincy, 20*, 95–108. https://doi.org/10.1080/08854726.2014.913876.

Rains, M., & McClinn, K. (2013). *Resilience questionnaire.* https://www.trauma-treatment-info.com/resilience-in-the-face-of-trauma/.

Rebadomia, F. M. L., Amparo, J. S. M. G., Reyes, J. P., et al. (2019). Effect of music with brainwave synchronizer on the performance of collegiate throwing athletes. *Sport Mont, 17*(2), 17–22. https://doi.org/10.26773/smj.190603.

Reiner, M., Rozengurt, R., & Barnea, A. (2014). Better than sleep: Theta neurofeedback training accelerates memory consolidation. *Biological Psychology, 95*, 45–53. https://doi.org/10.1016/j.biopsycho.2013.10.010.

Reinhold, M., Bürkner, P., & Holling, H. (2018). Effects of expressive writing on depressive symptoms—A meta-analysis. *Clinical Psychology: Science and Practice, 25*(1), e12224. https://doi.org/10.1111/cpsp.12224.

Ren, J., Friedmann, D., Xiong, J., et al. (2018). Anatomically defined and functionally distinct dorsal raphe serotonin sub-systems. *Cell, 175*(2), 472–487. https://doi.org/10.1016/j.cell.2018.07.043.

Rennemark, M., & Hagberg, B. (1997). Sense of coherence among the elderly in relation to their perceived life history in an Eriksonian perspective. *Aging & Mental Health, 1*(3), 221–229. https://doi.org/10.1080/13607869757100.

Rhéaume, A., Clément, L., & LeBel, N. (2011). Understanding intention to leave amongst new graduate Canadian nurses: A repeated cross-sectional survey. *International Journal of Nursing Studies, 48*(4), 490–500. https://doi.org/10.1016/j.ijnurstu.2010.08.005.

Rizvi, S. J., Grima, E., Tan, M., et al. (2014). Treatment-resistant depression in primary care across Canada. *The Canadian Journal of Psychiatry, 59*(7), 349–357.

Roche, M., Diers, D., Duffield, C., et al. (2010). Violence toward nurses, the work environment, and patient outcomes. *Journal of Nursing Scholarship, 2*(1), 13–22. https://doi.org/10.1111/j.1547-5069.2009.01321.x.

Rogers, C. R. (1959). A theory of therapy, personality and interpersonal relationships as developed in the client-centered framework. In S. Koch (Ed.), *Psychology: A study of a science. Vol. 3. Formulations of the person and the social context* (pp. 184–256). McGraw Hill.

Rogers, C. R. (1968). Interpersonal relationships. *The Journal of Applied Behavioral Science, 4*(3), 265–280. https://doi.org/10.1177/002188636800400301.

Rogers, C. (1986). *Carl Rogers on personal power.* Constable & Robinson.

Rogers, F. (2019). *The World According to Mister Rogers: Important Things to Remember.* (Revised ed.). Hachette Books.

Rogers, A. E., Hwang, W., & Scott, L. D. (2004). The effects of work breaks on staff nurse performance. *The Journal of Nursing Administration, 34*(11), 512–519. https://doi.org/10.1097/00005110-200411000-00007.

Rohr, R. (1999). *Everything belongs: The gift of contemplative prayer.* The Crossroad Publishing Company.

Rosen, C. S., Matthieu, M. M., Stirman, S. W., et al. (2016). A review of studies on the system-wide implementation of evidence-based psychotherapies for posttraumatic stress disorder in the Veterans Health Administration. *Administration and Policy in Mental Health and Mental Health Services Research, 43*(6), 957–977. https://doi.org/10.1007/s10488-016-0755-0.

Roth, G. (2008). Perceived parental conditional regard and autonomy support as predictors of young adults' self-versus other-oriented prosocial tendencies. *Journal of Personality, 76*(3), 513–534. https://doi.org/10.1111/j.1467-6494.2008.00494.x.

Rowan, J. (2015). Self-actualization and individuation. *Self & Society, 43*(3), 231. https://doi.org/10.1080/03060497.2015.1092332.

Rozman, R., Whitaker, T., & Beckman, D. (1996). A pilot intervention program which reduces psychological symptomatology in individuals with human immunodeficiency virus. *Complementary Therapies in Medicine, 4*(4), 226–232.

Rnic, K., Dozois, D. J. A., & Martin, R. A. (2016). Cognitive distortions, humor styles, and depression. *Europe's Journal of Psychology, 12*(3), 348–362. https://doi.org/10.5964/ejop.v12i3.1118.

Rudman, A., & Gustavsson, J. P. (2012). Burnout during nursing education predicts lower occupational preparedness and future clinical performance: A longitudinal study. *International Journal of Nursing Studies, 49*(8), 988–1001. https://doi.org/10.1016/j.ijnurstu.2012.03.010.

Rudman, A., Gustavsson, J. P., & Hultell, D. (2014). A prospective study of nurses' intentions to leave the profession during their first five years of practice in Sweden. *International Journal Nursing Studies, 51*(4), 612–624. https://doi.org/10.1016/j.ijnurstu.2013.09.012.

Ruiz, D. M. (1997). *The four agreements: A practical guide to personal freedom.* Amber-Allen.

Rumi, (1997). *The essential Rumi* (C. Barks, Trans.). Castle Books.

Ruotsalainen, J. H., Verbeek, J. H., Mariné, A., et al. (2016). Preventing occupational stress in healthcare workers. *Sao Paulo Medical Journal, 134.* https://doi.org/10.1590/1516-3180.20161341T1.

Rush, K. L., Adamack, M., & Gordon, J. (2013). *Expanding the evidence for new graduate nurse transition best practices.* Michael Smith Foundation for Health Research. http://www.msfhr.org/sites/default/files/Expanding_the_Evidence_for_New_Graduate_Nurse_Transition_Best_Practices.pdf.

Russ, V. (1998). Behind and beyond Kolb's learning cycle. *Journal of Management Education, 22*(3), 304–319. https://www.scribd.com/document/177429865/Vince-Russ-Behind-and-Beyond-Kolb-s-Learning-Cycle-1998-pdf.

Saakvitne, K. W., & Pearlman, L. A. (1996). *Transforming the pain: A workbook on vicarious traumatization.* W.W. Norton & Company.

Sabo Mordechay, D., Nir, B., & Eviatar, Z. (2019). Expressive writing—Who is it good for? Individual differences in the improvement of mental health resulting from expressive writing. *Complementary Therapies in Clinical Practice, 37,* 115–121. https://doi.org/10.1016/j.ctcp.2019.101064.

Salt, J., Cummings, G. G., & Profetto-McGrath, J. (2008). Increasing retention of new graduate nurses: A systematic review of interventions by healthcare organizations. *Journal of Nursing Administration, 38*(6), 287–296. https://doi.org/10.1097/01.NNA.0000312788.88093.2e.

Sanches, R. F., de Lima Osório, F., Dos Santos, R. G., et al. (2016). Antidepressant effects of a single dose of ayahuasca in patients with recurrent depression: A SPECT study. *Journal of Clinical Psychopharmacology, 36*(1), 77–81. https://doi.org/10.1097/JCP.0000000000000436.

Sanderson, C. (2015). *Counselling skills for working with shame.* Jessica Kingsley Publishers.

Sarabia-Cobo, C. M. (2015). Heart coherence: A new tool in the management of stress on professionals and family caregivers of patients with dementia. *Applied Psychophysiology Biofeedback, 40*(2), 75–83. https://doi.org/10.1007/s10484-015-9276-y.

Sardo, S. S. (2004). Learning to display emotional intelligence. *Business Strategy Review, 15*(1), 14–17. https://doi.org/10.1111/j.0955-6419.2004.00295.x.

Savage, B. M., Lujan, H. L., Thipparthi, R. R., et al. (2017). Humor, laughter, learning, and health! A brief review. *Advances in Physiology Education, 41*(3), 341–347. https://doi.org/10.1152/advan.00030.2017.

Schaufeli, W., & Buunk, B.P. (2003). Burnout: An overview of 25 years of research and theorizing. In M. J. Schabracq, J. A. M. Winnubst, & C. L. Cooper (Eds.), *Handbook of work and health psychology* (pp. 383–425). https://doi.org/10.1002/0470013400.ch19.

Schmidt, A., & Miller, J. J. (2004). Healing trauma with meditation. *The Buddhist Review: Tricycle, 1*(14). https://tricycle.org/magazine/healing-trauma-meditation/.

Schwabe, L., & Wolf, O. T. (2013). Stress and multiple memory systems: From "thinking" to "doing." *Trends Cognitive Science, 17,* 60–68. https://doi.org/10.1016/j.tics.2012.12.001.

Schwartz, J., & Gladding, R. (2011). *You are not your brain: The 4-step solution for changing bad habits, ending unhealthy thinking, and taking control of your life.* Avery.

Scott, E. S., Keehner Engelke, M., & Swanson, M. (2008). New graduate nurse transitioning: Necessary or nice? *Applied Nursing Research, 21*(2), 75–83. https://doi.org/10.1016/j.apnr.2006.12.002.

Seifi Ala, T., Ahmadi-Pajouh, M. A., & Nasrabadi, A. M. (2018). Cumulative effects of theta binaural beats on brain power and functional connectivity. *Biomedical Signal Processing and Control, 42,* 242–252. https://doi.org/10.1016/j.bspc.2018.01.022.

Seijts, G. H., & Latham, G. P. (2001). The effect of learning, outcome, and proximal goals on a moderately complex task. *Journal of Organizational Behavior, 22,* 291–307. https://doi.org/10.1002/job.70.

Sevlever, M., & Rice, K. (2010). Perfectionism, depression, anxiety and academic performance in premedical students. *Canadian Medical Education Journal, 1*(2), 96–104. https://doi.org/10.1155/2011/858497.

Shafran, R., Cooper, Z., & Fairburn, C. G. (2002). Clinical perfectionism: A cognitive–behavioural analysis. *Behaviour Research and Therapy, 40*(7), 773–791. https://doi.org/10.1016/S0005-7967(01)00059-6.

Shapiro, F. (2017). *Eye movement desensitization and reprocessing (EMDR) therapy: Basic principles, protocols and procedures* (3rd ed.). The Guilford Press.

Sherman, R., & Pross, E. (2010). Growing future nurse leaders to build and sustain healthy work environments at the unit level. *The Online Journal of Issues in Nursing, 15*(1). https://doi.org/10.3912/OJIN.Vol15No01Man01.

Sherman, R., Schwarzkopf, R., & Kiger, A. J. (2011). Charge nurse perspectives on frontline leadership in acute care environments. *International Scholarly Research Network Nursing, 2011,* 164052. https://doi.org/10.5402/2011/164052.

Shier, M. L., & Graham, J. R. (2015). Subjective well-being, social work, and the environment: The impact of the socio-political context of practice on social worker happiness. *Journal of Social Work, 15*(1), 3–23.

Siebert, D. C. (2006). Personal and occupational factors in burnout among practicing social workers. *Journal of Social Service Research, 32*(2), 25–44. https://doi.org/10.1300/J079v32n02_02.

Sifton, E. (1998). The serenity prayer. *Yale Review, 86*(1), 16. https://doi.org/10.1111/0044-0124.00193.

Silver, N. (2012). *The signal and the noise: Why so many predictions fail—but some don't.* Penguin Press.

Simard, S. W., Asay, A. K., Beiler, K. J., et al. (2015). Resource transfer between plants through ectomycorrhizal networks. In T. R. Horton (Ed.), *Mycorrhizal networks.* Springer.

Simon, C., & McFadden, T. (2017). *National Physician Health Survey: The process, preliminary data, and future directions* [Conference session]. Canadian Conference on Physician Health 2017, The Westin, Ottawa, ON, Canada.

Sloan, D. M., & Marx, B. P. (2018). Maximizing outcomes associated with expressive writing. *Clinical Psychology: Science and Practice, 25*(1), e12231. https://doi.org/10.1111/cpsp.12231.

Slomski, A. (2018). MDMA-assisted psychotherapy for PTSD. *The Journal of the American Medical Association, 319*(24), 2470. https://doi.org/10.1001/jama.2018.8168.

Slutsky, J., Rahl, H., Lindsay, E. K., & Creswell, J. D. (2016). Mindfulness, emotion regulation, and social threat. In J. C. Karremans & E. K. Papies (Eds.), *Mindfulness in social psychology.* Routledge.

Smallwood, J., & Schooler, J. W. (2015). The science of mind wandering: Empirically navigating the stream of consciousness. *Annual Review of Psychology, 66*(1), 487–518. https://doi.org/10.1146/annurev-psych-010814-015331.

Smith, B. S., & Zautra, A. J. (2002). The role of personality in exposure and reactivity to interpersonal stress in relation to arthritis disease activity and negative affect in women. *Health Psychology, 21*(1), 81–88. https://doi.org/10.1037//0278-6133.21.1.81.

Smyth, J. M., Johnson, J. A., Auer, B. J., et al. (2018). Online positive affect journaling in the improvement of mental distress and well-being in general medical patients with elevated anxiety symptoms: A preliminary randomized controlled trial. *JMIR Mental Health, 5*(4), e11290. https://doi.org/10.2196/11290.

Soares, V. P., & Campos, A. C. (2017). Evidences for the anti-panic actions of cannabidiol. *Current Neuropharmacology, 15*(2), 291–299. https://doi.org/10.2174/1570159X14666160509123955.

Soler, J., Cebolla, A., Feliu-Soler, A., et al. (2014). Relationship between meditative practice and self-reported mindfulness: The MINDSENS composite index. *PLoS One, 9*(1), e86622. https://doi.org/10.1371/journal.pone.0086622.

Solberg Nes, L. S., & Segerstrom, S. C. (2006). Dispositional optimism and coping: A meta-analytic review. *Personality and Social Psychology Review, 10*, 235–251. https://doi.org/10.1207/s15327957pspr1003_3.

Some, S. (2009). The seen and the unseen: Spirituality among the Dagara people. *Cultural Survival Quarterly Magazine.* https://www.culturalsurvival.org/publications/cultural-survival-quarterly/seen-and-unseen-spirituality-among-dagara-people.

Song, Y. Y., Simard, S. W., Caroll, A., et al. (2015). Defoliation of interior Douglas-fir elicits carbon transfer and defense signaling to ponderosa pine neighbors through ectomycorrhizal networks. *Scientific Reports, 5*(8495), 1–9.

Sone, T., Nakaya, N., Ohmori, K., et al. (2008). Sense of life worth living (ikigai) and mortality in Japan: Ohsaki study. *Psychosomatic Medicine, 70*(6), 709–715. https://doi.org/10.1097/PSY.0b013e31817e7e64.

Sounds True. (2018, July 24). *Father Greg Boyle: The answer to every question is compassion* [Podcast]. https://www.resources.soundstrue.com/podcast/father-greg-boyle-the-answer-to-every-question-is-compassion/.

Starcher, R. L. (2006). The new global system: Lessons for institutions of Christian higher education. *Christian Education Journal, 3*(1), 92–100. https://doi.org/10.1177/073989130600300107.

Statistics Canada. (2014). *Perceived life stress, 2014.* https://www150.statcan.gc.ca/n1/pub/82-625-x/2015001/article/14188-eng.htm.

Steege, L. M., & Rainbow, J. G. (2017). Fatigue in hospital nurses—'Supernurse' culture is a barrier to addressing problems: A qualitative interview study. *International Journal of Nursing Studies, 67*, 20–28. https://doi.org/10.1016/j.ijnurstu.2016.11.014.

Steger, M. F., Dik, B. J., & Duffy, R. D. (2012). Measuring meaningful work: The work and meaning inventory (WAMI). *Journal of Career Assessment, 20*, 322–337. https://doi.org/10.1177/1069072711436160.

Steger, M. F., Kashdan, T. B., & Oishi, S. (2008). Being good by doing good: Daily eudaimonic activity and well-being. *Journal of Research in Personality, 42*, 22–42. https://doi.org/10.1016/j.jrp.2007.03.004.

Stelnicki, A. M., & Carleton, R. N. (2020). Mental disorder symptoms among nurses in Canada. *Canadian Federation of Nurses Unions.* https://doi.org/10.1177/0844562120961894.

Stelnicki, A. M., Carleton, R. N., & Reichert, C. (2020). Nurses' mental health and well-being: COVID-19 impacts. *Canadian Journal of Nursing Research, 52*(3), 237–239. https://doi.org/10.1177/0844562120931623.

Stern, R., & Divecha, D. (2015). The empathy trap. *Psychology Today.* https://www.psychologytoday.com/ca/articles/201505/the-empathy-trap.

Stolovitch, H. D., & Keeps, E. J. (2011). *Telling ain't training* (2nd ed.). American Society for Training & Development, Workplace Learning and Performance.

Streb, M., Häller, P., & Michael, T. (2014). PTSD in paramedics: Resilience and sense of coherence. *Behavioral and Cognitive Psychotherapy, 42*(4), 452–463. https://doi.org/10.1017/S1352465813000337.

Sturgeon, J. A., & Zautra, A. J. (2015). Social pain and physical pain: Shared paths to resilience. *Pain Management, 6*(1), 63–74. https://doi.org/10.2217/pmt.15.56.

Sufi Healing Order. (2018). *The 5 element breath.* http://sufihealingorder.info/international-training-course/homework-seminar-1/five-element-breath/.

Sullivan, S., Mkabile, S. G., Fincham, D. S., et al. (2009). The cumulative effect of multiple trauma on symptoms of posttraumatic stress disorder, anxiety, and depression in adolescents. *Comprehensive Psychiatry, 50*(2), 121–127. https://doi.org/10.1016/j.comppsych.2008.06.006.

Sunderland, A., & Findlay, L. C. (2013). *Perceived need for mental health care in Canada: Results from the 2012 Canadian Community Health Survey–Mental Health* (pp. 3–9). Statistics Canada.

Super, A., Wagemakers, M. A. E., Picavet, H. S. J., et al. (2016). Strengthening sense of coherence: Opportunities for theory building in health promotion. *Health Promotion International, 31*, 869–878. https://doi.org/10.1093/heapro/dav071.

Superle, M. (2016). The United Nations convention on the rights of the child: At the core of a child-centered critical approach to children's literature. *The Lion and the Unicorn, 40*(2), 144–162. https://doi.org/10.1353/uni.2016.0017.

Suzuki, E., Tagaya, A., Ota, K., et al. (2010). Factors affecting turnover of Japanese novice nurses in university hospitals in early and later periods of employment. *Journal of Nursing Management, 18*(2), 194–204. https://doi.org/10.1111/j.1365-2834.2010.01054.x.

Swider, B. W., & Zimmerman, R. D. (2010). Born to burnout: A meta-analytic path model of personality, job burnout, and work outcomes. *Journal of Vocational Behavior, 76*(3), 487–506. https://doi.org/10.1016/j.jvb.2010.01.003.

Swift, J. K., & Greenberg, R. P. (2012). Premature discontinuation in adult psychotherapy: A meta-analysis. *Journal of Consulting and Clinical Psychology, 80*(4), 547. https://doi.org/10.1037/a0028226.

Tanzi, R. E., & Chopra, D. (2013). *Super brain: Unleashing the explosive power of your mind to maximize health, happiness, and spiritual well-being*. Harmony.

Taylor, C., & Dell'Oro, R. (2006). *Health and human flourishing: Religion, medicine, and moral Anthropology* (pp. 93–95). Georgetown University Press.

Taylor, E., & Cranton, P. (2012). *The handbook of transformational learning: Theory, research, and practice*. Jossey-Bass.

The Circle Way, (2019). *About*. https://www.thecircleway.net/about.

Thomas, K. W. (1992). Conflict and conflict management: Reflections and update. *Journal of Organizational Behavior, 13*(3), 265–274. https://doi.org/10.1002/job.4030130306.

Thomas, S., & Burk, R. (2009). Junior nursing students' experiences of vertical violence during clinical rotations. *Nursing Outlook, 57*(4), 226–231. https://doi.org/10.1016/j.outlook.2008.08.004.

Thunman, E. (2012). Burnout as a social pathology of self-realization. *Scandinavian Journal of Social Theory, 13*(1), 43. https://doi.org/10.1080/1600910X.2012.648744.

Tolle, E. (2005). *A new earth: Awakening to your life's purpose*. Plume.

Tonarelli, A., Cosentino, C., Tomasoni, C., et al. (2018). Expressive writing. A tool to help health workers of palliative care. *Acta bio-medica: Atenei Parmensis, 89*(Suppl 6), 35–42. https://doi.org/10.23750/abm.v89i6-S.7452.

Toussaint, L. L., Worthington, E. L., Jr.,& Williams, D. R. (Eds.), (2015). *Forgiveness and health: Scientific evidence and theories relating forgiveness to better health*. Springer.

Tracy, S. J. (2005). Locking up emotion: Moving beyond dissonance for understanding emotion labor discomfort. *Communication Monographs, 72*(3), 261–283. https://doi.org/10.1080/03637750500206474.

Travis, F. (2019). Temporal and spatial characteristics of meditation EEG. *Psychological Trauma: Theory, Research, Practice and Policy, 12*(2), 111–115. https://doi.org/10.1037/tra0000488.

Troy, A. S. (2015). Reappraisal and resilience to stress: Context must be considered. *The Behavioral and Brain Sciences, 38*, e123. https://doi.org/10.1017/S0140525X1400171X.

Troy, A. S., Wilhelm, F. H., Shallcross, A. J., et al. (2010). Seeing the silver lining: Cognitive reappraisal ability moderates the relationship between stress and depressive symptoms. *Emotion, 10*, 783–795. https://doi.org/10.1037/a0020262.

Tsamakis, K., Rizos, E., Manolis, A. J., et al. (2020). COVID-19 pandemic and its impact on mental health of healthcare professionals. *Experimental and Therapeutic Medicine*. https://doi.org/10.3892/etm.2020.8646.

Tuck, N. L., Adams, K. S., Pressman, S. D., et al. (2017). Greater ability to express positive emotion is associated with lower projected cardiovascular disease risk. *Journal of Behavioral Medicine, 40*(6), 855–863. https://doi.org/10.1007/s10865-017-9852-0.

Turner, K. A. (2010). *Spontaneous remission of cancer: Theories from healers, physicians, and cancer survivors*. ProQuest Dissertations & Theses Global. [Doctoral dissertation, University of California, Berkeley] (Publication No. 3444696).

Turner, E. H., Matthews, A. M., Linardatos, E., et al. (2008). Selective publication of antidepressant trials and its influence on apparent efficacy. *New England Journal of Medicine, 358*(3), 252–260. https://doi.org/10.1056/NEJMsa065779.

Unitarian Universalist Association. (2005). *Singing the journey*. https://www.uua.org/worship/music/hymnals/journey.

University of California, Berkeley. (2019). Raisin meditation: Why to try it. *Greater Good Science Center*. https://ggia.berkeley.edu/practice/raisin_meditation.

Uvnäs-Moberg, K., & Petersson, M. (2010). Role of oxytocin and oxytocin-related effects in manual therapies. In H. H. King, W. Jänig, & M. M. Patterson (Eds.), *The science and clinical application of manual therapy* (pp. 147–162). Elsevier.

van Oyen Witvliet, C., Ludwig, T. E., & Vander Laan, K. (2001). Granting forgiveness or harboring grudges: Implications for emotion, physiology, and health. *Psychological Science, 12*(2), 117–123. https://doi.org/10.1111/1467-9280.00320.

Vasiliadis, H. M., Dezetter, A., Latimer, E., et al. (2017). Assessing the costs and benefits of insuring psychological services as part of Medicare for depression in Canada. *Psychiatric Services, 68*(9), 899–906. https://doi.org/10.1176/appi.ps.201600395.

Venise, B. D., Lindo, J., Anderson-Johnson, P., & Weaver, S. (2015). Using Carl Rogers' person-centered model to explain interpersonal relationships at a school of nursing. *Journal of Professional Nursing, 31*(2), 141. https://doi.org/10.1016/j.profnurs.2014.07.003.

Vessey, J. A., Demarco, R., & DiFazio, R. (2010). Bullying, harassment, and horizontal violence in the nursing workforce: The state of the science. *Annual Review of Nursing Research*, *28*(1), 133–157. https://doi.org/10.1891/0739-6686.28.133.

Vestergaard-Poulsen, P., van Beek, M., Skewes, J., et al. (2009). Long-term meditation is associated with increased gray matter density in the brain stem. *Neuroreport*, *20*(2), 170–174. https://doi.org/10.1097/WNR.0b013e3 28320012a.

Vickers, P., & Moyers, R. (2020). Healing complex trauma 1: A unity of minds, hearts, and culture. *Journal of Indigenous Well-Being*, *5*(1). https://journalindigenouswellbeing.com/media/2020/05/126.139.Healing-Complex-Trauma-1-A-unity-of-minds-hearts-and-Culture.pdf.

Vitale, J., & Len, H. (2008). *Zero limits: The secret Hawaiian system for wealth, health, peace, and more*. Wiley.

Vlemincx, E., Van Diest, I., & Van den Bergh, O. (2016). A sigh of relief or a sigh to relieve: The psychological and physiological relief effect of deep breaths. *Physiological Behavior*, *165*, 127–135. https://doi.org/10.1016/j.physbeh.2016.07.004.

Wachholtz, A. B., Malone, C. D., & Pargament, K. I. (2017). Effect of different meditation types on migraine headache medication use. *Behavioral Medicine*, *43*(1), 1–8. https://doi.org/10.1080/08964289.2015.1024601.

Wagamese, R. (2016). *Embers: One Ojibway's meditations*. Douglas & McIntyre.

Wang, S., Wong, Y., & Yeh, K. (2015). Relationship harmony, dialectical coping, and nonattachment: Chinese indigenous well-being and mental health. *The Counselling Psychologist*, *44*(1), 78–108. https://doi.org/10.1177/0011000015616463.

Watkins, P. C., Emmons, R. A., Greaves, M. R., et al. (2018). Joy is a distinct positive emotion: Assessment of joy and relationship to gratitude and well-being. *The Journal of Positive Psychology*, *13*(5), 522–539. https://doi.org/10.1080/17439760.2017.1414298.

Watkins, L. E., Sprang, K. R., & Rothbaum, B. O. (2018). Treating PTSD: A review of evidence-based psychotherapy interventions. *Frontiers in Behavioral Neuroscience*, *12*, 258. https://doi.org/10.3389/fnbeh.2018.00258.

Watson, J. (1988). *Nursing: Human science and human care: A theory of nursing*. National League for Nursing.

Watson, J. (2003). Love and caring. Ethics of face and hand—An invitation to return to the heart and soul of nursing and our deep humanity. *Nursing Administration Quarterly*, *27*, 197–202.

Wei, M., Russell, D. W., Mallinckrodt, B., et al. (2007). The experiences in close relationship scale (ECR)-short form: Reliability, validity, and factor structure. *Journal of Personality Assessment*, *88*, 187–204. https://doi.org/10.1080/00223890701268041.

Welsh, D. (2009). Predictors of depressive symptoms in female medical–surgical hospital nurses. *Issues in Mental Health Nursing*, *30*(5), 320–326. https://doi.org/10.1080/01612840902754537.

Wenger-Trayner, E., & Wenger-Trayner, B. (2015). *Communities of practice: A brief introduction*. https://wenger-trayner.com/wp-content/uploads/2015/04/07-Brief-introduction-to-communities-of-practice.pdf.

West, M. A. (2020). Compassionate and collective leadership for cultures of high-quality care. In A. Montgomery, M. van der Doef, E. Panagopoulou, & M. P. Leiter (Eds.), *Connecting healthcare worker well-being, patient safety and organisational change: Aligning perspectives on health, safety and well-being* (pp. 207–225). Springer. https://doi.org/10.1007/978-3-030-60998-6_13.

Whitaker, R., & Cosgrove, L. (2015). *Psychiatry under the influence: Institutional corruption, social injury, and prescriptions for reform*. Springer.

Wieck, K. L., Dols, J., & Landrum, P. (2010). Retention priorities for the intergenerational nurse workforce. *Nursing Forum*, *45*(1), 7–17. https://doi.org/10.1111/j.1744-6198.2009.00159.x.

Wijk, C. H., & Waters, A. H. (2008). Positive psychology made practical: A case study with naval specialists. *Military Medicine*, *173*(5), 488–492. https://doi.org/10.7205/MILMED.173.5.488.

Wilber, K. (2001). *A theory of everything: An integral vision for business, politics, science, and spirituality*. Shambhala.

Wilkinson, H., Whittington, R., Perry, L., & Eames, C. (2017). Examining the relationship between burnout and empathy in healthcare professionals: A systematic review. *Burnout Research*, *6*, 18–29. https://doi.org/10.1016/j.burn.2017.06.003.

Williams, M. T., & Leins, C. (2016). Race-based trauma: The challenge and promise of MDMA-assisted psychotherapy. *Multidisciplinary Association for Psychedelic Studies*, *26*(1), 32–37. https://s3-us-west-1.amazonaws.com/mapscontent/news-letters/v26n1/v26n1_p32-37.pdf.

Wilson, S. D. (2015). *Hurt people hurt people: Hope and healing for yourself and your relationships*. Discovery House Publishers.

Wood, A. M., Joseph, S., Lloyd, J., et al. (2009). Gratitude influences sleep through the mechanism of pre-sleep cognitions. *Journal of Psychosomatic Research*, *66*(1), 43–48.

Wood, A. M., & Maltby, J. J. (2009). Gratitude predicts psychological well-being above the Big Five facets. *Personality and Individual Differences*, *46*(4), 443–447. https://doi-org.ezproxy.viu.ca/10.1016/J.PAID.2008.11.012.

WorkSafeBC. (2018). *Healthy workplaces*. https://www2.gov.bc.ca/gov/content/health/keeping-bc-healthy-safe/ healthy-communities/healthy-workplaces.

World Health Organization. (2019, May 28). *Burn-out an "occupational phenomenon": International Classification of Diseases*. https://www.who.int/mental_health/evidence/burn-out/en/.

Worthington, E. L., & Scherer, M. (2004). Forgiveness is an emotion-focused coping strategy that can reduce health risks and promote health resilience: Theory, review, and hypotheses. *Psychological Health, 19*, 385–405. https://doi.org/10.1080/0887044042000196674.

Xanthopoulou, D., Bakker, A. B., Demerouti, E., et al. (2007). The role of personal resources in the job demands-resources model. *International Journal of Stress Management, 14*(2), 121–141. https://doi.org/10.1037/1072-5245.14.2.121.

Yang, C., Barrós-Loscertales, A., Pinazo, D., et al. (2016). State and training effects of mindfulness meditation on brain networks reflect neuronal mechanisms of its antidepressant effect. *Neural Plasticity, 2016*, 1–14. https://doi.org/10.1155/2016/9504642.

Yates, J. (2015). *The mind illuminated: A complete meditation guide integrating Buddhist wisdom and brain science* (p. 6). Dharma Treasure Press.

Young, S. (2016a). *The science of mindfulness: How meditation works*. Sounds True.

Young, S. (2016b). *The icky-sticky creepy-crawly it-doesn't-really-hurt-but-I-can't-stand-it feeling*. https://www. shinzen.org/wp-content/uploads/2016/12/art_ickysticky.pdf

Yount, G., Church, D., Rachlin, K., et al. (2019). Do noncoding RNAs mediate the efficacy of energy psychology? *Global Advances in Health and Medicine, 8*. https://doi.org/10.1177/2164956119832500.

Zak, P. J. (2018). The neuroscience of high-trust organizations. *Consulting Psychology Journal: Practice and Research, 70*(1), 45–58. https://doi.org/10.1037/cpb0000076.

Zarrindast, M-R., & Khakpai, F. (2015). The modulatory role of dopamine in anxiety-like behavior. *Archives of Iranian Medicine, 18*(9), 591–603.

Zarshenas, L., Sharif, F., Molazem, Z., et al. (2014). Professional socialization in nursing: A qualitative content analysis. *Iranian Journal of Nursing and Midwifery Research, 19*(4), 432.

Zimmerman, B., Bandura, A., & Martinez-Pons, M. (1992). Self-motivation for academic attainment: The role of self-efficacy beliefs and personal goal setting. *American Educational Research Journal, 29*(3), 663–676. https:// www.uky.edu/~eushe2/Bandura/Bandura1992AERJ.pdf.

Zuardi, A. W., Rodrigues, N. P., Silva, A. L., et al. (2017). Inverted U-shaped dose–response curve of the anxiolytic effect of cannabidiol during public speaking in real life. *Frontiers in Pharmacology, 8*, 259. https://doi.org/10.3389/fphar.2017.00259.

Zukav, G. (2014). *Seat of the soul*. Simon & Schuster.

Zurmehly, J., Martin, P. A., & Fitzpatrick, J. J. (2009). Registered nurse empowerment and intent to leave current position and/or profession. *Journal of Nursing Management, 17*(3), 383–391. https://doi.org/10.1111/j.1365-2834.2008.00940.x.

Index

Page numbers followed by "*f*" indicate figures, "*t*" indicate tables, and "*b*" indicate boxes.

Relationship
  self-kindness, 123
  unconditional positive regard in, 112–114, 113*f*
Relaxation meditation, 198–199
Reorientation, sympathetic nervous system, 147
Reparenting, 213
Resilience, 17
  bolster, 17–18
  personal, 18, 22
Response, sympathetic, interrupting, 147–148
Rigid systems, thriving in, 53–54
Rituals, 189
  creation, 193–194
  sympathetic nervous system, 148
Rogers' theory, 52–53
Role modelling, 333
  leadership, 323–326
Root of desire, responding to, 156–159
Roots Theory, 21

S
Safety, as human need, 86
Sanctuary, finding, 156–159
Savouring
  cultivating gratitude by, 246
  fleeting pleasures, 245–248
Science of mindfulness, 186–187
Self
  cultivating and expressing gratitude for, 246–248
  disconnected, 165–166
  healing thy caregiving, 114–115
  meeting with real, 130–132
Self-actualizing
  activity, 38
  process, 38
Self-assessment, conflict, 327–329
Self-care, 119–129
  emotional, 122
  psychological, 121
  spiritual, 122–123
Self-compassion, 20, 46–47, 47*b*, 109–110, 174, 216, 229
  antidote to
    fight, 146
    workplace hostility, 116–117
  attuning practices, 120–121
  awareness without, 47*b*
  components of, 110
  curiosity and, 119
  as medicine, 114–115
  mindfulness and, 146
  pause for, strengthening practice, 124–125
  strengthening congruence with, 107
  weaving in, 117–118
  in workplace, 116
Self-conscious, 52–53
Self-destructive programming, 188–189
Self-efficacy, 19, 57–58, 290
Self-holding, 236–239
Self-integrity, 45, 114

Self-kindness, 110, 119–128
  assessment, 121–124
  physical, 121–122
  professional, 123
  relationship, 123
  workplace, 123
Self-oriented perfectionism, 170–171
Self-soothing, 216
  capacities, 228
Self-stigma, 191–192
Self-talk, negative, 120–121
Sense of coherence, 19–21, 20*f*, 23, 29*f*, 55–56, 179, 181, 187, 261, 341
  components of, 56–58, 183
    comprehensibility, 56
  development, 343
  and mindfulness, 183–186
  and thriving, 55–58
Sense of optimism, 183
"Shaking it off," stress reduction, 159–160, 169–170
Shame, 45, 82–83
Signal
  desire as, 156
  vs. noise, 142*t*
  to noise ratio, 141, 142*f*
Significant action, 141, 153, 240–244
Significant thing, 141, 148–149, 281, 288–289
  signal of, 153–154
Singing loving-kindness, 235
Skill development, to mindfulness, 192–194
Social capital, 314–315
Social cognitive theory, 289
Social connection, 318
Socialization, of caregivers, 331–332
Soothing
  with breath, 231*b*
  with forgiveness, 248–253
  with gratitude, 244–248
  with loving-kindness, 231–232
  with optimism, 239–244
  with touch, 236–239
Soul-eating emotion, 81
Spiritual distress, 25–26
Spirituality, 24
  and living our calling, 299–310
  in roots, 23–26
Spiritual self-care, 122–123
Stimuli, 39
Stress, 61–66, 100–101
  chronic, 9, 66
    impacts of, 87–88
  interrupting, 146–148
  management practices, 116
  physical, 65–66
  post-traumatic stress disorder (PTSD), 7–17, 69–70, 75, 144, 257, 259–260
  psychological, 65–66
  response, 63*f*, 64
  work, 64–66
  workplace, 241–243
Stress hormone, 65–66

Looking Back and Looking Forward: A Personal Note From the Author

When I look back on my childhood, no matter how many bright lights I try to shine on it, I cannot escape the grim reality that I spent my formative years feeling my way around in the dark. Childhood felt like a fight for survival, lacking safety and security on every plane of life. Even though people knew what was happening and saw the battle wounds, no one came for me. *Why didn't anyone come for me?* Through my eyes as a child, the only story that made sense to me was that somehow, for some reason, I didn't deserve any better. I hear and see the impacts of this same belief system played out by countless others.

You see, it wasn't the surface wounds that hurt me the most; that wasn't what broke my spirit. Instead, what broke me was the deep-seated belief that I was not loved and protected the way other children were because I was not worthy of it. Surely, if I had been worthy, someone would have sounded an alarm bell. But no one did. As a child, I interpreted the lack of effort from others as a confirmation of the scarlet letter I'd spend my life wearing.

From this place, I had to be both parent and child, caretaker and dependent. The requirements of surviving always took precedence over trust and play, causing a hypervigilant, even neurotic, need to mitigate the threats that swirled around me. This created a deafening static on the surface and an intolerable noise within. My brain learned to not only tend to actual threats, but also foresee all possible future threats too. That way, fixating at the level of the mind, I'd be sure to never be surprised, mitigating risks and minimizing any potential margins of error. After all, when all you've known is how to watch your own back, it's all you know how to do: Living with one eye open all the time.

The reality is, it was too painful to feel it at the time and it often still is. It was too hard to not get a break from the intensity of it all. My swirling mind and contracted gut became a haunting force that consumed every moment. I couldn't hold it in anymore. And so I gave way. And even today, when it's all too much, I still do. At that time, shutting down the inner noise was an act of mercy. The outer world was not a safe place for the noise to emerge. Separating from the desires of my heart and the pilot light that fuels meaning and passion in the world was like a crack in the foundation of my soul. I adapted to survive the hand I was dealt. Was it a choice? No way! It was a subconscious defence mechanism. My mind and body took charge, locking my spirit away, protecting my most vulnerable parts when no one else could.